LEADING THE WAY

LEADING THE WAY

EASTMAN AND ORAL HEALTH

Elizabeth Brayer

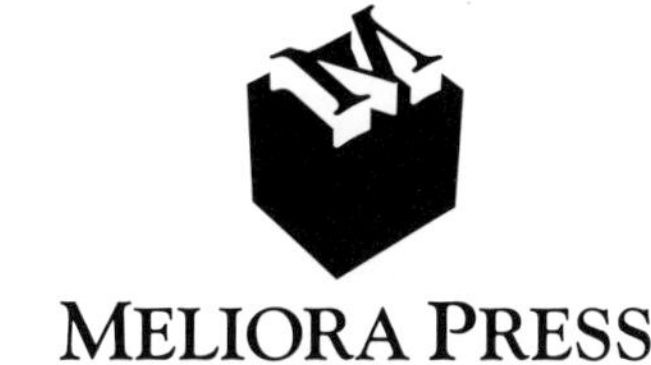

MELIORA PRESS

An imprint of University of Rochester Press

First published 2009

Meliora Press is an imprint of the
University of Rochester Press
668 Mt. Hope Avenue, Rochester, NY 14620, USA
www.urpress.com
and Boydell & Brewer Limited
PO Box 9, Woodbridge, Suffolk IP12 3DF, UK
www.boydellandbrewer.com

Cloth ISBN-13: 978–1–58046–311–9
Cloth ISBN-10: 1–58046–311–8
Paperback ISBN-13: 978–1–58046–332–4
Paperback ISBN-13: 1–58046–332–0

Library of Congress Cataloging-in-Publication Data

Brayer, Elizabeth.
    Leading the way : Eastman and oral health / Elizabeth Brayer.
        p. ; cm.
    Includes bibliographical references.
    ISBN-13: 978–1–58046–311–9 (hardcover : alk. paper)
    ISBN-10: 1–58046–311–8 (hardcover : alk. paper)
    ISBN-13: 978–1–58046–332–4 (pbk. : alk. paper)
    1. Eastman, George, 1854–1932. 2. Eastman Dental Center—History. 3. University of Rochester. School of Medicine and
Dentistry. 4. Dental public health—New York—Rochester—History. I. Title. [DNLM: 1. Eastman, George, 1854–1932.
2. Eastman Dental Dispensary. 3. University of Rochester. School of Medicine and Dentistry. 4. Dental Clinics—history—
New York. 5. Dental Health Services—history—New York. 6. Education, Dental—history—New York. 7. History, 20th
Century—New York. WU 11 AN6 B827L 2009]
    RK52.3.N7B73 2009
    362.19'7600974789—dc22
                                                                                                        2008055790

This publication is printed on acid-free paper.

Printed in the United States of America.

CONTENTS

PREFACE AND ACKNOWLEDGMENTS

ONE ROCHESTER CITY HISTORIAN DESCRIBED THE DECADE BEGINNING 1915 as "Rochester's golden age—because that was when George Eastman decided to part with the bulk of his fortune" for the betterment of his adopted city. During that window, Eastman, who as the head of the city's largest employer, the Eastman Kodak Company, was already considered the city's "boss," founded the Rochester Dental Dispensary, the Community Chest (an outgrowth of the city's War Chest), the Eastman Theatre and School of Music, the School of Medicine and Dentistry of the University of Rochester, and supported a host of other health, welfare, educational, and cultural organizations. The path of the rest of the century was set in that golden age. By the dawn of the twenty-first century, Kodak had been replaced by the University of Rochester as the area's largest employer, primarily because of its medical center, which Eastman sponsored in 1920.

Eastman didn't do it alone. The trustees of the Rochester Dental Dispensary were movers and shakers too: members of the families that founded Western Union, Bausch and Lomb, Michaels Stern and other the men's clothing companies, and the Ellwanger and Barry nurseries, as well as lawyers, congressmen, and prominent businessmen including Kodak executives. It was said they met for lunch at the Genesee Valley Club and plotted the city's future and that is not totally off the mark. In the beginning, each trustee had to pledge $1,000 a year to the dispensary for ten years, and that plus the building and endowment that Eastman gave, and a stipend from the city from 1915 to the 1970s, kept pediatric preventive dentistry, especially for the indigent, going for the next ninety-plus years. Along the way, community education was added—initially through hygienists and later postgraduate education for dentists—as was research beginning during the Bibby years. Later, boards of trustees took a more active role, for better or worse, in the day-to-day operations of the dental center.

NOTE ON THE NAME CHANGES

The institution founded in 1915 by George Eastman was originally named the Rochester Dental Dispensary (RDD). In 1941, it was renamed the Eastman Dental Dispensary (EDD). In 1965, it was renamed the Eastman Dental Center (EDC). This narrative reflects those name changes: when the institution is referred to as it existed 1941–64, it is called the Eastman Dental Dispensary (EDD) and so forth.

ACKNOWLEDGMENTS

I am especially indebted to Dr. Cyril Meyerowitz, who asked me to write an extended essay detailing George Eastman's motives in founding the Rochester Dental Dispensary and the School of Medicine and Dentistry how Eastman's intentions continued to impact the subsequent history of both institutions. He also asked that the ongoing tripartite and sometimes conflicting roles of research, education, and community service through clinical care be addressed throughout.

Dr. Stanley Handelman, professor emeritus, Eastman Dental Center; chairman, Department of General Dentistry, 1970–94; and research associate and clinical instructor, Eastman Dental Center, 1958–70, made many contributions to the work. He wrote, collected, and edited the important "Departments and Divisions" history chapter. We are indebted to all of the contributors too—Drs. David Levy, Ronald Billings, William Bowen, Stanley Handelman, J. Daniel Subtelny, Gerald Graser, Carlo Ercoli, and Bejan Iranpour. For the other chapters, Dr. Handelman pinpointed and described important research projects that have been carried out since the 1960s. His forty-year hands-on relationship with all aspects of this history project made his reading and correcting of the manuscript invaluable.

Larry Belle, project director and the manuscript's first reader, made many suggestions and revisions throughout our four-year odyssey and wielded a friendly scalpel to the ongoing direction of the manuscript without destroying a working relationship. Larry is also responsible for chapter heads and subheads.

Nancy Bolger read and edited that manuscript at an early stage.

Most of the illustrations may be found in the Basil G. Bibby Library at the Eastman Dental Center, University of Rochester Medical Center. Elizabeth H. Kettell, MLS, librarian, and Keith Bullis, media services manager, converted to digital files the images that we have used in this publication. I am grateful too for the assistance of Vanessa Buckholz, administrative assistant, office of Cyril Meyerowitz, director, who printed innumerable versions of the manuscript, and to Becky Herman, director of advancement and chief development officer for dentistry.

A year before I began to work on this narrative, Cathy Salibian interviewed the primary players at the Eastman Dental Center and the university's School of Medicine and Dentistry for their analysis of the interplay between dental research, education, and community dentistry. These interviews became a major source for this book.

All photographs, unless otherwise indicated, are found in the Basil G. Bibby Library, Eastman Dental Center, University of Rochester Medical Center, and are used by permission. The photographs printed from original negatives at the George Eastman House: International Museum of Photography and Film are used courtesy George Eastman House. So are the photographs that were originally obtained from the Business Information Center of Eastman Kodak Company before that archive closed and its Eastman photographs were transferred to the George Eastman Archive and Study Center at George Eastman House, where copies are available through Kathleen Conner, George Eastman House curator. Historical photographs of the London clinic are reproduced with the kind permission of the Eastman Dental Hospital in that city. Some photos were given to me or taken by me on visits to one of the European clinics.

Elizabeth Brayer
April 2009

INTRODUCTION

HISTORY OF THE EASTMAN DENTAL CENTER

CYRIL MEYEROWITZ, DDS, MS

The history of the Eastman Dental Center and the School of Medicine and Dentistry at the University of Rochester is a complex and interesting story that spans almost 100 years. It is a story of individuals with vision and foresight; a story of community and institution interactions; a story of philanthropy; a story of a successful public health venture; and a story of significant advancements in scientific research and clinical care. It is also a story of lost opportunities and unfulfilled possibilities, of personality conflicts, and of institutional ambiguity, conflict and rivalry. It is a human story after all. But in a larger sense it is the story of the people and organizations that have led the way to significant accomplishments in twentieth-century oral health. The University of Rochester and the Eastman Dental Center are, and have proven to be, extraordinarily fertile ground for dental education, clinical care, and research. And most gratifying, after ninety years we are poised to resolve the ambiguous role and status of dentistry within the University of Rochester Medical Center and allow it to achieve its true potential: to lead the way in making even greater contributions to oral health.

But how did this book come about? Subsequent to the merger of the Eastman Dental Center and the University of Rochester in 1998, the first strategic planning process for dentistry was held, and it included all faculty members involved in academic dentistry. As we moved through this strategic planning process, I became increasingly interested in the past events that shaped our thinking of the future. As I informally perused the archival collection of old documents and pictures housed in the Bibby Library, I was enthralled by the richness of our history and its complexity.

As George Eastman, philanthropist extraordinaire, played the central role in founding the Rochester Dental Dispensary, which now bears his name, I turned to the definitive work on Eastman, Elizabeth Brayer's *George Eastman: A Biography*. It includes a chapter on his interest and role in fostering dental care, and it occurred to me that our history deserved more than just one chapter. So, after consulting with a friend of mine with a doctorate in history, Larry Belle, I arranged to meet with Elizabeth Brayer to discuss the possibility of commissioning her to write this book. I was very pleased, after a number of meetings, to have sparked her interest sufficiently to have her agree to the project. I was also fortunate to have Larry Belle agree to coordinate this process. He has been instrumental in making this book a reality, as has Stanley Handelman, my friend and mentor, who contributed significantly in getting the divisional accounts, writing, and editing. Betsy Brayer has done a superb job. History is after all ultimately a story. Betsy Brayer does a wonderful job in telling the story, as I am certain you will discover in what follows.

The story she tells starts with the establishment of the Rochester Dental Dispensary in 1917. George Eastman was ahead of his time in understanding the importance of community involvement and philanthropy in the care for the indigent. He also was passionate about improving the oral health of children and saw the opportunity to do a "greater good" by adding education and research to the clinical mission (see chapter 1).

Following the establishment of the Rochester Dental Dispensary, Eastman, along with notable figures like Abraham Flexner, Rush Rhees, and George Whipple, played a significant part in the story with the establishment of the

School of Medicine and Dentistry. From the start, a pivotal question was dentistry's place and role in the School of Medicine and Dentistry (chapter 2). In chapter 2, William Bowen adds an outstanding section on the fellows program and the department of dental research, which later became the Center for Oral Biology.

The establishment of international clinics in London, Rome, Stockholm, Paris, and Brussels, which compose one of the unique dimensions of the Eastman Dental Center's history, is described in chapter 3. George Eastman's vision and ability to engage European municipal and national governments in the establishment of these institutions, designed specifically to improve the oral health of indigent children, is yet another example of his visionary philanthropy. The long tenure of the first director of the Rochester Dental Dispensary (renamed the Eastman Dental Dispensary in 1941), Harvey Burkhart, extended from the dispensary's founding in 1917 to 1946, when at age eighty-six, Burkhart died of a heart attack (chapter 4).

Basil Bibby, a New Zealander who had been among the first of the University of Rochester dental fellows and had gone on to lead the Tufts School of Dentistry, succeeded Burkhart as the second director of the Eastman Dental Dispensary (renamed the Eastman Dental Center in 1965). Under Bibby's leadership, Eastman Dental Center changed dramatically from being mainly a clinical service enterprise to one that included world-class education and research programs (chapter 5). The changes were of particular importance for the students at that time. As Stanley Handelman describes, "It was a period which placed young dental professionals at the heart of the learning process."

The complexity of the interactions between the Eastman Dental Center and the School of Medicine and Dentistry is explored in chapter 6. One can say that the story is marked by great accomplishments coupled with lost opportunities, dual and interweaving themes that characterize the relationship between the two institutions from their very founding. This recurrent theme, as described in chapter 7, is also evident during William McHugh's leadership of the Eastman Dental Center. This was a period when Eastman and the School of Medicine and Dentistry moved closer together as the dental center moved onto the Medical Center campus and clarified its affiliation with the Medical Center.

This closer physical and organizational linkage, begun in the 1980s, between the Eastman Dental Center and the university culminated in a formal merger of the two in 1998. As Thomas Jackson put it with considerable precision and economy, "The question is not why the merger happened but why it took seventy years" (chapter 8). Chapter 8 ends with the story of the establishment of the Eastman Institute for Oral Health in the fall of 2008, thus creating a new and fully integrated dental enterprise within the University of Rochester Medical Center while preserving the important academic relationships of dental research and education with the School of Medicine and Dentistry.

The establishment of the Eastman Institute for Oral Health under the unitary leadership of a director responsible for all dentistry at the university together with a vigorous and active Eastman Dental Center Foundation board, which has oversight over the endowment, is the contemporary realization of George Eastman's vision of dentistry as an integral and vital part of the university and the Rochester community.

From the inception of the Rochester Dental Dispensary to the establishment of the Eastman Institute for Oral Health, we have been a singular and extraordinary institution in the world of academic dentistry, combining as no other institution does a trinity of vigorous community engagement and service, advanced education and training, and leading edge oral health research. This unique combination of service, education, and research is clearly demonstrated in the work of the discipline-specific divisions with which our story ends—for now (chapter 9). Beyond question, our history and tradition now enhanced and consolidated in the Eastman Institute for Oral Health will ensure that Rochester will continue to lead the way in academic dentistry.

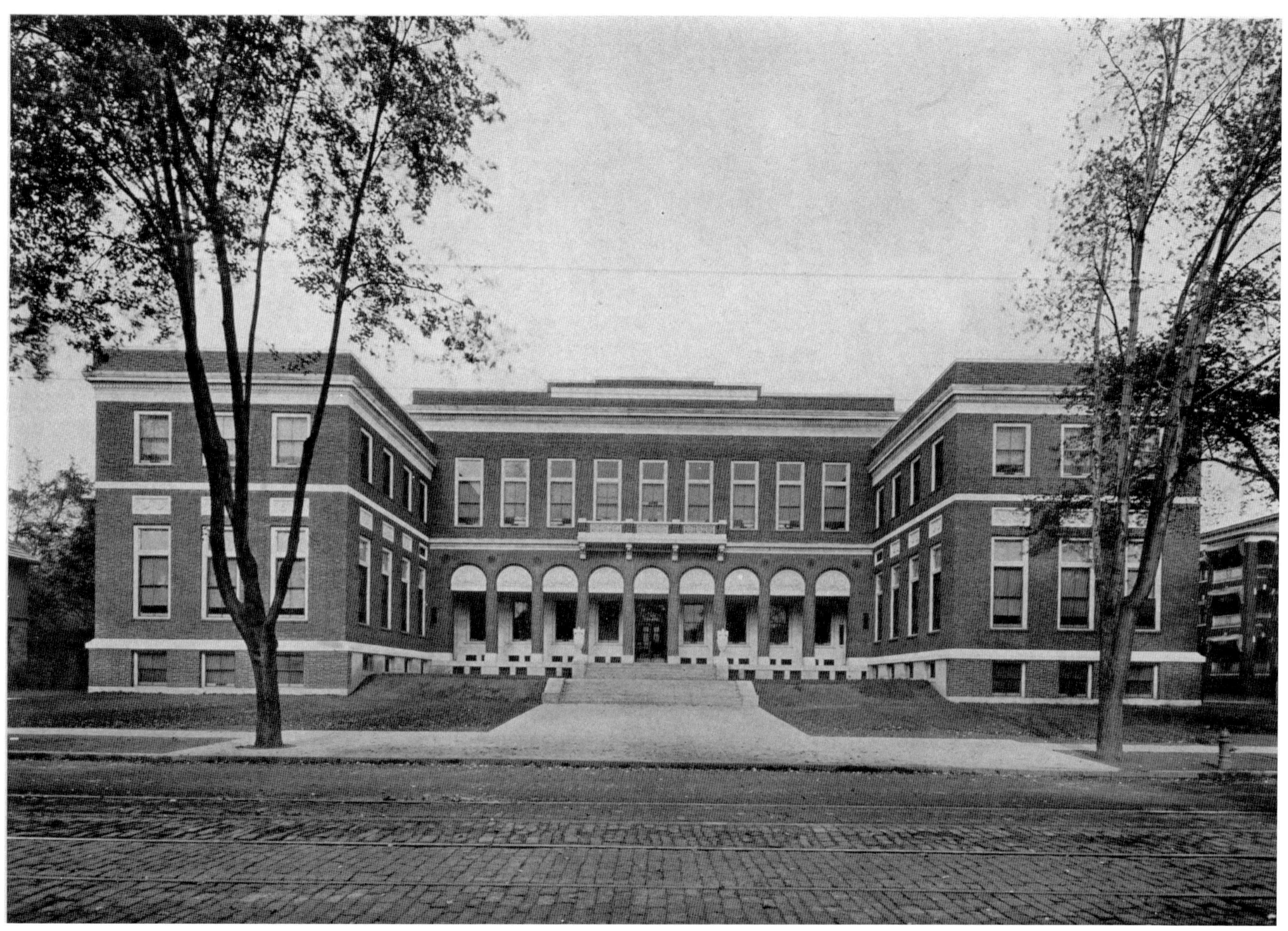

The Rochester Dental Dispensary at 800 Main Street, 1923

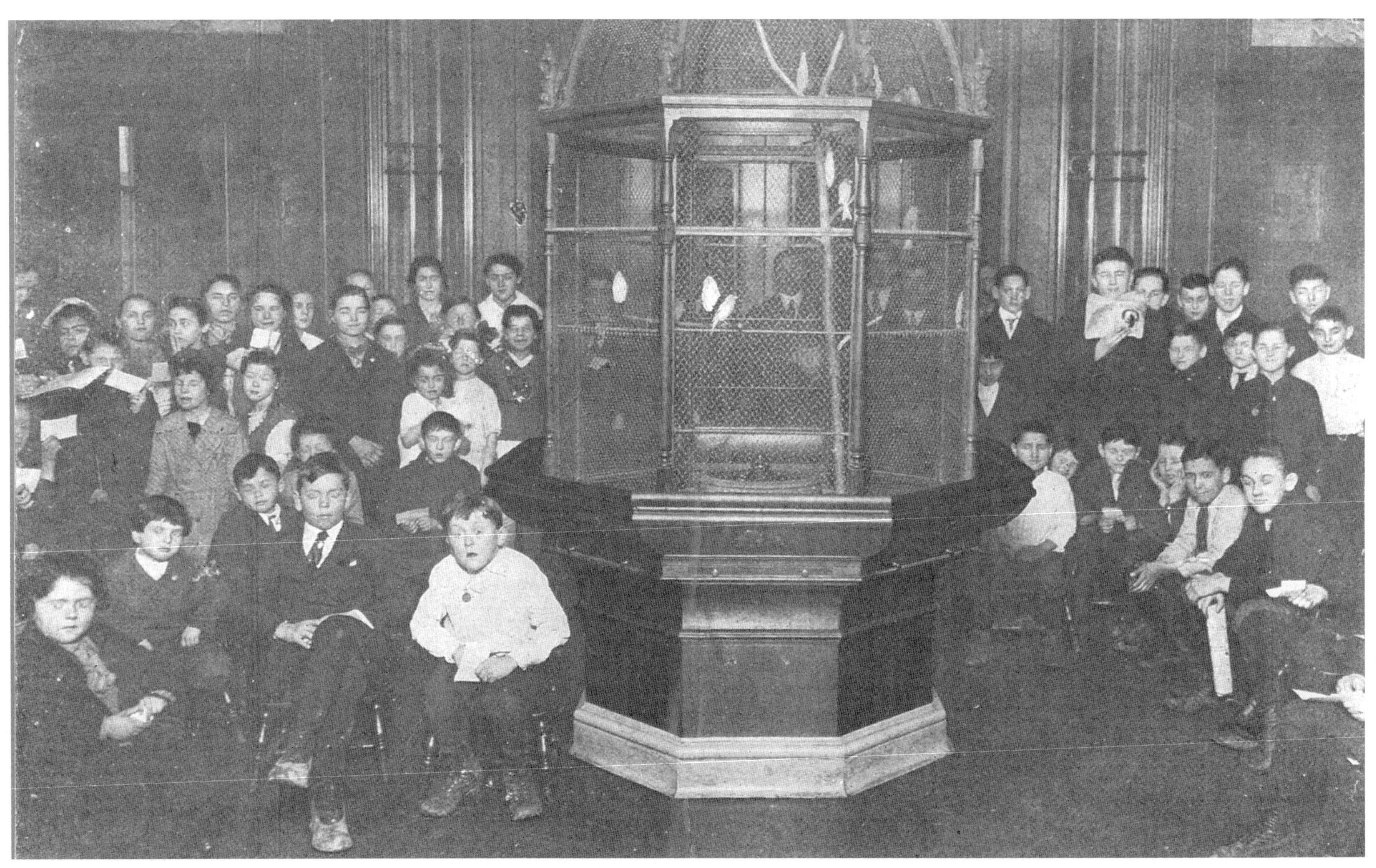

Scene in Children's Waiting Room of Rochester Dental Dispensary, ca 1920

Chapter One

REMAKING FACES

FOUNDING THE ROCHESTER DENTAL DISPENSARY

Eventually the poor will be able to chaw their food as well as the rich.

George Eastman

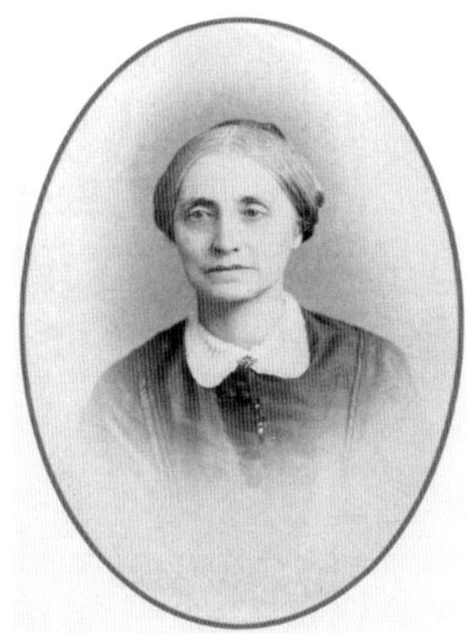

Maria Kilbourn Eastman (Courtesy George Eastman House)

BACHELOR GEORGE EASTMAN HAD HIS FIRST BIOGRAPHER, Carl Ackerman, describe his mother, Maria Kilbourn Eastman (1833–1907), as "the only woman in his life." As a young matron, Maria Eastman faced sleepless nights brought on by devastating toothaches. She described them in letters to her missionary sister in Ceylon, and her son vividly remembered the time the "toothpuller" came to his childhood home. He held his breath as he watched his mother sitting at the kitchen table while eight of her teeth were pulled—without benefit of anesthesia. "I never forgot the terrible pain she endured before, during and after" the extractions, her son said later.[1]

Most early toothpullers were itinerant medical men who extracted teeth with crude implements. Forceps were not invented until the 1840s, and it was then that dentistry and medicine began to separate, with each developing in different ways from craft to scientific profession by the end of the nineteenth century.

The year 1840 was also the beginning of the evolution of American dentistry as an autonomous profession, as David Levy has written in a paper of the same name.[2] Dentists Horace Hayden and Chapin Harris wanted to raise the level of dental education and tried to establish a dental department at the University of Maryland School of Medicine. They were unsuccessful and instead sought a charter from the state legislature for the Baltimore College of Dental Surgery, which would become the first college in the world devoted exclusively to dentistry.[3]

The refusal to include a chair in dentistry at Maryland has been called medicine's "historical rebuff"[4] of dentistry by most commentators, but Levy presents another point of view. The mid-nineteenth century physician's practice, as a contemporary wrote, centered on "the lame, the blind, the halt, the poor,"[5] while dental clients were for the most part wealthy persons. Levy explains how dentists during this early period were actually the elite practitioners:

Unlike the physician of the day whose treatment was risky and whose results were uncertain, the dentist had a technique that was predictable. Most oral surgery, while admittedly painful, did not depend on aseptic technique. Complications from properly or improperly conducted oral surgery were transitory and self-limiting. Restorative techniques were even more certain.[6]

In this view, the new direction that dentistry took with the opening of the Baltimore College of Dental Surgery signaled that the dental profession no longer wanted simply to be a branch of medicine.

EARLY ADVANCES

Nitrous oxide as anesthesia was first successfully used (in 1844) by Hartford dentist Horace Wells, but the public demonstration of its use was generally considered a failure because the patient cried out during the operation. In 1846, William Morton, who had enrolled in the Baltimore College of Dental Surgery but left before graduation to become Wells's partner, conducted the first successful public demonstration of the use of ether as an anesthesia for surgery.[7]

In 1839, *The American Journal of Dental Science*—the world's first dental journal—began publication. That same year, Charles Goodyear invented the vulcanization process for hardening rubber. The resulting vulcanite, an inexpensive material easily molded to the mouth, made an excellent base for false teeth and was soon adopted for use by dentists. In 1864, the molding process for vulcanite dentures was patented, but the dental profession fought the onerous licensing fees for the next twenty-five years.

James B. Morrison patented the first commercially manufactured foot-treadle dental engine in 1871. Morrison's inexpensive, mechanized tool supplied dental burs with enough speed to cut enamel and dentin and revolutionized the practice of dentistry. Unfortunately it was a laborious process, and patients experienced a great deal of vibration. Beatrice Bibby, wife of Dr. Basil Bibby, would recall in the course of an interview the foot treadles (similar to those on old sewing machines) on the prophylactic machines brought to the Rochester schools by hygienists.[8]

The collapsible metal tube that produced significant changes in toothpaste manufacturing and marketing was introduced in the 1880s. Dentifrice had been available only in liquid or powder form, usually made by individual dentists and sold in bottles, porcelain pots, or paper boxes. Tube toothpaste, in contrast, was mass-produced in factories, mass-marketed, and sold nationwide; in twenty years, it became the norm. The Colgate family—distant cousins and good friends of George Eastman—ran one of the best-known toothpaste factories. Indeed, in 1873, Colgate mass-produced the first toothpaste in a jar. In 1892, Dr. Washington Sheffield of Connecticut manufactured toothpaste in a collapsible tube; his product was marketed as "Dr. Sheffield's Creme Dentifrice." In 1896, Colgate Dental Cream was packaged in collapsible tubes, imitating Sheffield's innovation. A few years after the end of World War II, Colgate began adding fluoride to toothpaste.

Willoughby Miller, an American dentist in Germany, noted the microbial basis of dental decay in his 1890 book *Micro-Organisms of the Human Mouth.* Miller's book generated an unprecedented interest in oral hygiene and started a worldwide movement to promote regular tooth brushing and flossing. Later studies showed that while brushing did have a positive effect on preventing periodontal disease, no relationship could be detected between brushing and tooth decay. Allegedly, most Americans did not brush their teeth until returning World War II soldiers brought their acquired habits of tooth brushing home. Lack of brushing may not have caused George Eastman to lose his teeth at an early age, but that loss became another reason for his interest in preventive dentistry for children.

In 1895, German physicist Wilhelm Röntgen discovered a mysterious ray that he identified as an "x-ray." He also discovered that x-rays would expose film without light. Professor Röntgen was the first to behold what no other human had ever seen, a perfectly clear outline of the bones in his wife's hand, visible through the flesh. For this great discovery, he received the Nobel Prize for physics in 1901. Röntgen refused to patent his discovery, saying it was free for the benefit of mankind.

Design plans for x-ray generators were immediately published in journals, and scientists around the world soon had their own machines working. The speed at which x-rays were accepted was remarkable. The Eastman Kodak Company was soon manufacturing dental x-ray films. Cynics said this was the real reason for George Eastman's great interest in dentistry.

EARLY DENTISTRY IN ROCHESTER

Dentistry in the 1840s was neither organized nor recognized as a profession. And the technology was primitive. Dentist's offices lacked electricity, gas, and plumbing.

William Tichenor was one of fifteen dentists who practiced in Rochester during the 1840s. Because his descendants saved so much memorabilia, now housed at the Rochester Museum and Science Center, we have a good idea of the kind of dental services Maria Kilbourn Eastman found when her terrible toothaches occurred.

Three dentists shared Tichenor's office in the Reynolds Arcade, Rochester's glass-enclosed marketplace and community center. The city's library and post office were in the arcade, along with daguerreotype studios and Eastman's Commercial College, run by George Eastman's father, George Washington Eastman. John Jacob Bausch and Henry Lomb opened one of those daguerreotype studios in 1853. Tichenor advertised that his was an "improved dental practice" and that teeth were "prepared on plate is such a manner as to warrant them useful, durable, and natural." His advertisement read:

Advice free, and all operations warranted durable.

He also prepares and keeps constantly on hand a superior article of Dentifrice for beautifying and preserving the teeth and gums. References given if desired

Tichenor's business card read:

Natural Teeth carefully treated, and Artificial Teeth usefully and beautifully inserted from one to an entire set, without the attendance of the patient more than ten minutes.

Tichenor would have had a chair for his patients—either one designed for the purpose or one pressed into service. At that time, portable head-rests were available that could adapt regular chairs to the dentist's use. Handles made of ivory, ebony, pearl, steel, and horn identified each of the instruments as to their use. (Ivory was for one type of instrument, ebony for another, and so forth.) Tichenor would have kept his instruments in a portable case, since commercially manufactured dental cabinets were not available until the 1860s.

Of the 471 treatments listed in Tichenor's daybook, 108, or 23 percent, were extractions, while 207, or 44 percent, involved plugging or filling teeth by relatively crude methods. The 1840s drilling method involved twirling a steel drill between the fingers at 100 rpm. In contrast, the foot-treadle drill that came into use in the 1860s could achieve speeds of 2,000 rpm. (Modern drill speeds are in excess of 350,000 rpm.) It took about thirty minutes in the 1840s to drill and fill a medium-sized cavity, so many patients opted to have

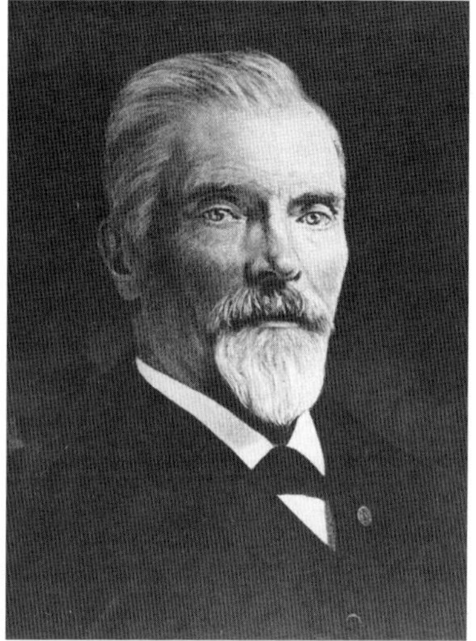
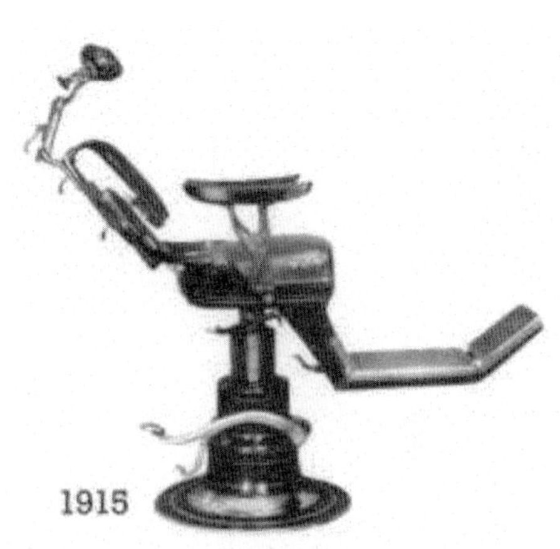

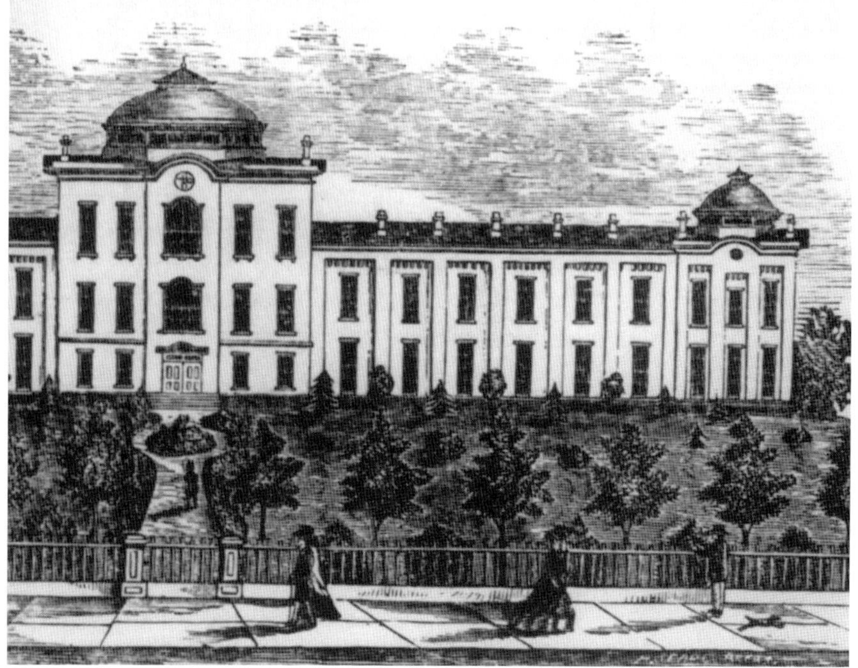

Henry Lomb; Ritter Dental Chair, 1915; City Hospital

the problem tooth extracted. Tichenor's practice was not confined to his office or home. His correspondence indicates that he also traveled to patients' homes throughout the state.

Rochester dentists and businessmen were an especially inventive lot. Until 1844, when Elijah Pope & Co. Surgical Instrument Makers opened for business, there was no firm manufacturing dental instruments and supplies; dentists made their own instruments and apparatuses, including chairs. Dr. John B. Beers made the first gold crown used in capping a broken tooth, and Frank Ritter helped revolutionize the dental equipment industry.

THE DENTAL CHAIR

The dental chair metamorphosed throughout the eighteenth and nineteenth centuries. In 1790, Josiah Flagg attached an adjustable headrest to a wooden Windsor chair; an arm extension held instruments. Portable headrests could adapt regular chairs in the homes that the toothpullers visited.

In 1832, James Snell invented the first reclining dental chair. In 1848, Waldo Hanchett patented his version of a dental chair, and the first pump-type hydraulic dental chair was introduced in 1877. Three nineteenth-century Rochester firms manufactured dental chairs. Robert W. Archer & Bros. made chairs as early as 1868, including a portable black metal dental chair.

Rochesterian Frank Ritter produced the all-in-one modern dental chair, leading to the formation of the Ritter Dental Company, for many years the world's leading manufacturer of chairs, dental units, and x-ray machines.

Frank Ritter (1844–1915) was born in Bavaria, where he apprenticed as a cabinetmaker. He emigrated to New York City in 1870 and, after experiencing the heat of summer there, moved to Rochester in 1872 where he hoped the climate would be more like that of his native Bavaria. The 1848 revolutions in many of the German states resulted in a massive exodus, and the largest immigrant population of both Rochester and the United States as a whole came from the German states. Ritter joined many of his countrymen in their move to Rochester, including John Jacob Bausch and Henry Lomb, who had closed their Daguerrean studio and were building a little lens shop into a thriving business. In 1873, Ritter started his own business, at first producing ornamental carvings for parlor furniture. The business grew, and by 1883 Ritter had a large stone and brick factory building. In 1887, Dewell Stuck came from Michigan with an idea for a new type of dental chair; Stuck persuaded Ritter to manufacture it.

Dentistry was just then emerging as a profession. The era of the itinerant toothpullers was passing. Higher educational standards were demanded and more dental schools were being opened. Preventive as well as operative dentistry was being recognized. With these advances came the demand for more modern equipment.

From Stuck's blueprints, Ritter produced the all-in-one modern dental chair. The "Stuck Chair" was the first to have a disk base; other dental chairs of that day were supported on four legs. The firm's first fifty chairs were shipped and warmly received by the profession. In 1890, experiments began on a new dental chair, which when marketed in 1891 was called the "Celebrated Columbian Chair."[9] It soon picked up the nickname the "jack-knife chair." Two features made this chair distinctive. First, it used hydraulic pressure for the raising and lowering mechanism. Second, it had the greatest range of any chair produced at that time: it could be raised higher and positioned lower than others on the market. In all, 215 of the Celebrated Columbian Chairs were produced and sold. The first chair, finished toward the end of 1893, featured telescoping tubes for raising and lowering; it also had roller bearings. As soon as it was exhibited, it was widely acclaimed. It was this chair that revolutionized the dental business and established the Ritter Dental Company firmly as the leader in its field. More than 6,500 of these chairs were manufactured and sold.

By 1895, Ritter's factory had abandoned the manufacture of furniture. That year, the brothers O. H. and A. F. Pieper joined Ritter and soon harnessed the new magic of electricity into a pioneer electric engine. The dental electric lathe was added to the line in 1896. In 1914, the electrically operated air compressor was introduced. The distributing panel was added in 1915; this incorporated electrical and air appliances necessary for a more modern dental practice. In 1917, the company introduced the first units combining the services of air, water, gas, and electricity in one compact assembly, bringing all operating essentials to the side of the chair.[10]

The convergence of Rochester inventiveness in several fields helped set the stage for the first free dental clinic in the United States, which opened in 1901 in Rochester, New York.

THE NATION'S FIRST
FREE DENTAL CLINIC

Preventive dental care for children was all but unknown until the twentieth century. If they were lucky or had a good diet and genes, children might keep their teeth until maturity. More likely, decaying teeth or receding gums might start in early adulthood and the toothpuller would be called. This is what happened to George Eastman and his mother, painful events that primed the budding philanthropist to undertake a project in preventive dental care for children.

At the turn of twentieth century, Rochester had an enlightened dental profession. "Rochester is justly entitled to the credit for the establishment of the first free dental clinic in the United States, which was started by the Rochester Dental Society in 1901," Harvey J. Burkhart, DDS LD, wrote in the "Centennial History of Dentistry in Rochester" in 1934. "This service was rendered in the City [now Rochester General] Hospital, but discontinued after a trial of two years." The problem seems to have one of location rather than concept, because in 1904 the clinic was restarted at Public School No. 14.

Captain Henry Lomb (1828–1908), cofounder of Bausch and Lomb, made an initial donation of $600 for instruments and appliances. A charter was obtained from the State Board of Charities, and the dispensary opened to the public on Washington's birthday, February 22, 1905. Through cooperation with school principals, children were sent to the clinic from different schools. If dental service was required, they were told to consult their dentists. The clinic treated those children whose families could not afford a dentist. The organizers soon found that "voluntary medical and dental services are usually not very reliable. So it was decided to employ a regular dentist, whose salary was paid by Captain Lomb up until his death in 1908."[11]

Henry Lomb's contribution to dentistry followed his success in the field of optical instruments in Rochester. He and John Jacob Bausch (1830–1926) had opened a daguerreotype parlor and shop in the Reynolds Arcade in 1853. Lomb provided the $60 capital. His investment of $60 in Bausch's optical venture earned him part interest in the firm. Unlike Bausch and his sons, William and Edward, Lomb was not a scientist but served the company as sales agent.

The shop offered horn-rimmed spectacles as a sideline. Bausch imported the horn from an older brother in Germany, then cut and polished it. Legend has it that one day when Bausch was kicking stones while walking to work, one stone unexpectedly bounced. It turned out to be a piece of hard rubber, and Bausch wondered if hard rubber would make good frames for spectacles. In 1866 he signed a contract with the India Rubber Comb Company for the exclusive right to make microscopes, telescopes, and other optical instruments from its vulcanite product. (Contemporaneously, dentists were using vulcanized rubber for plates.) Newer and cheaper spectacle frames led to increased sales, and a new factory on St. Paul Street for the grinding of optical lenses opened in 1874. Vulcanite soon made Bausch & Lomb the premier optical company. By 1889, it was the largest optical factory in the world.

John Jacob Bausch was a role model for George Eastman. According to a letter he wrote to Bausch in the 1920s, Eastman as a child, ever the entrepreneur, hung around the Bausch and Lomb factory on North Water Street, picking up disks of discarded hard rubber punched from eyeglass frames. He then used a jackknife to cut them into finger rings to sell to childhood companions.[12] At some point, Eastman decided that one day he, like Messrs. Bausch and Lomb, would be a captain of industry. (If the Kodak camera had not done it, he would have tried something else.)

Bausch and Lomb's venture echoed the story of other Rochester immigrants. Foreign-born Rochesterians, particularly Germans fleeing the repressions that followed the collapse of the revolutions of 1848, brought skills and trades that enabled them to develop specialized shops that would free Rochester from its reliance on flagging flour mills. Two-thirds of the Germans immigrating to Rochester were engaged in manufacturing, and many of them fabricated products used in dentistry. For example, brewer John Pfaudler, who founded the Pfaudler Vacuum Fermentation Company in 1902, later produced glass-lined metal tanks for liquids. Other Rochester firms, such as the Taylor Instrument Company, which made thermometers and gauges, or the Wilmot Castle Company, which manufactured sterilizers, would contribute to dentistry. Members of the Rochester families who founded and managed these companies intermarried over the generations, so that when the Rochester Dental Dispensary opened in 1917, the chairs, engines, instruments, sterilizers, lantern slides, x-ray plates and films equipping it, and portable equipment that prophylactic squads took to the schools often came as gifts from this extended family.[13] The contributions of the foreign-born to dentistry in Rochester continue to the present time.

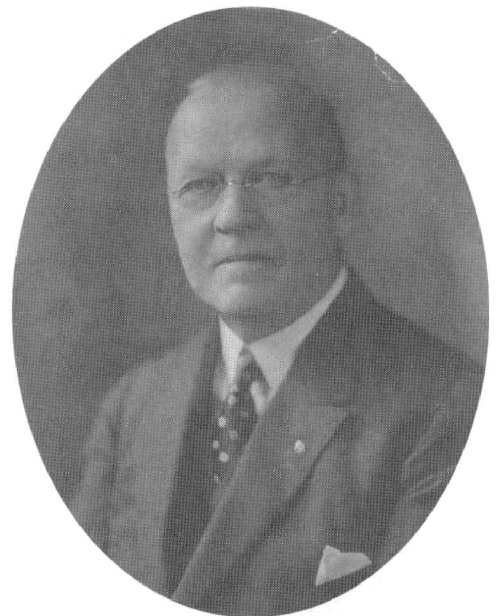

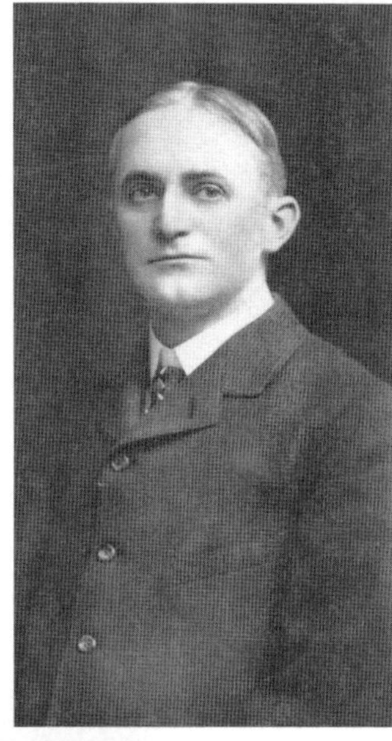

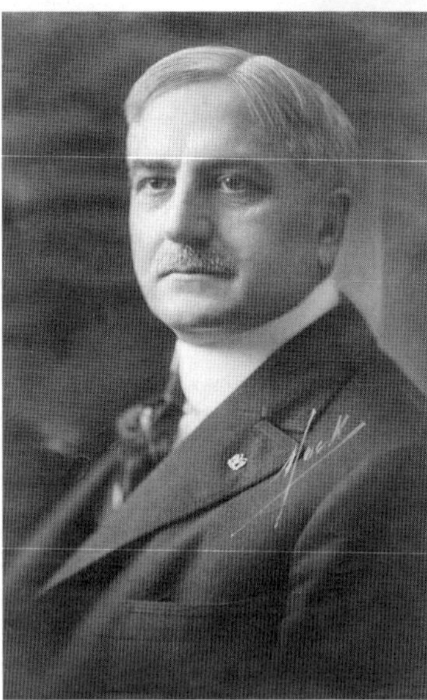

Clockwise from top, left: William Bausch, George Eastman (Courtesy George Eastman House), Harvey Burkhart

Shortly after the dental clinic was established at School No. 14, Henry Lomb persuaded Eastman and William ("Billy") Bausch (1861–1944), son of the other founder of Bausch and Lomb, to join him in furnishing a second clinic. This new clinic was established at School No. 26, where children in the immediate neighborhood could be treated.

According to the National Academy Press in *Dental Education at the Crossroads,* "The first dental inspection of schoolchildren began in 1906 in Rochester, New York. These inspections were undertaken primarily as part of the oral hygiene movement. This movement also included the founding of children's dental clinics with funding from George Eastman in Rochester and the Forsyths in Boston. Both clinics evolved into leading centers of dental research and postgraduate education."[14]

In 1909, Eastman was one of ten Rochesterians who contributed $200 a year toward the maintenance of the Free Dental Dispensary of the Rochester Dental Society. After Henry Lomb's death in 1908, William Bausch had picked up the gauntlet, and he may have asked Eastman, a close friend, to take Lomb's part in the project. These clinics carried on until 1917, when the Eastman-sponsored dental dispensary opened its doors.

The early free clinics supported by the Bausches and Lombs had a national impact, according to Harvey Burkhart, the first director of the Rochester Dental Dispensary:

> To the dentists of Rochester, who were instrumental in the organization of the first dental clinic, is no doubt due the credit for the far-reaching effect in calling the attention of the profession and the public to the value of early attention to the teeth. The pattern set here in the organization and maintenance of the clinic was followed in many other towns and cities throughout the land and also adopted in some places abroad.

When continuation of these clinics was threatened by lack of funds, Eastman, foreshadowing conditions he would employ in the future, offered to fund the dental project on three conditions:

1. That treatment be rendered in a central clinic

2. That the city provide $12,000 annually for dental prophylaxis in schools

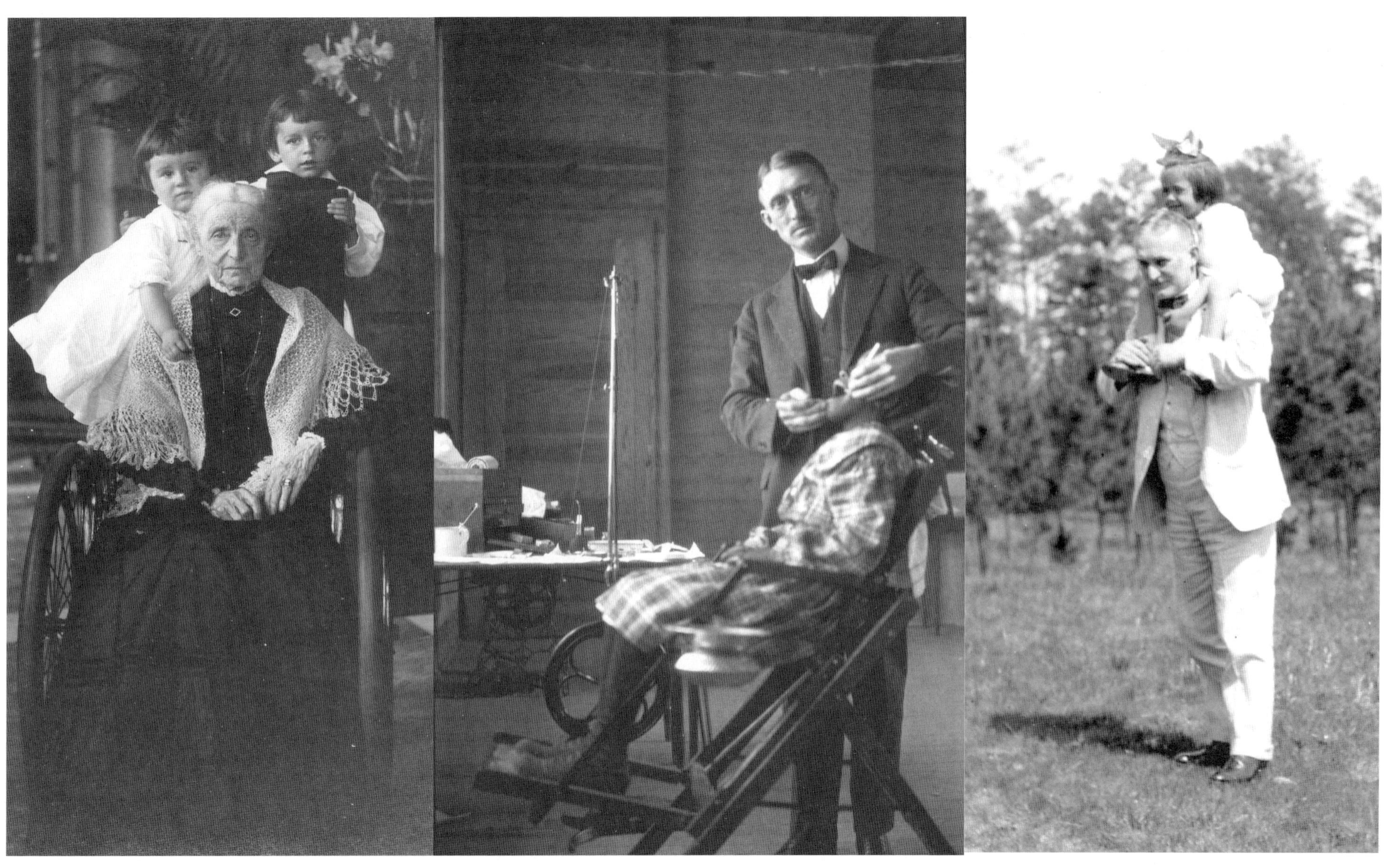

Maria Kilbourn Eastman and great-grandchildren (Courtesy George Eastman House);
Dentist treats child at Oak Lodge, George Eastman's Carolina farm (Courtesy George Eastman House);
George Eastman with grandniece Ellen Maria Dryden (Author's collection)

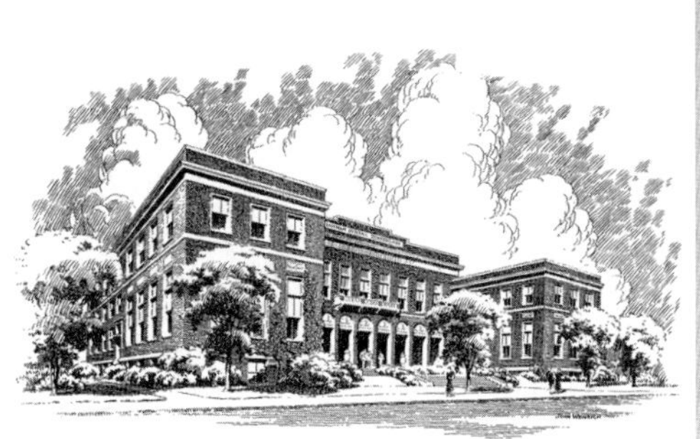
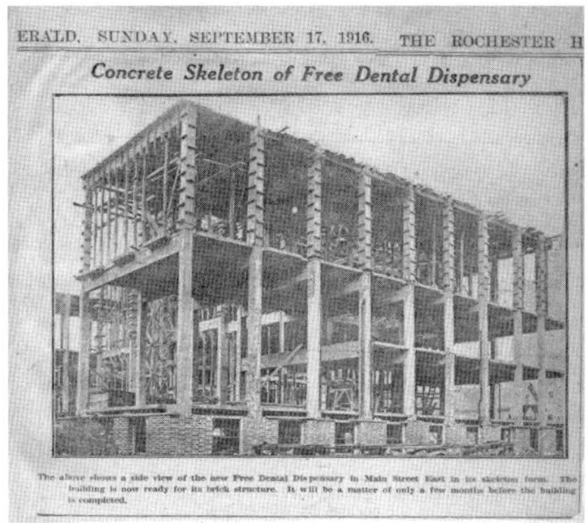

*Delineation of the proposed Rochester Dental Dispensary;
Concrete skeleton of the building under construction*

3. That ten citizens contribute $1,000 a year for five years for an operating budget

These citizens became the board of directors; Eastman himself was not a member of the board. When his conditions were met, Eastman would single-handedly undertake the responsibility of erecting and furnishing the dispensary. Decades later, Eastman would broaden the program to pilot clinics in key cities around the world to demonstrate the importance of dental care for children. For one who occasionally grumbled about the evils of socialism, Eastman was about to embark on his own great experiment in socialized medicine.

FORESHADOWING THE
ROCHESTER DENTAL DISPENSARY

That Eastman, a bachelor, had an abstract interest in children is evident from his long-term involvement in the Rochester Orphan Asylum and from his support of the Children's Aid Society, Children's Shelter, Children's Playground League, Playground and Recreation Association of America, and the National Child Labor Committee. And in 1913, Judge George Carnahan solicited Eastman for help in building a Children's

Shelter. Carnahan told Eastman that if he wasn't interested to say so quickly. "But I am interested," Eastman countered. "What is your plan?" Carnahan returned with a plan and Eastman quietly wrote out a check for $43,000, the entire amount needed.

The health of children interested Eastman enormously. He frequently asked Dr. Albert D. Kaiser, a pediatrician and for many years the city's esteemed medical officer, how this or that disease common to children might be controlled. He was at his best with children and never felt the need to put on his icy public mask with them. The children he knew best were his grandnephew and grandniece. George Eastman Dryden remembers visits to his great uncle at Eastman House as a halcyon time in his life.[15] As snapshots attest, their summers were spent romping through the gardens, pulling wagons, racing about with glee, dabbling in the heated lily pond, lunching on the east terrace porch, playing hide and seek around hydrangea pots, and careening on brick paths in great-grandmother Maria's wheelchair—all while Uncle George snapped their pictures with his latest Kodak camera. Eastman made 900 East Avenue a magic place for the young. Perhaps the most poignant communication of this period was the telegram that arrived from young Dryden in 1920: "PASSED ENTRANCE EXAMINATIONS . . . CAN I COME TONIGHT AND HAVE BRACES PUT ON TEETH?" Chances are the youth got his wish. Other people's children were easier to deal with: dental care did not turn them into houseguests.

THE FORSYTH DENTAL INFIRMARY

Boston's Forsyth Dental Infirmary for Children served as both an inspiration and a model for Eastman. In 1913, Nelson Curtis, the Boston photographic paper manufacturer who supplied the raw stock for the Velox paper that Kodak manufactured, sent Eastman pamphlets about the Forsyth Dental Infirmary then proposed for Boston. In 1914, while visiting Cambridge to check on the Massachusetts Institute of Technology buildings, which he was funding anonymously, Eastman slipped off to look over the infirmary construction incognito. "During the rest of that year," an Eastman biographer reports, "Eastman reflected upon the possibilities of a similar project in Rochester without revealing his thoughts to anyone."[16] The Boston clinic was the first such experiment in centralized dental care for children in the

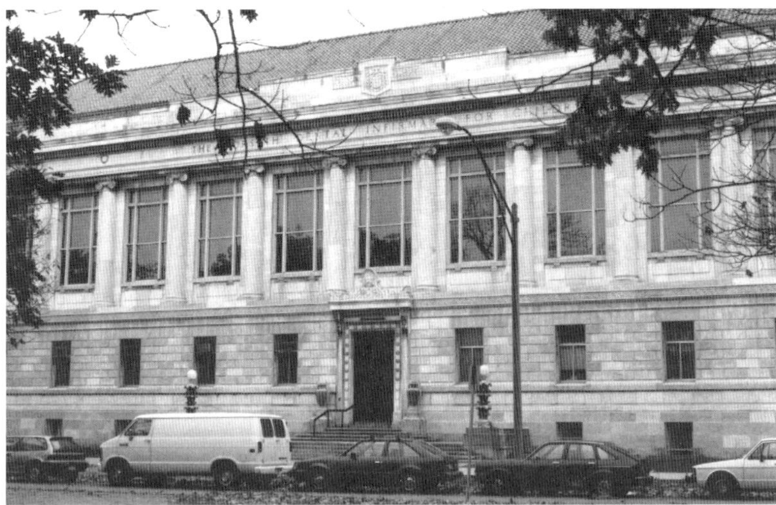

"Boston's Temple to Dentistry": the Forsyth Dental Infirmary
(Author's collection)

country, perhaps in the world.[17] A second visit to the clinic in 1914 confirmed Eastman's commitment.

William Forsyth, who emigrated from Scotland in the 1830s, was, like William Bausch, a pioneer in the manufacture of vulcanized rubber goods. His four sons continued his business interests in the production of vulcanized rubber, creating substantial wealth for the family. Before his death, James Bennett Forsyth had begun discussions pertaining to establishing a dental clinic for the children of Boston. In 1910, James's two surviving brothers, Thomas and John, along with their sister Mary, fulfilled his dream by founding the Forsyth Dental Infirmary for Children, an outwardly imposing and beautifully designed facility constructed of white Vermont marble. Opening its doors in 1914, the new clinic was charged with providing complete oral therapy for children, with an emphasis on prevention of dental caries. Dental interns and graduate dentists staffed the clinic. Thomas Forsyth remarked at the dedication ceremony, "It has been my wish that the infirmary should be a home to the children, beautiful and cheerful; a protector of their health, a refuge in their pain." In its first ten years, the infirmary treated over 150,000 children for dental and craniofacial problems.

Believing that oral hygiene and early detection were key factors in controlling disease, Forsyth established the Forsyth School for Dental

Hygienists in 1916, the same year that Eastman and Burkhart established a school for dental hygienists as an integral part of the Rochester Dental Dispensary. Forsyth scientists also pioneered important research in the dental field and eventually became a research-only institution, dropping the clinical treatment facilities entirely.

MORE FREE CLINICS

In the spring of 1915, William Bausch chaired a committee of citizens and dentists that proposed more free dental clinics in locations throughout Rochester in addition to those that had been established earlier. Eastman greeted the proposal with his usual protracted silence and voluminous research. Four months later, he presented his own solution: a centralized clinic with trained hygienists, paid by the city but under the control of an independent board of trustees. The hygienists would visit the Rochester schools twice a year to clean and check children's teeth and refer the serious cases to the central clinic. With his proposal came his offer to build the clinic if these conditions were met. Eastman's letter to Bausch said, in part:

> I should not care to have anything to do with this affair unless a scheme be devised which will cover the whole field and do the work thoroughly and completely and in the best manner. Basing my opinion on all the information that has come to me up to the present time, I do not think that the work of treating children's teeth, outside of prophylactic work to be done by the hygienists, can be satisfactorily done and supervised at clinics distributed over the city.[18]

It's possible that Eastman read a report to the Carnegie Foundation on medical education in the United States prepared by Abraham Flexner in 1910. Flexner's survey concluded that "graduates . . . are lamentably lacking in knowledge and technique and need a postgraduate training before they go into general practice." If this was true for fledgling doctors, Eastman may have reasoned, it would also apply to fledgling dentists. A centralized clinic would provide this postgraduate year. Another argument for a single clinic was that "it is necessary to have as operators young, immature dentists who cannot be allowed to work without first-class supervision." It would be easier to provide supervision in a centralized clinic.

MATCHING FUNDS REQUIRED

Along with centralization, Eastman's other key requirements were financial: "A corporation to be managed by trustees . . . to provide for the raising of . . . not less than $10,000 yearly for five years." William Bausch organized a board of fifteen trustees who each agreed to contribute $1,000 a year to the operation of the dispensary. Eastman proposed to "build and equip a suitable central building and contribute . . . $30,000 per year for five years." Then, "if the institution is . . . performing its mission satisfactorily I will endow it with . . . $750,000. If . . . $40,000 is not enough for running expenses . . . I will furnish the same proportion of any additional sum." In the publicity, Eastman's name was not mentioned, and the clinic was incorporated as the Rochester Dental Dispensary on October 26, 1915. Its purpose: the prevention and curing of diseases of the ear, nose, mouth, and throat. Eastman contributed the budget for the first year and then resigned as a trustee. The choice of a director was left to the trustees, hardly any of whom had not heard about a wonderfully comfortable set of false teeth that Dr. Burkhart had provided for Mr. Eastman. Harvey Burkhart was the unanimous selection.

The central clinic was not the be-all and end-all of Eastman's project, however, as his letter to a Columbus, Ohio, correspondent indicates:

> The Dispensary is only incidental to the main scheme, which is prevention of trouble in the teeth. The Di\spensary will devote its attention to repairing the trouble which has already occurred and the education of the prophylactic force which will operate in the schools. The expectation is that eighty per cent of the teeth trouble can be prevented by this work, which will be very systematically done.

From the start, Harvey Burkhart hoped that a dental school would augment the dispensary. Instead of waiting five years to endow the dispensary with $750,000 as he had promised if the institution lived up to expectations, Eastman decided to make it a nice round $1 million after just three years. During his lifetime and by bequest, Eastman donated about $3 million to the Rochester Dental Dispensary. His generous gift has been carefully managed, and in 2000, the nearly $50 million endowment provided support for the Eastman Dental Center, the Eastman Department of Dentistry, and the Center for Oral Biology at the University of Rochester's School of Medicine and Dentistry.

Critics saw Eastman's central clinic as a monument to himself and his sudden (to the outside world) interest in dentistry as a marketing device to sell x-ray film and plates. Sensitive to the second charge (the first he considered silly, since he was opposed to monuments), Eastman had his biographer, Carl Ackerman, refute it in a long note that began: "He had long since made it a definite policy not to mix business and philanthropy." (Nevertheless, the income from the dispensary doing x-ray work for Rochester dentists at reasonable rates would amount to about $54,000 per year during Eastman's lifetime.)

The project began with a set of architectural renderings entitled "Suggestions for the Rochester Dental Dispensary." In July 1915, Eastman sent Edwin Gordon, architect, a Dr. Burns, dentist, and William Bausch to Boston to meet Thomas A. Forsyth. Gordon came home with drawings, blueprints, and pictures of the Beaux Arts Forsyth building, which he carefully pasted in his growing Eastman-projects scrapbook. Gordon's first renderings featured a limestone facade with classical pilasters and a red tile roof, strongly reminiscent of the Boston clinic. The name, Rochester Dental Dispensary, chosen by Eastman, would remain until 1941, nine years after his death. At that time, the trustees chose to honor the founder be renaming it Eastman Dental Dispensary.[19]

A note from Thomas Forsyth included in the package of blueprints and drawings of the Forsyth institution that Gordon brought back from Boston said in part:

> When that day arrives that the United States shall be dotted with similar institutions, then I shall be content that the Forsyth Infirmary has actually accomplished ALL that it was founded for; i. e. not alone that the children of Boston be benefited, but that our cities and towns, observing the good that we are daily accomplishing, should pattern similar buildings for their own use. The greater the number of such institutions, the less the need for insane hospitals, sanitariums and prisons.[20]

THE NEW ROCHESTER DENTAL DISPENSARY OPENS

On October 15, 1917, the doors of the new dispensary opened at 800 East Main Street, two city blocks from the University of Rochester's Prince Street campus. The functional, U-shaped building of rough-textured brick with white Venetian marble trim patterned after Italian Renaissance architecture, two stories plus basement, restrained yet handsome in proportion and detail, had cost George Eastman $402,972.88 for property, architects, models, and construction. For the dedication, the dental society provided music and flowers, and Eastman furnished the fifty-cent luncheons for 500 guests. As was usual with this shy man, he managed to be out of town for the dedication, to the dismay of William Hall Walker, his business partner, who came from Great Barrington, Massachusetts, to attend the festivities. When Eastman learned that the state dental society had appropriated $500 for a testimonial gift to him, he grumbled sternly, "I don't want any loving cup. I wish you'd take the money and buy something for the dispensary instead."

The second floor "operatory," a large room with floor-to-ceiling windows along the two long sides to take advantage of daylight and space for sixty-eight operating units specially designed by the Rochester-based Ritter Dental Company, appears amazingly light, airy, and modern in vintage photographs. The daughters of the late Frank Ritter,[21] Mrs. Adeline Ritter Shumway and Mrs. Laura Ritter Brown, gave thirty of the thirty-seven motorized units consisting of a chair and attached equipment, which were installed in 1917 in memory of their father, inventor of the modern dental unit. By this time, Adeline Ritter Shumway was president of the company. The units were designed by Otto Pieper, Ritter engineer, with tips from Eastman, and served as models for the manufacture of similar units elsewhere. Later, Eastman and Burkhart would devise an improved dental cabinet with a wash stand at one end and a sterilizer at the other so that the operator did not have to waste steps by leaving to wash his or her hands or to sterilize instruments. According to Dr. William McHugh, former director of the dental center, "At his [George Eastman's] suggestion, the Ritter Company developed a single unit to combine such dental equipment as drills, spittoon, gas and water supply."[22]

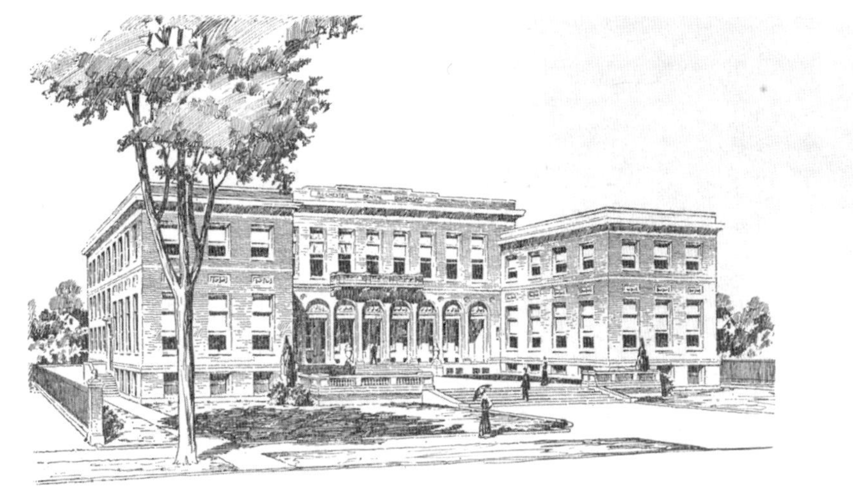

Invitation to the dedication of the Rochester Dental Dispensary

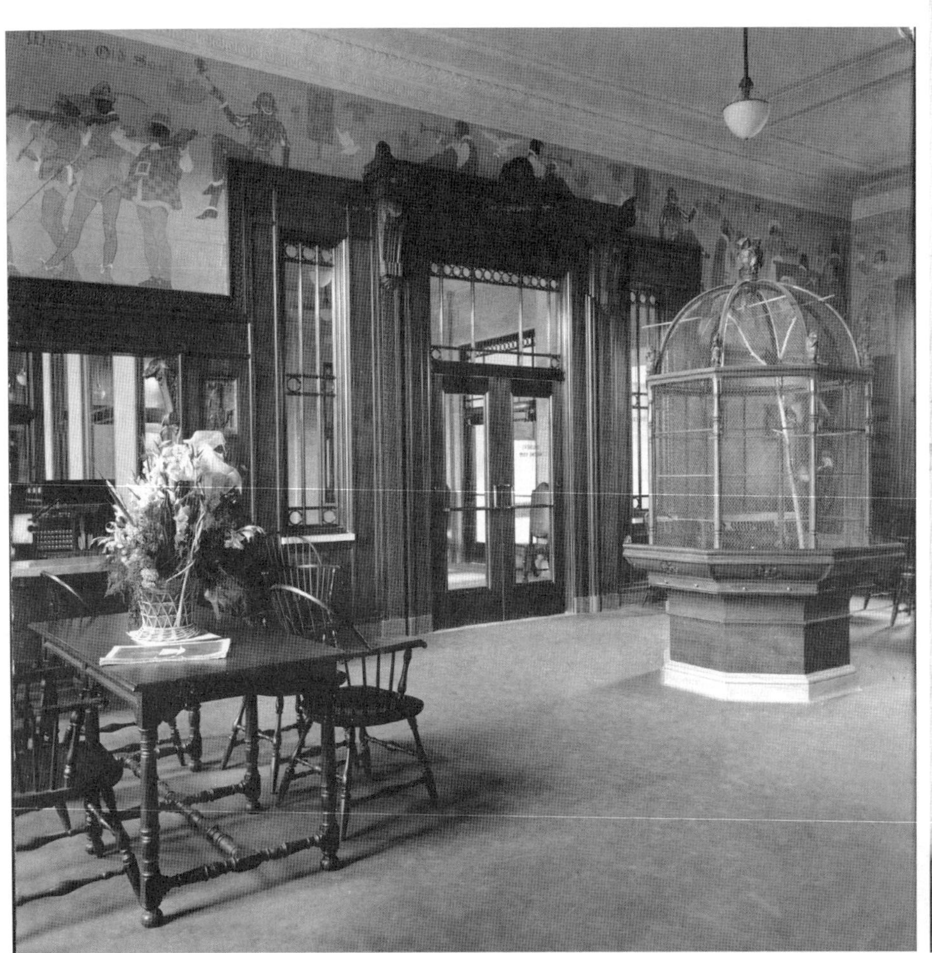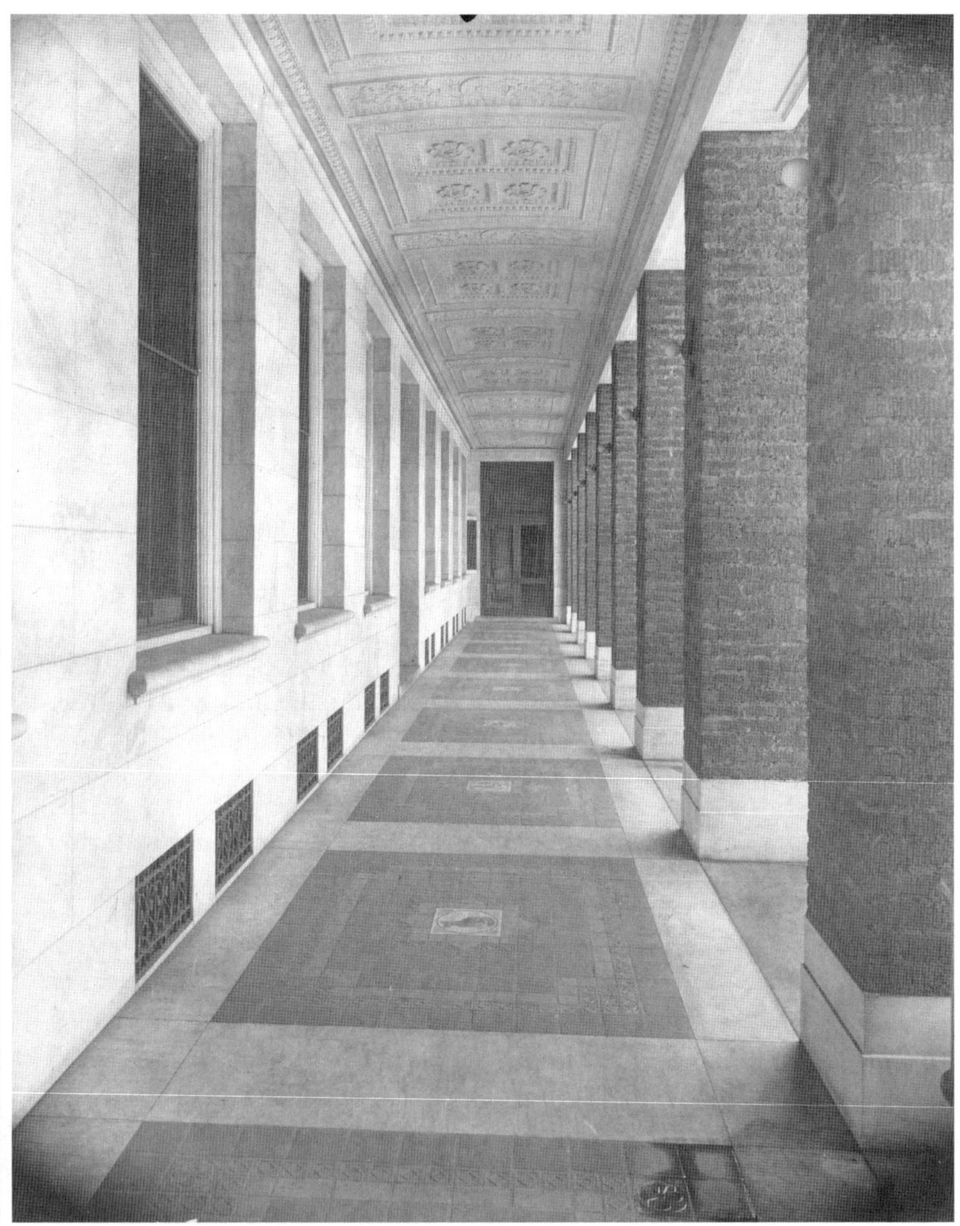

Aviary in Children's Waiting Room and dispensary arcade

MR. GEORGE EASTMAN
THE PRESIDENT AND DIRECTORS
OF THE
ROCHESTER DENTAL DISPENSARY
EXTEND A CORDIAL INVITATION
TO THE MEMBERS
OF THE DENTAL PROFESSION
TO AVAIL THEMSELVES OF THE FACILITIES PROVIDED
AT THE DISPENSARY
TO CARRY ON EXPERIMENTAL AND RESEARCH WORK

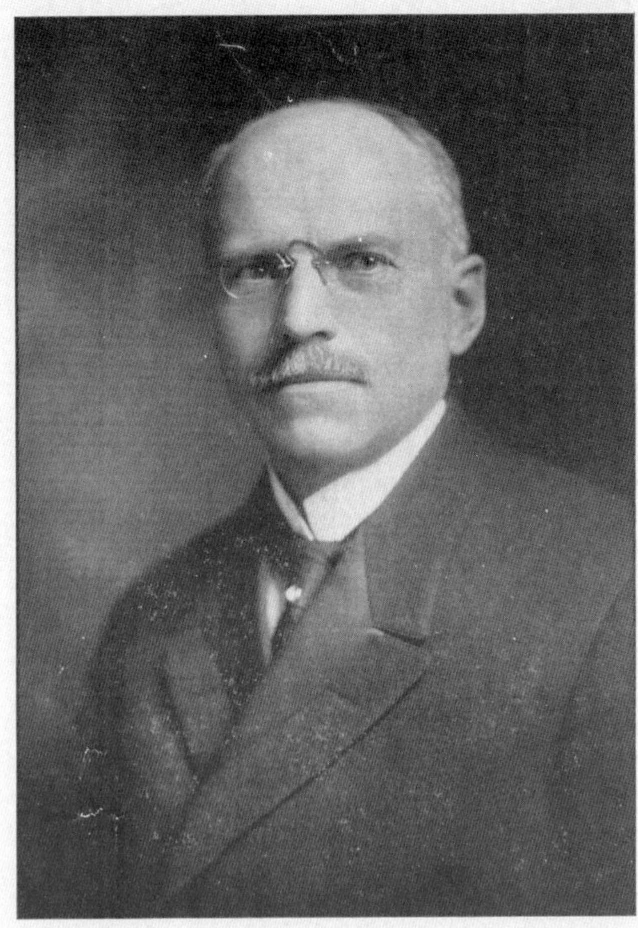

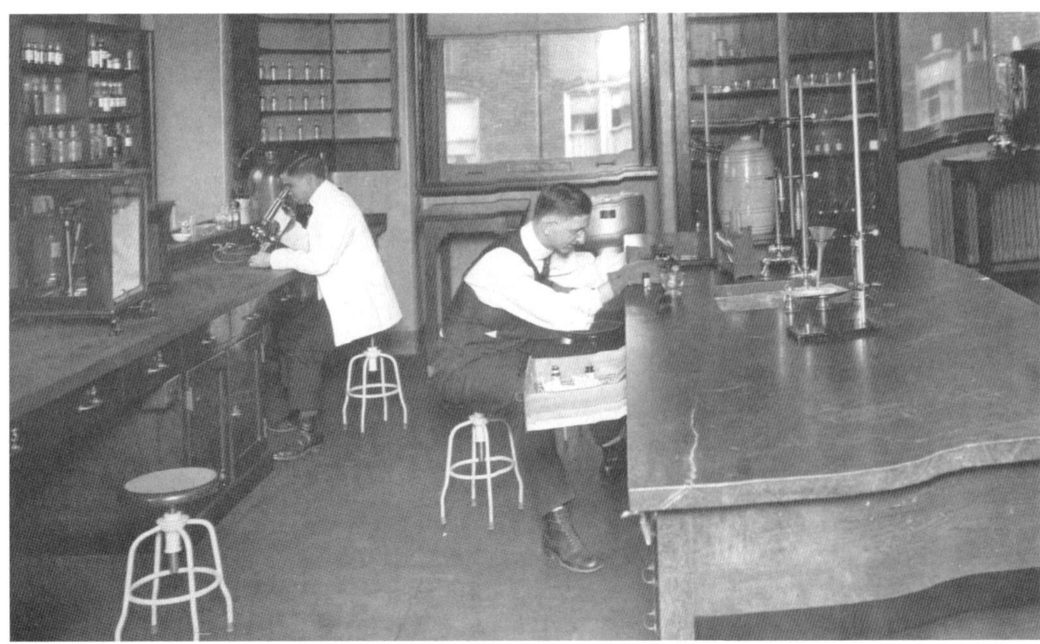

The early research department was dedicated to the memory of Dr. Rudolph Hofheinz.

"And incidentally," Carl Ackerman wrote, "the construction of those units, largely designed for this institution, served as models for the manufacture of units which in succeeding years were in use in practically all of the leading dental offices in the United States.[23]

The most notable feature of the new building was the children's waiting room provided by William Bausch. Oak brackets were carved in the form of elephants, sheep, and dogs, and oak paneling had animal figures sculpted in high relief. Above the paneling were whimsical murals by Clifford Ulp, head of the art department at Mechanics Institute, depicting Mother Goose scenes of "Goosie Goosie Gander," "Sing a Song of Sixpence," and "Little Jack Horner" (in a corner, of course). Behind the drinking fountain was a ceramic mosaic wall in bronzed tiles with frogs and lily pads. (Eastman went along with the brightly colored murals but had architect Ed Gordon repaint the outdoor arcade a pristine white.) In the center of this large and cheerful space was a handsome aviary with live birds. The room represented Bausch and Eastman's effort to encourage the children of Rochester not to fear dentistry. The birdcage would become the logo for Eastman dental clinics and when more were built in Europe, they too had birdcages in the waiting rooms. (In the beginning, parrots lived in the aviary. They were found to be too raucous, too frightening to small children, and combative to the point of nastiness, so they were replaced by mild-mannered canaries.)

The east wing contained the research department, the library of the dental society, and a museum of skulls, both human and animal (some animals shot by the donor himself), illustrating dental formations. The west wing housed the x-ray and photographic departments and rooms for special examinations and root canal work. Dr. Rudolph Hofheinz, Captain Lomb's dentist, had been named principal of the Dental Hygiene School but died suddenly before it opened. Mrs. Hofheinz donated the laboratory equipment in her husband's memory and contributed additional funds for dental research. The mezzanine was arranged as a children's hospital for oral surgery patients. Besides the main operatory, the second floor contained the orthodontia department to the west and the extracting and oral surgery rooms to the east. The basement was given over to the kitchen and lunchroom. Twenty to thirty dental interns (all male at this time) every year each had his own chair, equipment, and patients; interns in oral surgery were assigned to hospitals. Standard surgical, x-ray, and laboratory techniques and procedures were put into operation.

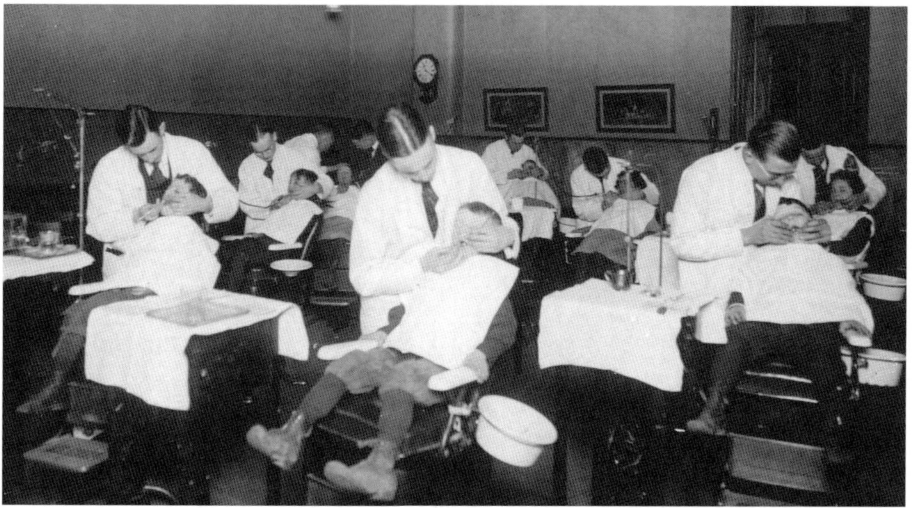

Interns at work, 1917

Work was limited to children under sixteen, unless the family income was five dollars per week or less; then, children could come until they were twenty-one years old.[24] To insure appreciation of services, at least five cents per visit was charged. In 1920, in consideration of 1,000 shares of Kodak stock from Mr. Eastman, reduced rates were extended to children of Kodak employees. By 1970 the general fee was only fifty cents, and a fee schedule was established for patients not receiving Medicaid at 30 to 50 percent of the prevailing private insurance rate. If financial necessity required, the fee could be reduced. However, this was mostly academic since there was actually little effort expended to actually collect fees. The rate of collection ran between 25 percent and 50 percent.

In addition to being given dental care, the children were also examined for nose, throat, and mouth defects. Ackerman noted, "An astonishingly large number had hypertrophied tonsils and adenoids to such a degree as to cut down nasal respiration to a point that very markedly interfered with the normal development of the jaws." On his initial visit to the Forsyth Dental Infirmary for Children in 1914, Eastman had been allowed to stand in the operating theater and watch a tonsillectomy performed on a young girl. The experience left an indelible impression about the efficacy of this operation as a prophylactic measure.

The charter Eastman approved for the dispensary in 1915 described its purposes as "to own, maintain, and operate a dispensary for the prevention, treatment, and cure of diseases of the eye, ear, nose, mouth, throat, and any part of the head by medical, surgical, or prophylactic methods." Interestingly, although everyone knew that Mr. Eastman's primary interest was preventive dental care for the indigent children of Rochester, the words "teeth," "dental," "children," "indigent," or "Rochester" do not appear in the charter or bylaws.

MASS PRODUCING DENTAL CARE

Ackerman wrote, "The dispensary was on a 'mass production' basis. Within three years the records were formidable."[25] Eastman had pioneered in mass production and standardization of parts into photographic manufacturing, so it was natural that he would apply similar techniques to dentistry. Within a few years, the dental department reported the advantages gained by standardization of filling materials and methods made possible by the centralized clinic. The department of orthodontia reported even more miraculous results: "Not only were the appearance and comfort of many children improved," but Eastman further claimed, without any basis in fact, that "improvements in speech were obtained by widening the arch, and frequently children who were below normal mentally were helped by the removal of nerve pressure usually found in a crowded jaw."

In 1921, Eastman himself, ever the tinkerer and inventor, would go back into the Camera Works and design a special orthodontia camera for the "remaking of faces," as he called the straightening of teeth, with the hope of improving a person's bite and appearance. The unit led to a new department—dental photography. Next to tonsillectomies, "remaking faces" seemed to be his primary interest. Pictures were taken periodically of the front view and profile of patients' faces. With the Eastman camera, there were no variations in position or size; orthodontic progress thus became reproducible.

As for more routine dental care, prophylactic squads were galvanized and dispatched to public and parochial schools with portable chairs, instruments, sterilizers, and lantern slides proselytizing oral hygiene. (The city paid for this until the 1960s.) Toothbrush drills were de rigueur. Follow-up cases were referred to the dispensary. To train the squads as well as the hygienists who worked at the dispensary, Burkhart engaged two instructors at $100 a month,

an assistant to teach the toothbrush drill, a social service worker, a matron, and a principal. Pamphlets printed in English, Italian, Yiddish, and Polish were sent to Rochester parents, instructing them to bring their babies to the dispensary as soon as the first tooth erupted and to keep them on the rolls for follow-ups until age sixteen. (Sixteen remains the top age for pediatric dental patients at the University of Rochester Medical Center (URMC), as compared to eighteen or twenty-one for pediatric medical patients.) Thus, while Eastman's main object was clinical community dentistry for children whose families could not afford dental care, the role of education—for children, parents, and young dental school graduates—began to evolve immediately through the emphasis placed on the hygienist. Burkhart's hope of founding a school to train dentists would have to be deferred.

ROCHESTER'S SCHOOL FOR DENTAL HYGIENISTS

Female dental assistants were first hired in the nineteenth century when "Lady in Attendance" signs were routinely seen in the windows of dental offices. Their duties included chair-side assistance, instrument cleaning, and inventory. Cyrus M. Wright established the first formal training program for dental nurses at the Ohio College of Dental Surgery in 1910. The program was discontinued in 1914 mainly due to opposition from Ohio dentists. In 1913, Alfred C. Fones opened the Fones Clinic for Dental Hygienists in Bridgeport, Connecticut, coining the term *dental hygienist* and establishing the world's first oral hygiene school. Most of the twenty-seven women graduates of the first class were employed by the Bridgeport Board of Education to clean the teeth of school children. The claim of greatly reduced incidence of caries among these children gave impetus to the dental hygienist movement. As the first to use the term *dental hygienist,* Dr. Fones would become known as the father of dental hygiene.

In 1924, female dental assistants were further organized and codified when Juliette Southard and her female colleagues founded the American Dental Assistants Association.[26] One of the first places to subscribe to the new hygienist movement was Rochester. In establishing the Rochester Dental Dispensary in 1915, George Eastman listed as one of his conditions

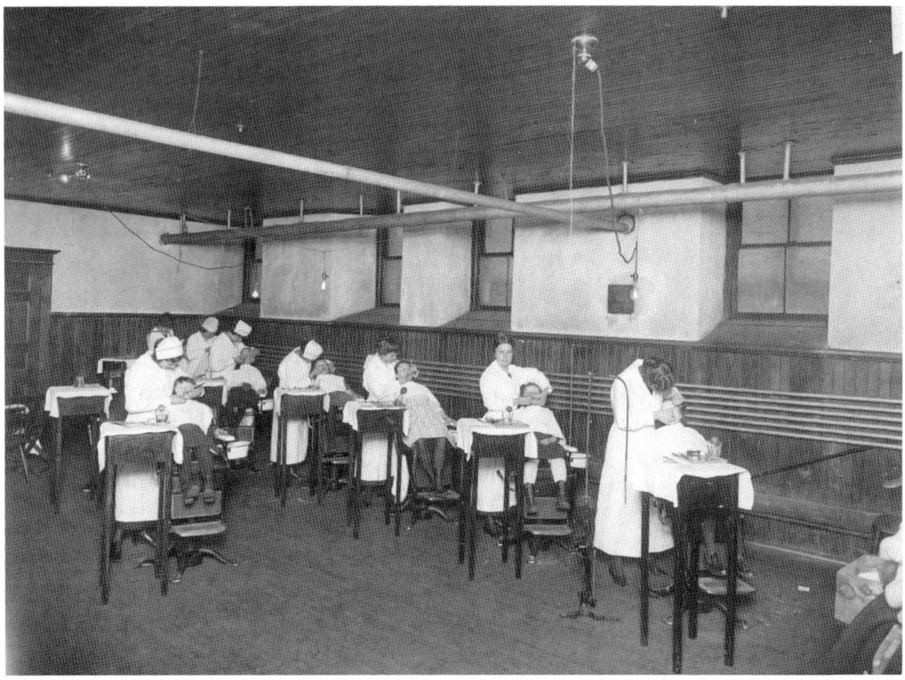

Hygienists at work

recruiting "the services of a sufficient number of dental hygienists and material to clean and examine the teeth of the school children twice a year."

The School for Dental Hygienists (SDH) of the Rochester Dental Dispensary opened in 1916 in borrowed rooms of the University of Rochester's Catharine Strong Hall.[27] By starting the school for oral hygiene in a university building, Eastman may have been suggesting that an affiliation between the Rochester Dental Dispensary and the university should be established. Perhaps the student hygienists could receive instruction in the Eastman Laboratory for physics and biology, which had opened in 1904. Perhaps a dental school would someday be part of the university. When Eastman purchased land on which to erect a beautiful state-of-the-art dental dispensary, it would be two blocks from the university. But then, as we shall see, when the School of Medicine and Dentistry was formed, it would be many miles away on the other side of town. Almost immediately, the men's undergraduate campus would follow, leaving the women's campus, the Memorial Art Gallery, the Eastman Theatre and School of Music, the dental dispensary, and the school of oral hygiene in the older, more central section of Rochester.

In 1917, according to American Dental Association (ADA) histories, Irene Newman in Connecticut received the world's first dental hygiene license. However, Rochester Dental Dispensary histories assert that the first diplomas from the School for Dental Hygienists of the Rochester Dental Dispensary were distributed in January 1917. This is because there were two terms of study. Short Term Girls, who already had their RN degree or experience in dental offices, attended classes and lectures from September to January or January to June and then could take their examination. Long Term Girls starting from scratch attended classes from September to June. Nineteen hygienists graduated in the June ending the first short term, thirty-six the second year, forty-one the third, and fifty-five the fourth. Tuition began at $60 in the first year and increased to $105 by the fourth year.

The second condition of Eastman's proposal, to prepare "trained dental hygienists," possibly suggested by Harvey Burkhart, was controversial. "At that time," Burkhart would write, "this was regarded in the light of an experiment and many doubts were expressed about the wisdom of creating a new vocation for women." Eastman had no doubts and lobbied mightily in Albany to obtain legislation to amend the state charter so as to legalize the practice of oral prophylaxis by women. As a result, the School for Dental Hygienists of the Rochester Dental Dispensary was the first such school to be established by legal authority. An early catalog explains:

> The aim of the institution is to educate young women to do prophylactic work in dental offices, the schools, and public institutions. Ample facilities are provided for careful training and instruction in the various branches taught.

> With the enactment of the law making possible a school for the instruction of young women in oral prophylaxis, a new avenue of employment was opened to them. The opportunities for engaging in a work, which will be agreeable, helpful and remunerative, have induced many young women to take up this new work.

> With the education of the public in the necessity for the care of the teeth in order to promote good health, the recognition by school authorities of economic value of good teeth, and the desire on the part of the dental profession to give more time and attention to oral prophylaxis in private practices, a splendid opportunity is presented to young women to gain immediate and

steady employment. There should be little difficulty for any capable dental hygienist to secure a position.

Positions can be assured to at least forty graduates.

The course of instruction at the SDH was divided into theoretical and practical. The theoretical course included lectures in anatomy, physiology, bacteriology, histology, sanitation, sterilization, dental pathology, special anatomy of the head, teeth, and jaws, dental prophylaxis, foods nutrition, skin diseases, mouth hygiene. A few years later, roentgenology, or the study and use of x-rays, was added, so named for the inventor of x rays, Wilhelm Röntgen. Later, possibly during the de-Germanization that occurred in this country during World War I, the course was renamed radiology.

The practical course was devoted to the teaching of values and the use of instruments in the various operations. The catalog for the School for Dental Hygienists, 1927–28, states: "Abundant clinical material will be available in the Dispensary and the public schools. Lectures will be given in the dispensary forenoons, five days in the week, and practical work afternoons in the dispensary or public schools." The licensed hygienists who joined the licensed dentists in cleaning the teeth of children in the schools were trained at the SDH. The prophylactic squads were provided with portable equipment, probably provided free by Rochester industries and consisting of chairs, engines, instruments, sterilizers, and so on. Under careful and strict supervision, hygienists made the rounds of the schools twice a year. A school lecturer was employed by the dispensary to deliver illustrated lantern slide lectures on oral hygiene and other health subjects. After the teeth had been cleaned, a survey was made of the mouth and any pathological conditions that were observed. If additional dental work was necessary, duplicate records were made, one for the teacher and parents and the other for the dispensary, so that all these cases could be followed up.

It didn't take long for the School for Dental Hygienists to acquire the trappings of a finishing school or junior college. By 1920, a student had composed an alma mater. A yearbook, *The Scaler,* was being published with prophesies, class wills, a sorority, and jokes about students, faculty, and dentistry—but not about Dr. Burkhart or the redoubtable Dr. Ruth Vann, the school director. There were dates and proms, convocations and graduations in Catherine Strong Hall. After the Eastman School of Music opened in 1921, graduations were held in Kilbourn Hall.

An opportunity to broaden the educational component of the dispensary occurred in 1919 when Burkhart read about the Rockefeller-supported General Education Board that was granting money to start medical schools. Thinking that the Flexner mentioned as general secretary of the project was Simon Flexner, MD, Burkhart wrote and invited him to visit the dispensary. The doctor passed the letter on to his brother, Mr. Abraham Flexner, who was not a doctor or dentist but was often assumed to have a degree and who did visit Rochester with one of his patrons—John D. Rockefeller Jr. This would bear more medical than dental fruit.

THE TONSILLECTOMY MARATHON

"The tonsil clinic . . . is the one thing that really interests me nowadays," Eastman wrote in 1920. The oral surgery department of the dispensary had been established, according to Dr. Burkhart, to deal with parts of the mouth other than teeth: "cleft palate, harelip, and most notably, defective nasal respiration caused by enlarged tonsils and adenoids." Operating three days a week with eighteen beds, the oral surgery department also "removed tonsils and adenoids when symptoms from these parts seemed to have a direct bearing on dental work." In addition, "during the routine examination of dispensary cases, many were found to have diseased tonsils which were not strictly obstructive, but which were detrimental to the children's good health."[28]

Children with infected tonsils and adenoids were thought to be more susceptible to infectious diseases; it was believed that removal of the culprits would prevent whooping cough, measles, scarlet fever, rheumatism, and heart and kidney disease. Burkhart wrote, "Many children can't breathe, can't digest, can't grow or learn because of the poisoned excretions from diseased tonsils and adenoids."[29] George Eastman, with his great respect for scientific experts, was no skeptic. If the doctors said tonsils caused illness, then, by George, he would remove every diseased and enlarged tonsil from every Rochester schoolchild. "If we do what we ought to do," the publicity stated, "what an example Rochester could set before the world! Will we do it? Will we rid our children of tonsils and adenoids? Of course we will!"

Special clinics were set up at the dispensary and procedures were systematically scheduled. Dr. Albert D. Kaiser (1887–1955) organized and supervised the history-taking and medical exams and eventually wrote a book,

Tonsils In or Out?, about the exercise. Dr. Edwin S. Ingersoll was the chief pediatric laryngologist, with three other surgeons doing the bulk of the operating. As a University of Rochester undergraduate, Kaiser had been a tutor for George Eastman's grandnephew and grandniece. He would go on to be chief of pediatrics at Rochester General Hospital and a professor at the University of Rochester Medical School, and finally the eminent City of Rochester health officer from 1945 to 1955.[30] Ingersoll and Eastman were good friends who competed in a friendly fashion in deciding who baked the best lemon meringue pie. Kaiser and Ingersoll would take their tonsillectomy statistics on the road to medical conventions.

Children selected for tonsillectomies were brought to the dispensary during the late afternoon, given supper and shown a movie chosen by Eastman. They spent the night at the clinic, underwent the operation in the morning, and were sent home the following day. Those who had no transportation were picked up by taxi or by the free transport provided by the Women's Motor Corps of the Red Cross, supervised by Eastman's good friend, Netta Ranlet, who was equally involved in another Eastman project, the Rochester Philharmonic Orchestra. The public campaign for tonsillectomies was heartily endorsed by the newspapers and promotions could be seen in shop windows, in going-to-the-hospital posters, and lantern slide shows in movie theaters, and could be heard from the pulpits of the city. Physicians at Johns Hopkins, Cornell University Medical College, and the University of Rochester department of physiology, along with George Goler, the city's health officer, concurred that "the benefit from tonsillectomy is a change for the better in growth and development of the child." Schools and agencies such as the Hillside Children's Center agreed that there had been "an increase in weight, considerably fewer sore throats, and many more smiling countenances because the aggravation has been removed.... All the children recovered quickly, with no set-backs."[31] Donations of toys, games, and phonograph records represented a new concept in making the hospital experience less scary for the patients.

As the "operable cases of tonsil and adenoid defects reached an alarming total" and the small in-house clinics began waiting lists, it was decided to hold an emergency clinic. Two hundred operations a week were scheduled for seven weeks. "As a matter of record," Eastman reported proudly, "it may be stated that operations were performed on 1,470 children without a single fatality."

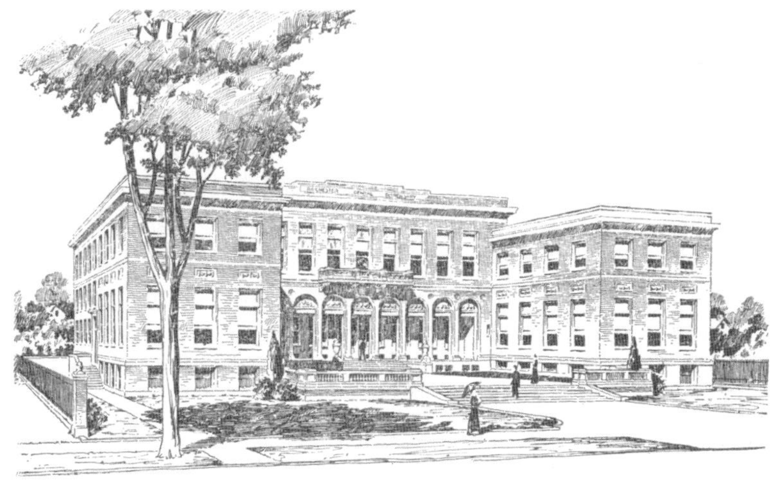

ROCHESTER DENTAL DISPENSARY

FOUNDED BY GEORGE EASTMAN

SCHOOL FOR DENTAL HYGIENISTS

COMMENCEMENT EXERCISES

THURSDAY, JUNE FOURTEENTH

NINETEEN HUNDRED AND SEVENTEEN

School for Dental Hygienists catalog

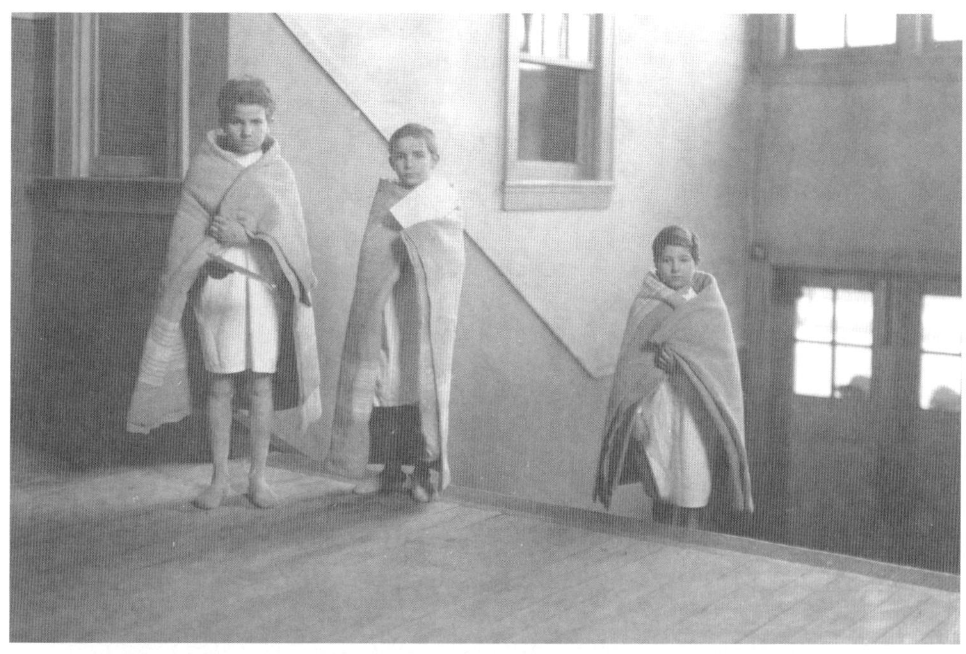
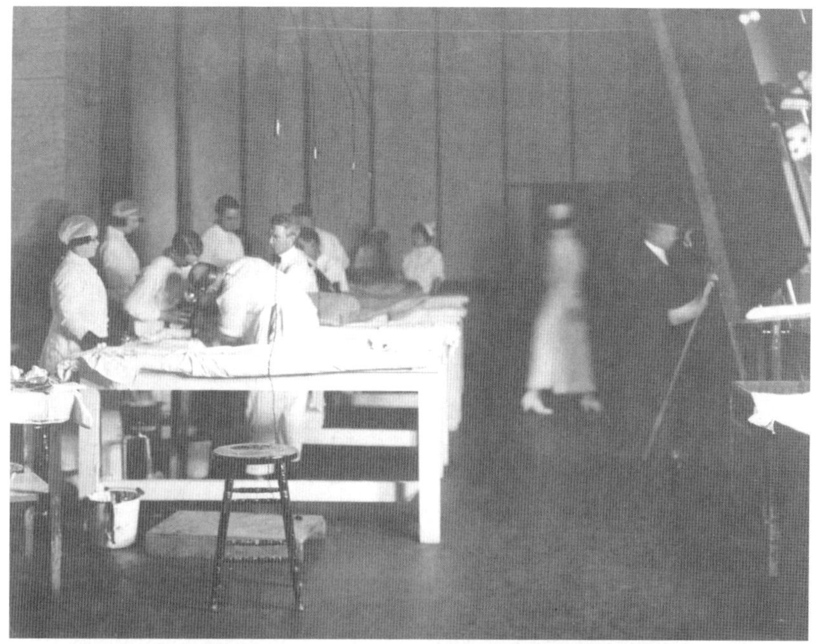
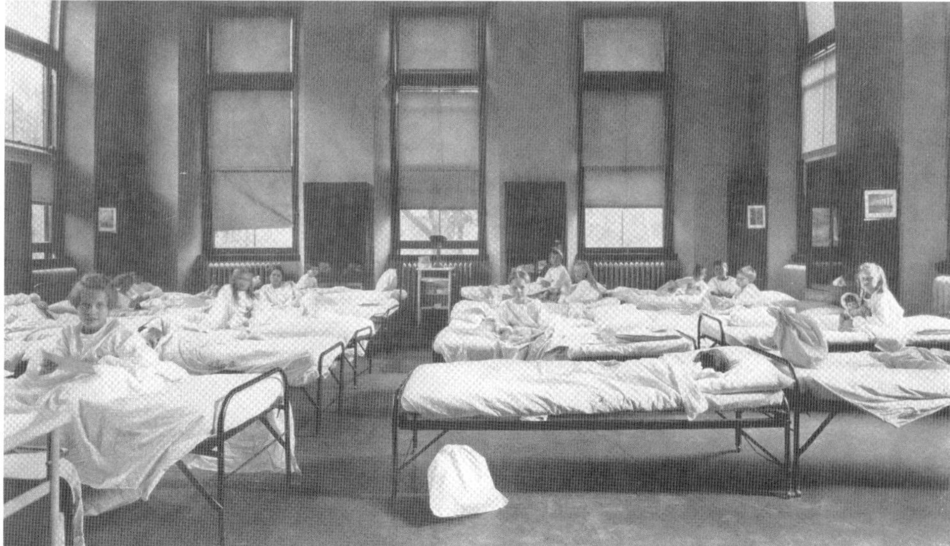
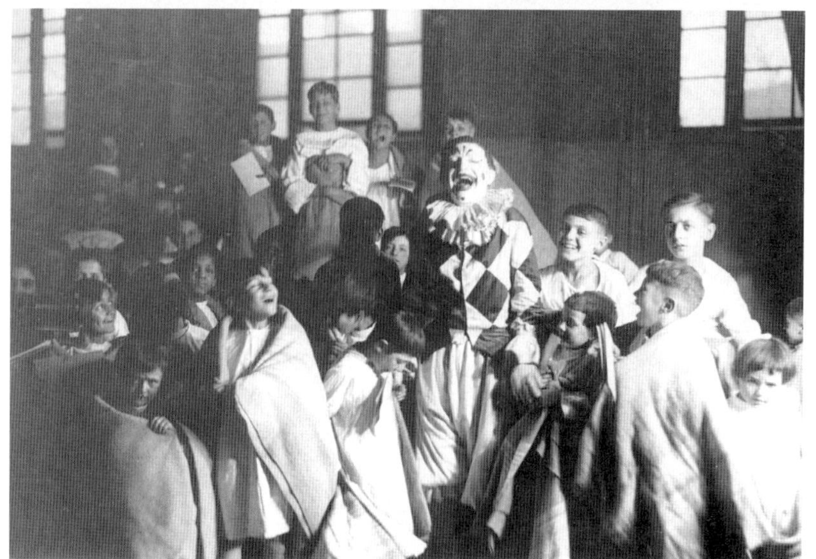

Scenes from the Great Tonsillectomy Marathon

To Dr. Rhees, president of the University of Rochester, who was vacationing in Maine, Eastman wrote: "Herewith I am sending you a newspaper clipping containing an account of the Dental Dispensary clinic. The first forty-one, which were operated on yesterday, were all ready to go home at eight o'clock this morning. They began operating again about a quarter of nine this morning and the two men who did the whole forty were done by a quarter before eleven." With the cooperation of the dispensary and four city hospitals, Goler and Ingersoll organized an even more intensive tonsil clinic for the following winter, January to April, 1921. The surgeons and "x-ray men" were sent to the Rockefeller Institute to learn about "the new tonsil treatment" from Dr. Simon Flexner, Abraham Flexner's brother. The planners met at Eastman House, 900 East Avenue, where "Mr. Eastman spoke briefly of the great desirability of continuing the campaign begun last summer for the removal of diseased tonsils and adenoids," the minutes recorded. It was then that Eastman commissioned nine thousand tonsillectomy/adenoidectomy operations to be performed in two months. Eastman provided funds and executive direction, prodded school authorities and hospital staffs into cooperating, borrowed the city's convention hall annex for a mass operating theater, and moved in long rows of tables and cots. "The ensuing 'round-the-clock tonsillectomy marathon alarmed and fascinated the whole medical world," well-known author Roger Butterfield wrote in recalling his own childhood participation in the marathon. "Streets around the hall teemed with anxious parents propelling their even more anxious offspring toward the ether cones and surgical tools."[32]

"The tonsil clinic . . . is running finely," Eastman said after this incredible happening was underway. "The only thing that worries us is getting consents from the parents. Out of the 18,000 children that have been diagnosed as needing the operation, we have only 7,500 consents, which, at the rate we are operating, will only give us fodder until the first of April; so we are working every scheme to get after the parents." More than any other single incident, the tonsillectomy marathon reflects the arbitrary power one individual once wielded over an entire community. No other Rochesterian before or since could have closed all the schools for half a day and moved their populations en masse into a makeshift operating theater where 7,833 sets of tonsils were summarily removed. Eastman may not have fully understood the extent of his influence and power. He thought he was just doing his job to promote good health among children, starting in Rochester.

The children whose teeth and tonsils were treated have a different memory of the dental center and tonsillectomy marathon than the philanthropist did. Many remember the tears they shed and the fear and anger they felt toward the mythical George Eastman, blaming the unseen cause of their discomfort for the sore throats and mouths they suffered. "He helped the poor whether they liked it or not—medically, culturally, in every way," recalled Martha Gould Axelrod, who had both a tooth and her tonsils removed. Thanks to Eastman funding, she was also diagnosed and treated for an enlarged thyroid. (Rochester's drinking water from Hemlock Lake was so pure it had no trace elements such as iodine or fluorine.) Many of these same children also received musical instruments from Mr. Eastman through the Rochester public and parochial schools and date their love of music to playing an Eastman instrument during their schooldays.[33]

The dispensary remained Eastman's favorite project up to the end of his life. The following is typical of the panegyrics he conjured up when describing it: "The Rochester Dental Dispensary has succeeded in abolishing in the child's mind the association of dentistry with pain and fear. To the children of Rochester, dentistry is akin to play. They frolic to and from the institution as if they were on an outing."[34]

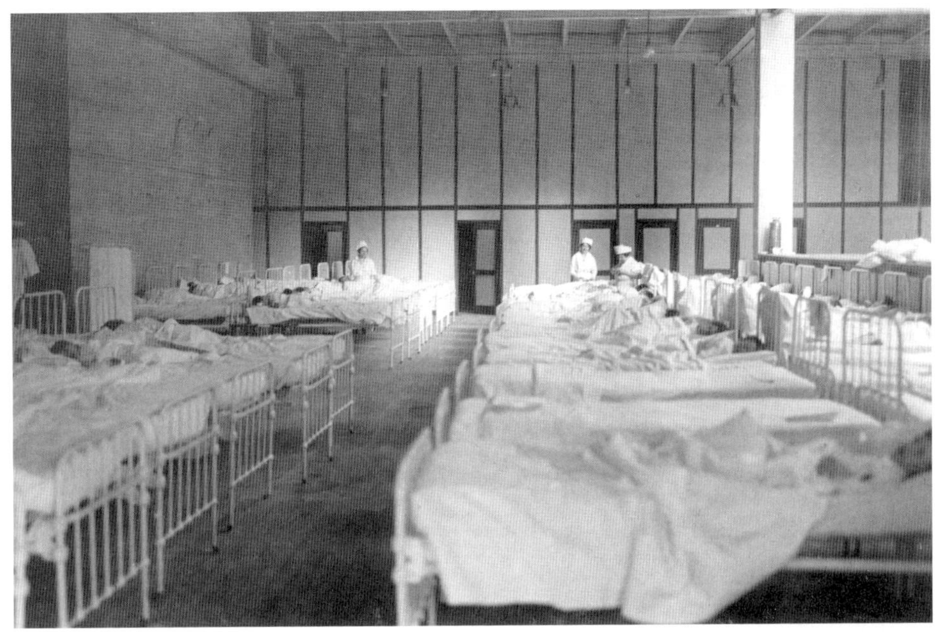

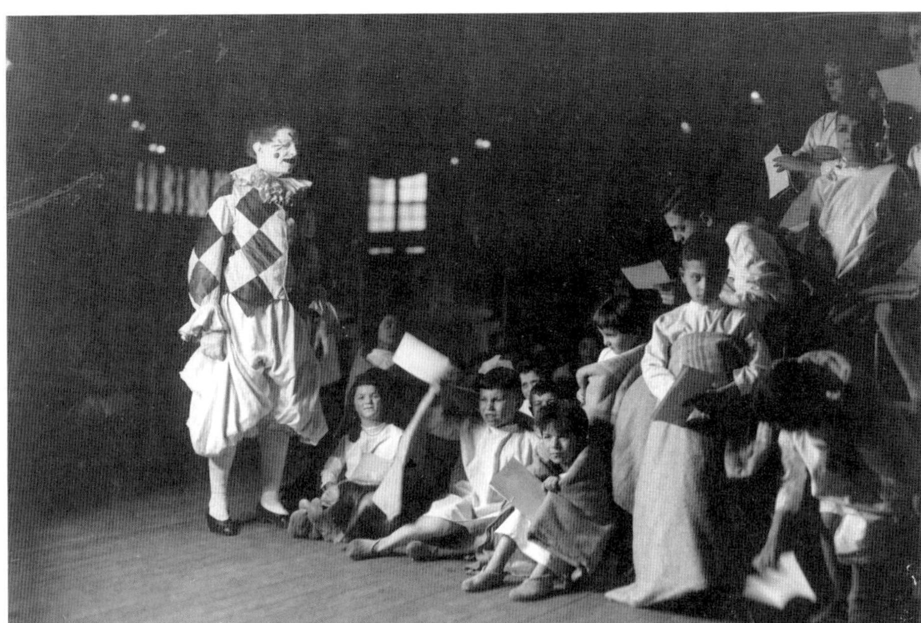

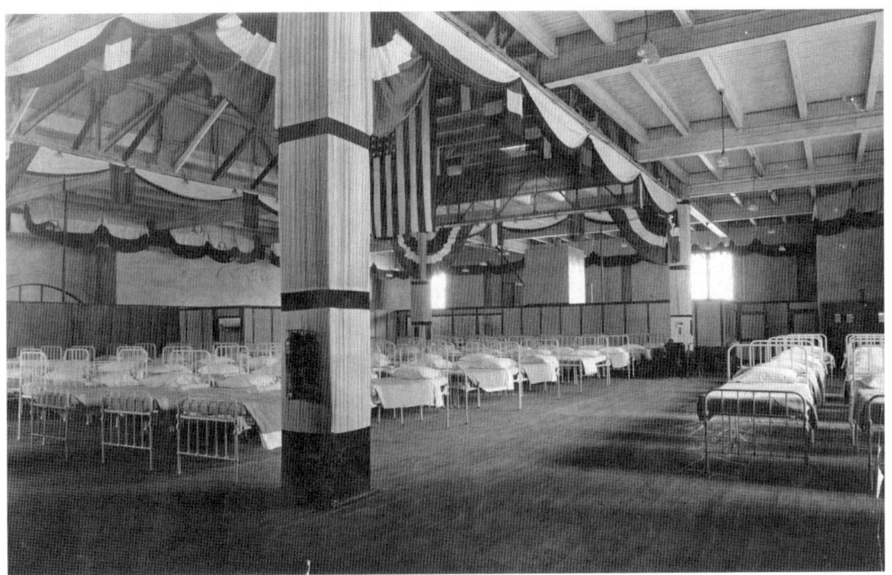

Scenes from the Great Tonsillectomy Marathon

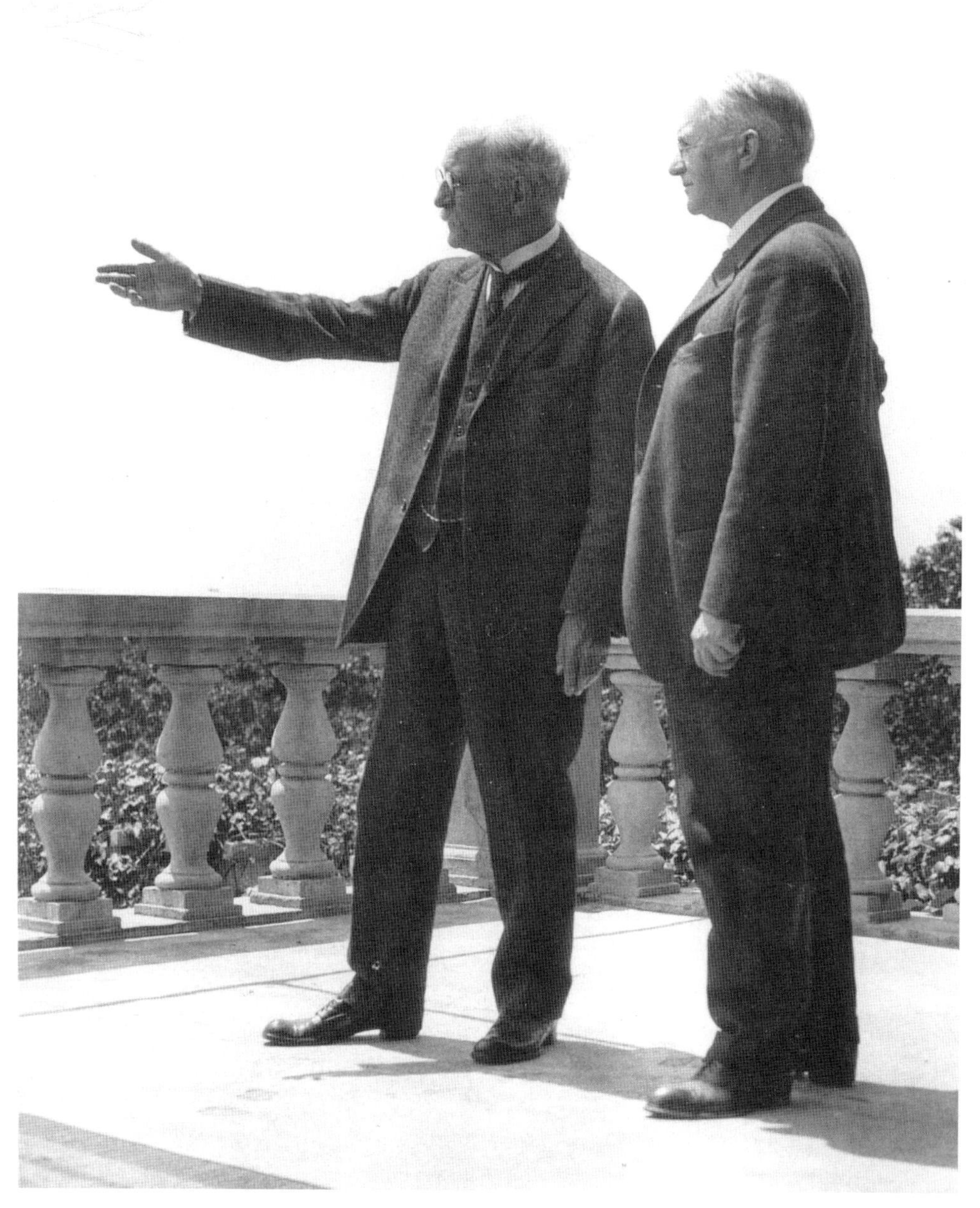

Rush Rhees and George Eastman (Author's collection)

A DREAM DEFERRED

THE SCHOOL OF MEDICINE AND DENTISTRY

Mr. Eastman has given the city a fine dental dispensary . . . a beautiful and efficient institution.
It seems to me his interest might be extended to the medical field.

Abraham Flexner

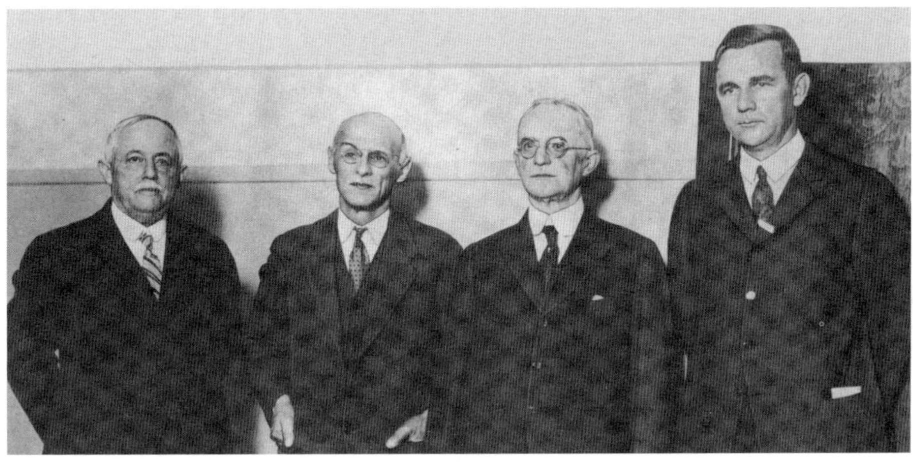

Rush Rhees, Abraham Flexner, George Eastman, and
George Hoyt Whipple were the team most responsible for
the founding of the School of Medicine and Dentistry

THE EASTMANS ORIGINALLY ESPOUSED HOMEOPATHY.[1] As developed and promoted by Dr. Samuel Hahnemann of Leipzig about 1800, the homeopathic theory was that a drug that will produce certain disease symptoms in a healthy person would cure a sick person who has the same symptoms. Homeopaths also believed that small doses of a drug are best; in an era of aggressive treatment often using mercury and arsenic, this moderate therapeutic system at least caused little harm. Before more scientific treatments became available, Hahnemann had a following among the leading families of Rochester.

The years 1880 to 1920 were the heyday of homeopathy in Rochester. Hahnemann (later Highland) Hospital opened in 1889. Eastman financed a fireproof surgical center and a new nurses' wing at the hospital, and established the Maria Eastman Nurse Fellowship in his mother's memory, contributing $500 a year for the rest of his life. Although health care became a primary Eastman philanthropic interest, he did not believe in endowing hospitals, just as he did not believe in endowing orchestras. He said that if people wanted a hospital or an orchestra, they should support it.

The Sibley and Watson families, who rode to prominence as founders of Western Union, built the Homeopathic Hospital (later called Genesee Hospital) on the east side of Rochester. George Eastman was one of the few on the hospital board who was not a Sibley or a Watson. This was the hospital where Maria Eastman had successful surgery for uterine cancer in 1890. Eastman's gratitude led to benevolences in the form of buildings and endowments. In 1907, Eastman endowed another Maria Kilbourn Eastman Nurse Fellowship, this time at the Homeopathic Hospital, and soon built nurses' residences for the Hahnemann Hospital and the Homeopathic Hospital.

In 1908, Eastman provided the lion's share in a fund drive to enlarge City (later named Rochester General) Hospital, an institution founded in 1856 by the Rochester Female Charitable Society and the only local hospital that did not follow Hahnemann's theories.[2] City Hospital was where, in 1901, members of the Rochester Dental Society had established the first free dental clinic in the United States. By 1908, Eastman was disillusioned with homeopathy. His support of City Hospital, which already had a tie to dentistry, mirrored the move of many community leaders toward what they considered more "scientific" medicine. Whether any of them read Abraham Flexner's 1910 report on the state of medical education is not known, but they were certainly aware of its conclusions. Eastman was being primed for Flexner's assault on his pocketbook a decade later.

THE FLEXNER REPORT

In 1910, Abraham Flexner startled medical and educational circles with his scathing report to the Carnegie Foundation on the weaknesses of medical education in the United States. Flexner, who was not a physician himself, saw that the problem stemmed from the American emphasis on the trade-school-style apprentice training of physicians rather than on a scientifically based program in which medical school staffs devoted themselves exclusively to instruction and research. Of the nearly 150 medical schools Flexner reviewed, he praised only five. On the basis of the report, the Rockefeller-supported General Education Board put Flexner on staff in 1912; by 1917 he was the board's secretary and chief executive, empowered to spend millions on improving medical education in the United States.

Flexner's 1910 report on medical education is notable for its absence of any mention of dental education. This omission was probably one reason that the Carnegie Foundation would commission William Gies in 1926 to study and report on dental education. By then it was too late, Gies concluded, to make "dentistry . . . a specialty of the conventional practice of medicine, but [it] should remain a health service of equal recognition with other specialties of medicine." Gies would also feel impelled to state: "Dentistry is an important branch of health service and cannot longer be ignored in the training of general [medical] practitioners. . . . Antagonism between medicine and dentistry is unworthy of both and has no justifiable basis from the standpoint either of scientific progress or of the public interest."

Did this remarked-upon and long-lasting antagonism between medicine and dentistry foretell the later relations between the Eastman Dental Center and School of Medicine and Dentistry?[3] Backed by $100 million from John D. Rockefeller, Flexner had the clout to make or break a medical school.

He planned to achieve his reforms by reconstructing existing institutions and creating new ones. Flexner encountered little difficulty arm-twisting smaller schools to adopt "clinical full-time," as the system was called. Johns Hopkins, Yale, and Washington (St. Louis) universities reformed according to the Flexner formula. But Harvard, Columbia, and Cornell, though hungering for Rockefeller money, all had prominent practitioners doing their clinical teaching. These schools, Flexner decided, were not "half as much interested in scientific medicine as in the persons who held posts from which they would have to be dislodged." It was impossible, Flexner tried to explain, to carry on a modern medical school "which did its laboratory teaching at 59th Street and Ninth Avenue and its clinical teaching with practicing consultants in the Presbyterian Hospital at 70th Street and Madison Avenue." The situation was similar at Cornell. "So for the moment New York [City] seemed impossible [to reform]."

Flexner then decided, "The situation might be taken in the flank"[4] and he looked upstate. Albany and Buffalo had medical schools loosely affiliated with universities, and Syracuse had one that might be raised to what Flexner considered "a true university level." His first proposal was to close the Albany and Buffalo medical schools and throw all the support to Syracuse. But he came to feel that Syracuse could not provide either the adequate leadership for reorganization or the local funds to match the Rockefeller grant.

By a strange coincidence, if not for that letter from Harvey Burkhart to Simon Flexner extolling the assets of the new dental dispensary, Rochester may never have had a major center of healing, teaching, and research.

"PLANTING" A MEDICAL SCHOOL IN ROCHESTER

George Eastman and the John Rockefellers, senior and junior, had diametrically opposite approaches to philanthropy. Eastman believed in hands-on philanthropy during his life span. He often said, "I want to see the action during my lifetime." His major philanthropies, including his gifts to local educational institutions and anonymous gifts to MIT, were examples of this philosophy. He regularly stopped by the Rochester Dental Dispensary and the Eastman Theatre between Kodak and home to check on the happenings and receipts of the day. He hired and fired theater managers and architects, picked the movies to be shown, and stood in to observe tonsillectomies.

The Rockefellers preferred to do their good works through surrogates, establishing foundations that would carry on beyond their lifetimes. Since the Rockefellers were good Baptists, their surrogates were too—notably Dr. Frederick Gates and Dr. Wallace Buttrick, who ran the Rockefeller General Education Board and who were both graduates of the Baptist-affiliated Rochester Theological Seminary. When Rush Rhees, a little-known professor of New Testament theology and ordained Baptist minister, became president of the University of Rochester in 1900, very few knew that one of the great academic executives of the twentieth century had arrived on the scene. Gates, Buttrick, and Rhees were all members of a Baptist old-boy network. Flexner, a Canadian Jew, knew this and saw his opportunity. He explained the chronology in his autobiography:

> As [Dr. Buttrick and I] sat together in a Pullman car one day, I said to him quite casually, "The University of Rochester is a modest but good institution, isn't it?"
>
> "Yes," he replied. "I know it well. Gates and I are graduates of the Rochester Theological Seminary. I know Rhees well—a fine college head. Why do you ask?"
>
> "It has occurred to me that if we could help to plant a first-rate medical school there, perhaps New York City would wake up."
>
> "Why Rochester?" Buttrick asked.
>
> "There are medical schools at Buffalo, Syracuse, Albany; it won't be easy to find money or men to reorganize them. Rochester has a clean slate; and besides there is Mr. Eastman."

Buttrick was surprised. "Do you know him?" Buttrick wondered. "No," replied Flexner, though Flexner had earlier visited the Rochester Dental Dispensary at Harvey Burkhart's invitation and in the company of his patron, John D. Rockefeller Jr., "but I do know that he has given the city an endowed dental clinic. It seems to me not unlikely that his interest might be extended to the medical field."

Flexner described the dispensary to colleagues as "a beautiful and efficient institution." After the conversation dropped, Flexner continued to reflect that the dispensary could prove a step toward achieving his goals for medicine. Soon, he had decided to "plant" his new school in Rochester. Within a week after the train conversation, Rhees had a scheduled meeting with colleagues in New York. Flexner asked for a minute of his time. He remembers:

> Our interview was brief.
>
> "President Rhees, there is no medical school in Rochester; would you like to have one?"
>
> "Only if we could have a first-rate one."
>
> "We are not interested in any other kind. Do you know Mr. George Eastman?"
>
> "Oh, yes, intimately."
>
> "Can you arrange a meeting between us in Rochester?"
>
> "I think so."

Within forty-eight hours, Rhees telegraphed Flexner an invitation to an Eastman breakfast. Via the Twentieth Century Limited overnight from New York to Rochester, Flexner arrived at George Eastman's palatial home on East Avenue by taxi about 8:00 A.M.

> As I entered I was greeted by the strains of organ music. After laying aside my hat and coat, I was ushered into a large reception room, where I was met by Mr. Eastman—a pallid gentleman in the sixties, well dressed, his thin white hair covered by a skullcap. The music continued. Before me was the organ, banked with flowers, the organist himself being almost invisible. A butler whispered in my ear, asking what I wished for breakfast. "Orange juice, eggs, and coffee," I replied. Mr. Eastman followed the music intently; not a word was spoken. . . . Promptly at ten the music ceased, and the organist made his way out through the fragrant flowers. Thereupon Mr. Eastman rose and asked me to his study. Before a wood fire, the ashes of which were snow-white, we seated ourselves on a sofa. Mr. Eastman, lighting a cigarette, turned to me with the words "President Rhees tells me you wish to talk with me."

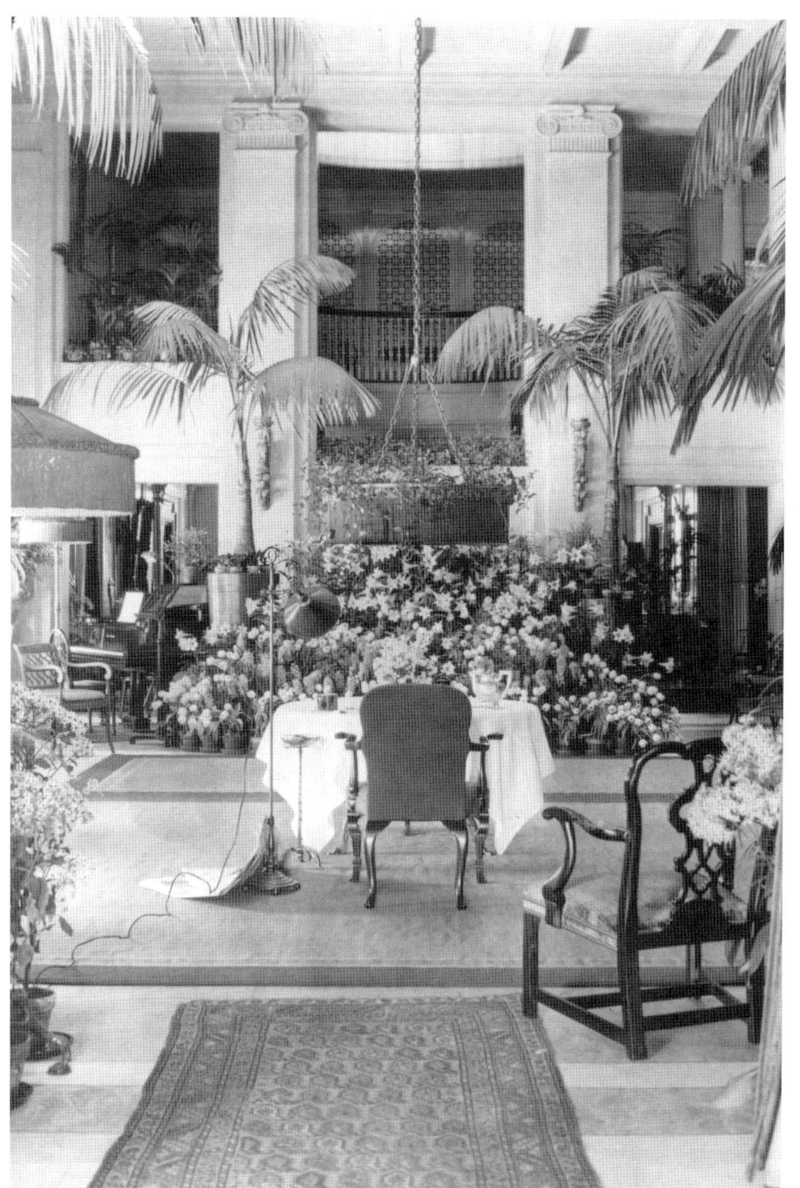
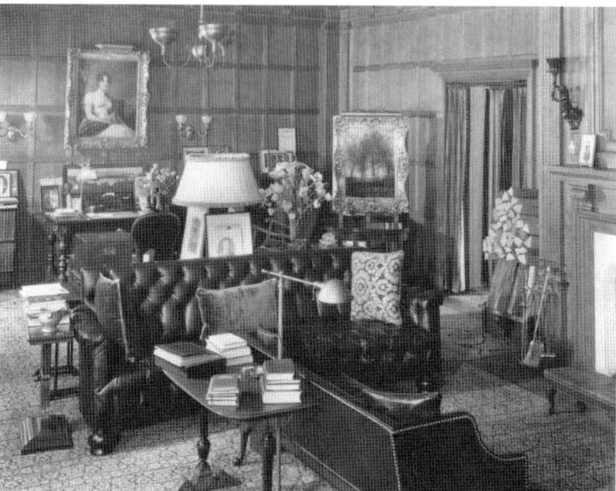
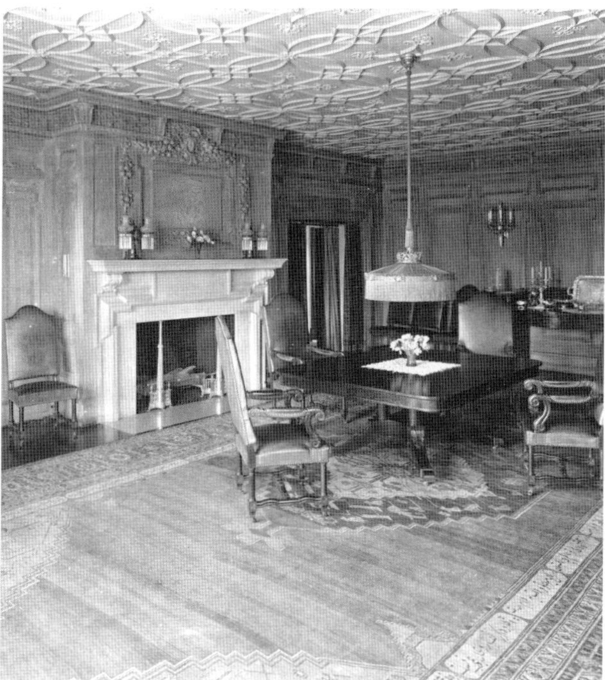

Flexner arrived at Eastman's house for breakfast in the conservatory, discussion in the billiard room, and stayed for lunch and dinner in the dining room (All courtesy George Eastman House)

I might have been embarrassed, but his gentle smile and soft voice were disarming and reassuring. I asked if I might tell him the story of medical education in the United States.

Eastman listened silently but intently as Flexner outlined his plan. As noon approached, the taciturn host pressed a button to order lunch. Flexner felt he was making progress.

There was a time when major projects were initiated and carried to completion not by boards or committees or interminable studies or blue-ribbon panels but by just one, two, or three persons. And sometimes, important decisions were made with startling alacrity—in the space of a few days.

We can only surmise what was going through Eastman's mind. A healing institution of the finest quality, he appreciated, would make his adopted city a better place in which to live. As with the Eastman Theatre and School of Music, then under construction, it would be an asset in attracting and keeping superior personnel for his Kodak operations. Both Eastman and Burkhart were thinking along the lines of a university affiliation for the dental dispensary.

In mid-afternoon, Eastman announced that he had to go to the office, but he invited Flexner and Rhees to return for dinner so that discussions could continue. In the billiard room after dinner Eastman asked:

"How much will it cost?"

"Eight to ten million."

"Let's say ten then. I have recently distributed thirty-one million so can only offer two-and-one-half."

"Where will the rest come from?"

"From the Rockefellers."

"Then it will be our school, not yours."

"That is the best I can do now."

"There's no hurry. Wait till you sell more Kodaks."

On that note Flexner departed on his train, but a few days later a telegram from Eastman brought him back to Rochester. This time Eastman offered $3.5 million—to the same objections. "I'd like to do this thing," Eastman said, "and I should like to see it settled before I go to Japan."

"You shouldn't have said that," Flexner shot back with satisfaction before heading for the door, "for now I know you will go higher."

A few weeks later a handwritten note invited Flexner to lunch at Kodak Park. "I can see him now as he rose behind his desk, smiling and pointing his finger at me," Flexner wrote years later describing Eastman, who then said: "'I shall make you one more offer and then I never want to see your face again,'" Flexner regretted that the friendship was over but asked for the offer anyway. "I'll give five million dollars, including the dental clinic valued at one million, if the [Rockefeller-sponsored General Education] Board will give five million," Eastman responded.

Before Eastman could reconsider, Flexner accepted the offer. Eastman, of course, had no legal authority to offer this, having placed the Rochester Dental Dispensary in the hands of trustees. But his standing as Rochester's primary employer meant that he had the political means to achieve his goals. Flexner, of course, also had no legal authority to accept the offer, as Frederick Gates reminded him when he reported back to the General Education Board that he had successfully planted a new medical school.

"ONE OF THE HEALTHIEST COMMUNITIES IN THE WORLD"

Eastman's goal in founding the School of Medicine and Dentistry and Strong Memorial Hospital (later incorporated under Dean Donald Anderson as the University of Rochester Medical Center) was, he said, nothing less than producing in Rochester "one of the healthiest communities in the world." The emphasis was on prevention in both medicine and dentistry, and it is clear that he expected a dental school to develop within the medical school complex. Another Eastman focus was indigent children, an underserved population. In 1921, the Democrat and Chronicle quoted him as saying that "the time is near when it will be possible for the poorest family in Rochester to have the benefits of all that modern medicine and surgery afford in the treatment

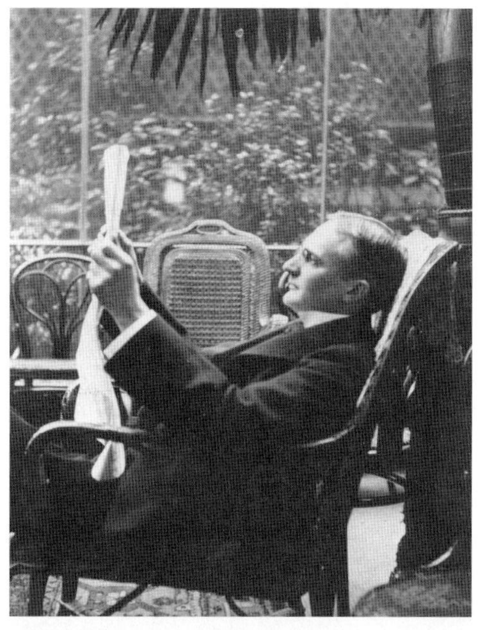

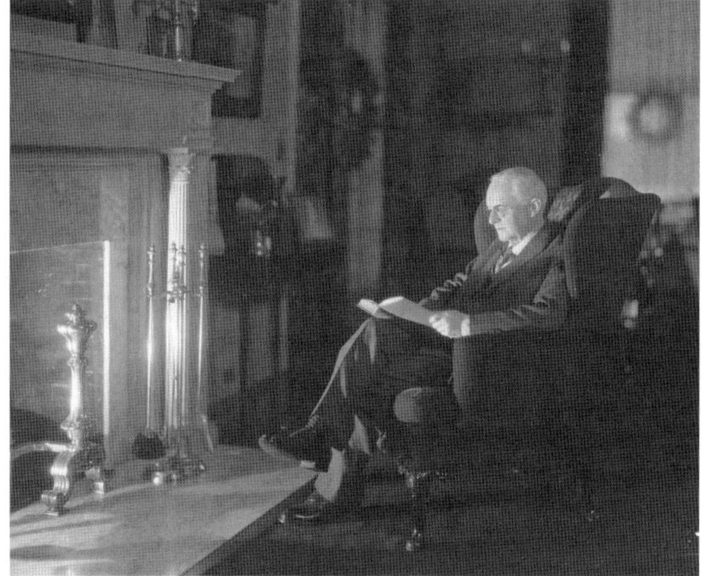

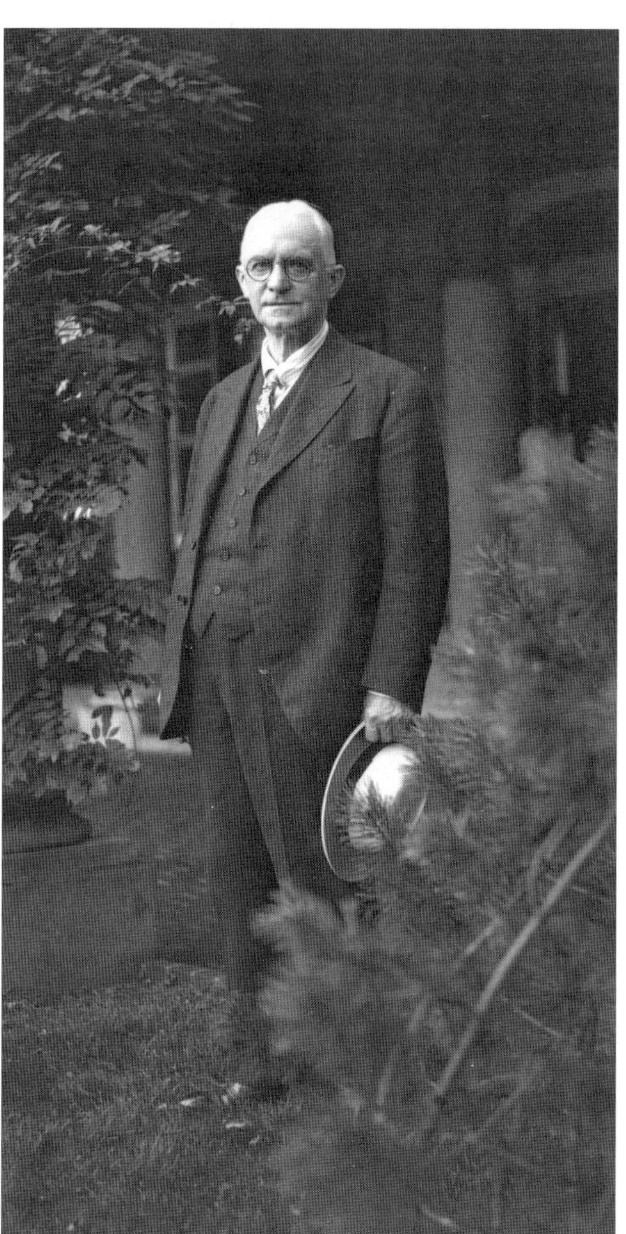

George Eastman at home in 1897 and 1931 (All courtesy George Eastman House)

of cases of sickness and in preservation of health. . . . There are many people in Rochester who haven't the means to send their sick friends to such
medical centers as Baltimore, Rochester, [MN], or Boston for treatment by
specialists," Eastman continued, and once the School of Medicine and Dentistry was complete, he maintained, "no such need will exist, for treatment of
equally high order will be obtainable in this city."

Lauding city health officer George Goler for his "safeguarding of public
health" through groundbreaking and widespread preventive measures, Eastman noted, "there are two distinct phases to activity in behalf of public health.
First is disease prevention, in which the city physicians and school nurses play
an important part. Second is the placing of the most effective curative forces
within the reach of all citizens, regardless of their financial status."

DENTISTRY TO BE ON A
PAR WITH MEDICINE

After negotiations, Eastman formally proposed the following to President
Rhees: "To aid the University to establish a school of medicine, surgery,
dentistry, I will turn over to the University 5,000 shares of Eastman Kodak
stock [valued at $4 million], if you secure the cooperation of the trustees
of the Rochester Dental Dispensary in turning over the plant and endowment to the University and secure an additional $5 million for establishing
and maintaining said school." The donor understood that his gift would form
an endowment and that the expected grant by the General Education Board
would cover the costs of construction and equipment.

Eastman dealt with his problem through a critically important letter to the
dispensary trustees, written on June 25, 1920:

The main object in mind when the Dispensary was founded was the care of
teeth of children in Rochester and its vicinity. . . . I did not foresee that it
might have an opportunity to become a part of a greater project for a higher
grade of dental education than had before been attempted. Since the opening
of the Dispensary, I have, on several occasions, discussed with our director,
Dr. Burkhart, the growing necessity of such dental education, but neither of
us could see clearly a way of bringing it about. When the plan to establish a
great medical school in connection with the University of Rochester came up,
I welcomed the opportunity. . . .

I feel that an alliance of this sort can be effected in such a way that it will not
interfere with the present work of the Dispensary and will, at the same time,
enable it to accomplish a much larger work than we had in mind when it was
founded. The carrying out of such an alliance will call for a very high degree
of cooperation between the Trustees of the Dispensary and the Trustees of the
University, and under present conditions I have no fear of such cooperation,
but new conditions may arise which will render it more difficult. It is in view
of this that I should like to put forward on record my wishes as far as they can
be formulated.

Eastman assured the trustees of the dental dispensary that allying with the
medical school would not interfere with the dispensary's work, but rather
would pave the way for expanded service. "If the dispensary's utility is ever
ended or so diminished that a separate institution was no longer required,"
Eastman wrote, its property and endowment would pass to the university
"for the benefit primarily of dental education, but if they cannot be advan-
tageously so used, for the benefit of general medical education." The donor
fully appreciated that the alliance would "call for a very high degree of cooperation between the two sets of trustees." Although the two institutions did
ally to equip the projected dental education program with clinical facilities,
the university did not appropriate the dispensary.

Flexner accepted the proposal that dentistry as well as medicine should
be taught in the projected school and that the dispensary should be affiliated in some fashion. (Since the dispensary was valued at more than $1
million, Eastman's total commitment amounted to more than $5 million.)
Flexner's remarks on the occasion of the announcement of the Rockefeller
fund for the project clearly suggests that the money was for a dental as well
as a medical school:

In one very important respect the Medical Department of the University of
Rochester will try to make a novel contribution to education. . . . The new
School of Medicine will, it is hoped, undertake to place training in dentistry
on the same academic and scientific level as training in medicine and surgery
and to this end will seek the cooperation of the Trustees of the Dental Dispensary and the practicing profession of the city.[5]

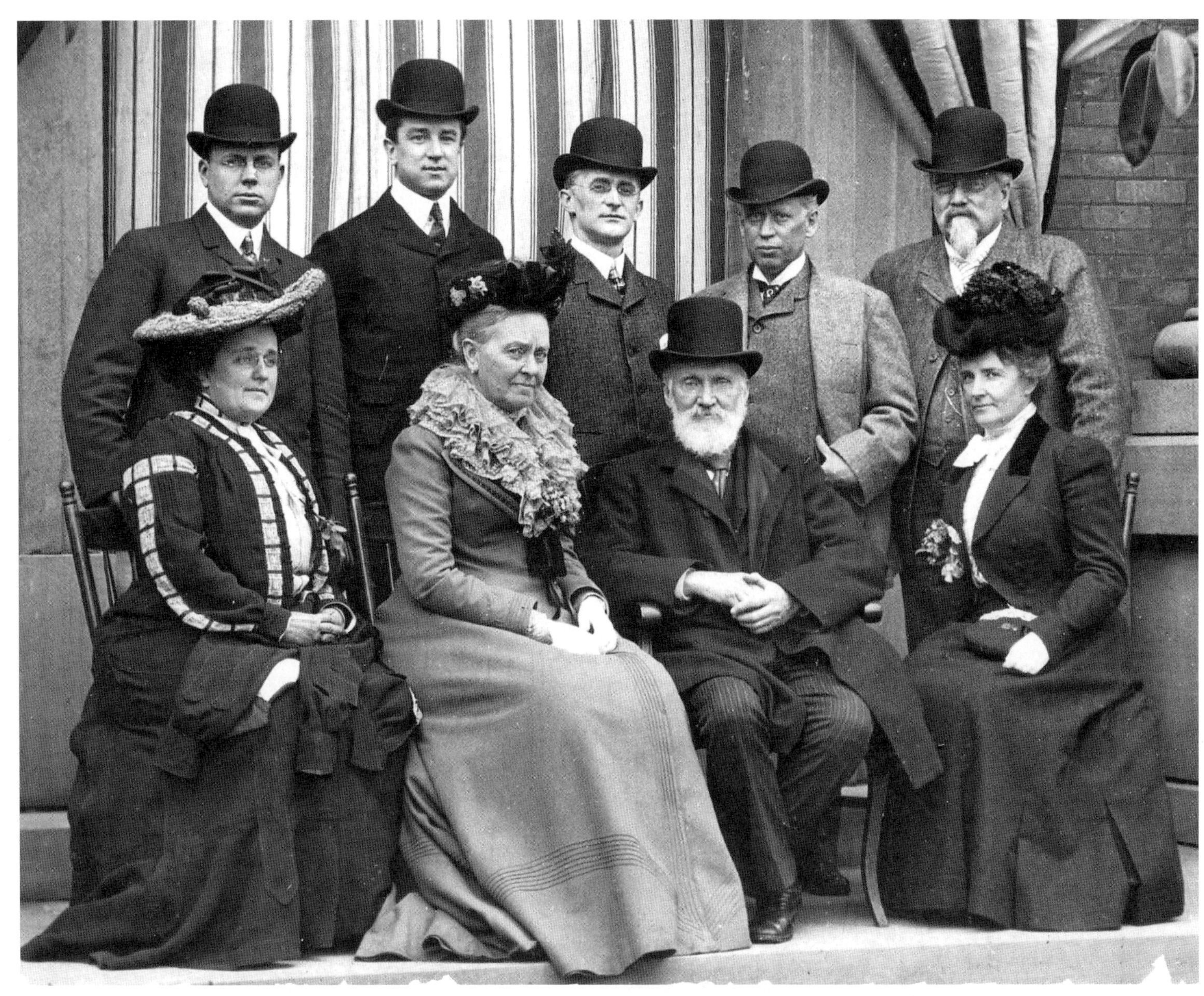

Rare 1902 photo of Helen Strong Carter (first row, left) and her father, Henry Strong (back row, right), with Kodak officials and Lord and Lady Kelvin (Courtesy George Eastman House)

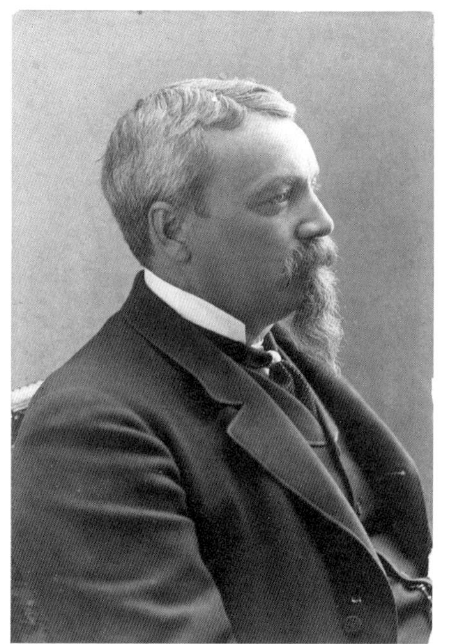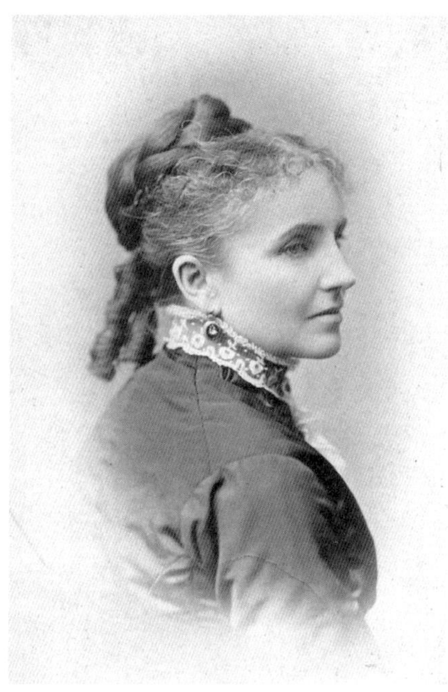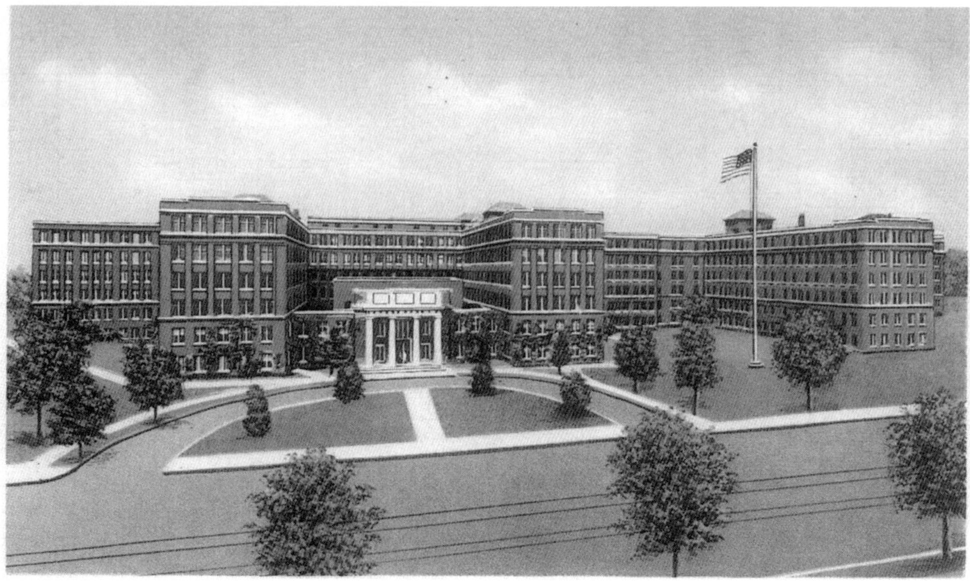

Henry Strong and Helen Phoebe Griffin Strong, in whose memory Strong Memorial Hospital was given (Author's collection)

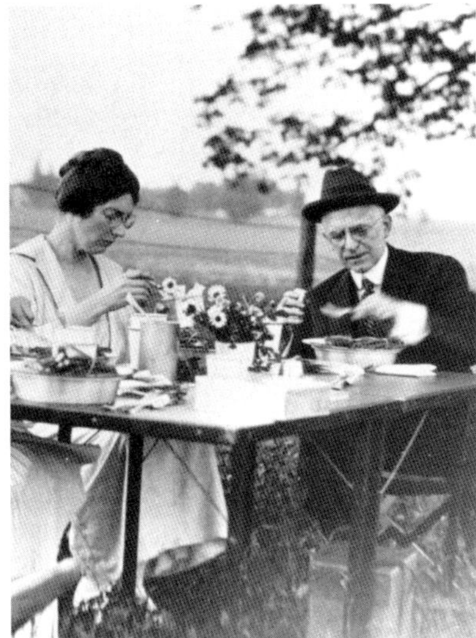

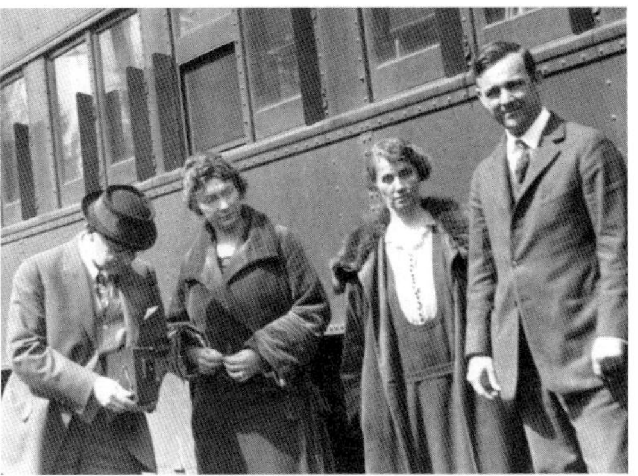

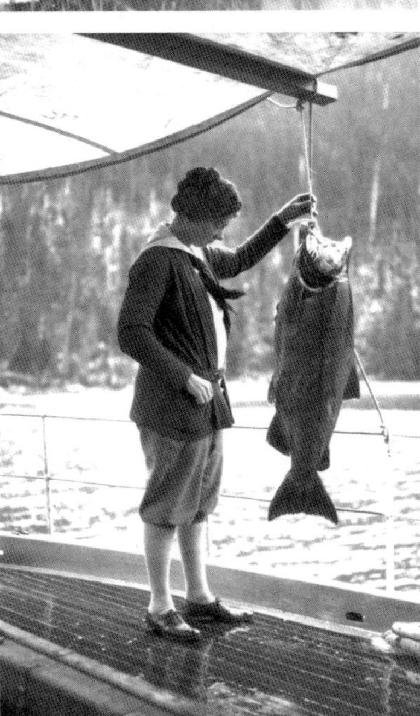

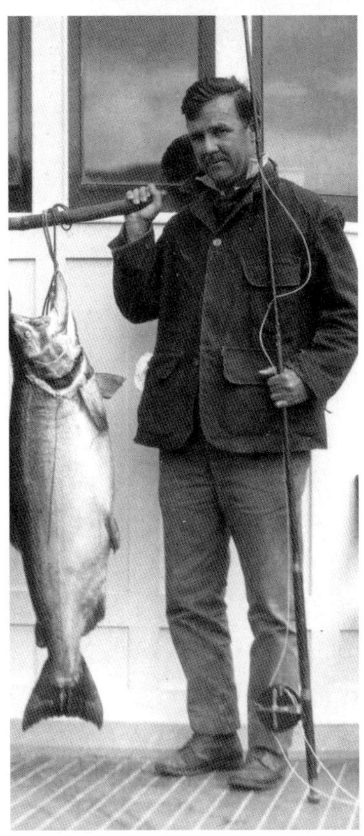

*The Whipples often vacationed with George Eastman.
Sometimes they caught big ones. (All courtesy George Eastman House)*

According to one anonymous, undated history found in the Bibby Library archives of the Eastman Dental Center, "the dental school was never formed and was limited to a department within and subordinate to the medical school. . . . The basic reason for failure to establish a dental school was that decisions for such an undertaking were greatly influenced by the medical school administration." Nevertheless, because of the influence of the Flexner report, research funds from the Rockefeller Foundation, the dean of the medical school's interest in research, and the hard work of several devoted dentists, a graduate program emphasizing dental research and basic sciences was developed in 1929 by Dean George Hoyt Whipple.

Eastman further prevailed upon the two daughters of Henry A. Strong, his original business partner, to donate funds for a teaching hospital. Gertrude Strong Achilles and Helen Strong Carter pledged $500,000 each to erect such a hospital in memory of their parents. (Helen, who was married to the governor of the Hawaiian Islands, planned to found a dental dispensary in Honolulu. Instead, she partially funded Strong Memorial Hospital.[6]) Since their brother, Henry Griffin Strong, was recently deceased, Eastman provided the third $500,000 for the hospital, declining to have his name placed upon the donor plaque. On Flexner's recommendation, the Rockefeller-funded General Education Board pledged $5 million to establish a new school in Rochester for medical and dental education and research.

Eastman, Flexner, and Rhees unveiled the project in June 1920 at a large community dinner at the Genesee Valley Club. The press recounted how, amidst immense enthusiasm, the "curious mystification" of many weeks' duration was explained and new vistas of fame, influence, and beneficence for Rochester were unfolded. Flexner, the star of the occasion, told the audience, which included many influential Rochester physicians and dentists, that the enterprise's success depended on the cooperation of the city's medical and dental fraternity. Accounts of the meeting in the *Rochester Democrat and Chronicle* carried photographs of John D. Rockefeller and George Eastman side by side. Eastman expressed pride in being associated with the oil magnate in the creation of a great medical complex. Rockefeller, in turn, indicated his appreciation to Eastman for "all you have done and are doing for good."

At the same time, Eastman asked the dispensary trustees to cooperate fully with the new School of Medicine and Dentistry in the teaching of dentistry but he did not publicly call for the corporate union of the two institutions. Still, sources indicate that Burkhart knew about the caveat pertaining to the dispensary property and

endowment and the possibility of their passing to the university if a separate institution was no longer required. The rest of Burkhart's life was devoted to seeing that
that his institution remained separate and intact.

GEORGE HOYT WHIPPLE

In October 1920, George Hoyt Whipple, pathologist, researcher, director
of the Hooper Foundation in San Francisco, and dean of the University of
California Medical School, took it for granted that his career would keep
him permanently in California. So when Rush Rhees's letter arrived asking
Whipple to come east with the view of heading a new medical school, he
gave many reasons for staying where he was.

Whipple, while indicating reluctance at first, was the unanimous first choice
of Rhees and both Simon and Abraham Flexner, and thus of Eastman, for the
post of dean of the new medical school. Whipple explained that research, not
administration or developing a laboratory or building a medical school, "is and
always will be the field of greatest interest to me."[7] Rhees was not daunted by
the refusal. "Far from closing the case," he said, "it intensifies my impression
that he is the man we ought to get." Eastman told Rhees to stop writing letters and go get his man.[8] Instead of purchasing a train ticket for Whipple, he
bought one for Rhees, who decreed: "I am not returning until George Whipple
says 'yes.'"[9] In Rochester "they now have $10 million available," Whipple
noted, with "no strings tied to the gifts, and the desire to develop a school of
the type of [Johns] Hopkins. . . . The trustees expect President Rhees and the
dean to develop the policies of the school and determine the choice of men for
the various chairs in the medical school faculty."

The die was cast. On January 29, 1921, Whipple wrote to his mother that
"evidently there is a great opportunity there and it has a strong appeal for
me. I . . . hope to come to a decision . . . Katharine [Whipple's wife] is much
excited." On February 25, the University of Rochester trustees unanimously
appointed Whipple dean of the new school and professor of pathology. In
early April, Whipple accepted the appointment to begin July 1, 1921. Rhees,
Flexner, and Eastman had won.

"From all we can learn, he is the man best fitted for the job of organizing
the faculty of the new Medical School that there is in the country," Eastman
wrote his lifelong confidant on philanthropic matters, Frank Babbott.[10] As

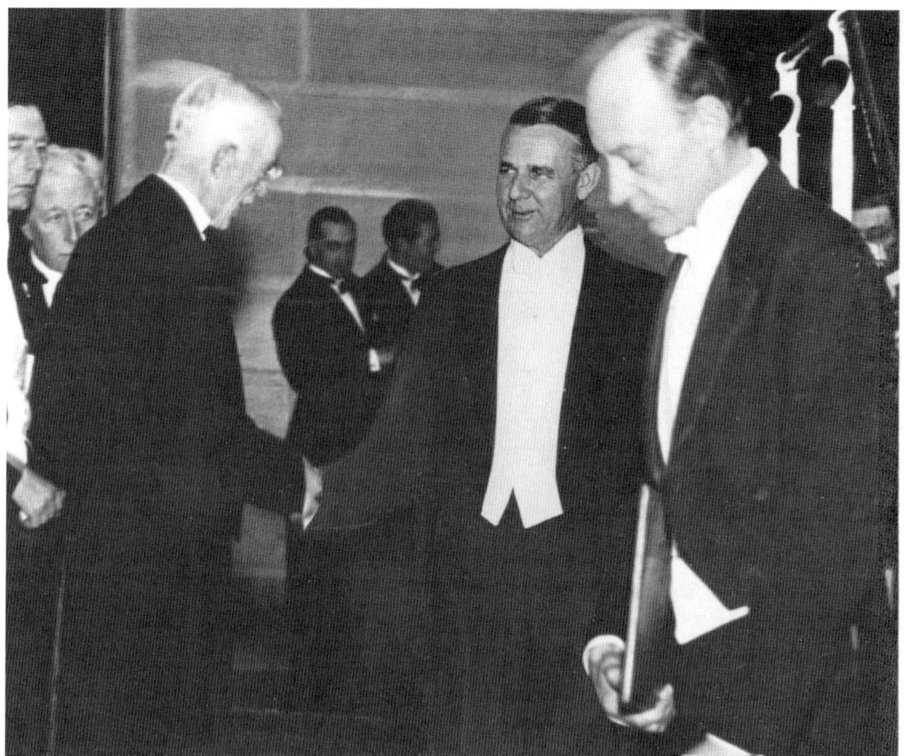

George Hoyt Whipple receives the Nobel Prize

part of the agreement, Rhees assured Whipple that the medical school was
to be physically a part of the university, with buildings and grounds paid for
out of income from the Eastman and Rockefeller gifts.

GEOGRAPHY IS DESTINY

Where to put the new School of Medicine and Dentistry? The University
of Rochester, before Eastman's munificent gifts, was a university in name
only. But since its move in 1860 to Azariah Boody's farm on Prince Street
(so named for Boody's horse) and University Avenue, the university had
grown to include a library, several science buildings, an art gallery (1913),

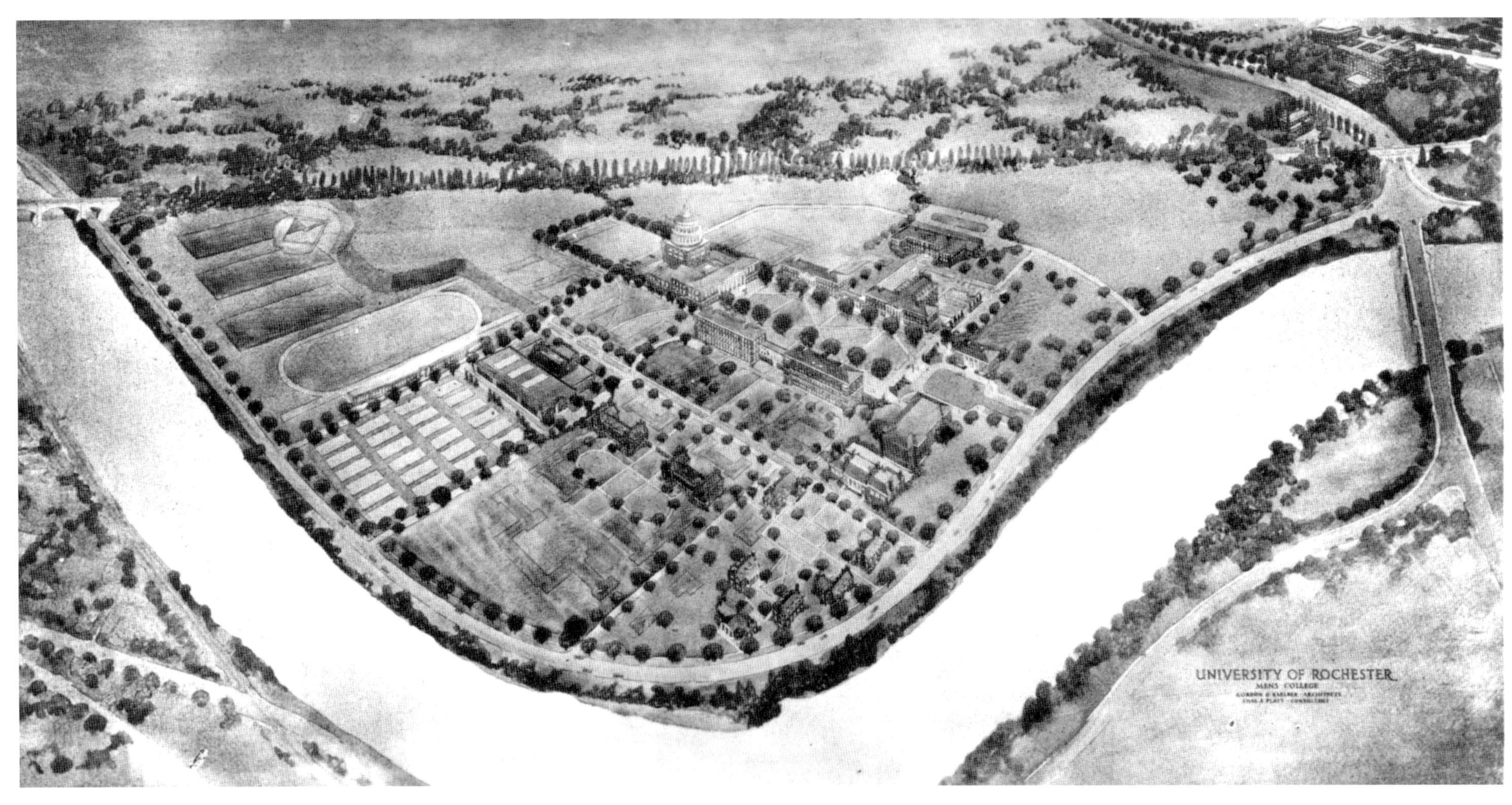

The men's undergraduate campus of the University of Rochester; the medical center upper right.

dormitories, and a gym (1901). Nearby were the women's classrooms and dormitory and, beginning in 1921, the Eastman School of Music with its theater and dormitories. But there was no room in this increasingly crowded older section of Rochester for the new School of Medicine and Dentistry.

The Crittendon farm five miles away on the southern outskirts of the city became available at a good price. There was plenty of room there not just for the School of Medicine and Dentistry but also for a university-based teaching hospital, a municipal hospital, and a school of nursing. All were built there. But the then-rural site meant that any dental students "going on together [with medical students] during the first two years and then . . . going into the dispensary for dentistry training" (as Whipple defined the school's "initial plan") would have a five-mile daily trip for their clinical work.

A campaign for "ten million dollars in ten days" ensued in 1924 following the decision to build the undergraduate men's River Campus on newly purchased golf club land across the railroad tracks from the medical school being erected on the Crittendon farm. Eastman reminded Rhees that the $10 million campaign to buy Oak Hill Golf Club was "mainly to buy clothes for the baby [the medical and dental school] which the General Education Board left on our doorstop. If I had known the baby would grow so fast, I should probably have told Flexner to take it back home in the beginning, but it is such a pretty baby that one does not want to give it up now without a struggle to help support it."[11] Rhees was unable to persuade the money managers of the General Education Board to meet the Eastman offer.

The undergraduate campus of the whole university remained divided between Prince Street and the River Campus until 1955 when the women joined the men on the River Campus. It would be another twenty years before the Eastman Dental Center moved to the School of Medicine and Dentistry campus. This long separation worked against any thoughts of merger or even of affiliation.

A SCHOOL OF MEDICINE
BUT NOT DENTISTRY

Flexner's landmark 1910 report on the state of medical education was the fourth in a series on professional education in the United States sponsored by the Carnegie Foundation for the Advancement of Teaching. Almost a century later, it still shapes medical and dental school curricula.

A report focusing on dental education was published in 1926, the tenth in the series of Carnegie reports. Its author, William Gies, was a Columbia University professor of biochemistry with a particular interest in dental research. Gies visited every existing dental school, then spent five years evaluating them in 250 pages of text and a 450-page appendix. His five conclusions were the following:

1. Dental education deserves the same attention by universities as medicine. It should not be regarded as a trade school or profit center for funneling funds to medical schools. Dentistry is the oral specialty of medicine, autonomous because of its mechanical emphasis. Research should not be ignored and dental libraries should be upgraded.

2. Dental teaching and research should be as good as in other university departments and remuneration should be raised to attract full-time educators. Endowments should be established to provide income.

3. Preparatory education of dentists should equal that of physicians.

4. Undergraduate dental curriculum should be devised for intensive preparation for duties of general practice only.

5. An optional full-year graduate curriculum . . . including dispensary and hospital experience and encouragement in research should be provided for all specialties in oral science especially those of practice, public health administration, teaching, and investigation.[12]

Many of Gies's conclusions reflect existing—if not yet uniformly accepted—arguments and conclusions. For example, one result of the Gies report was that proprietary (privately owned) dental schools were virtually eliminated and dental education in the United States came under the auspices of universities. But the backlash against proprietary schools had predated the report, and the economic realities of bringing these schools up to standard hastened their demise.[13]

Gies, like Flexner, forcefully supported a strong basic science curriculum and influenced many dental schools to strengthen their programs. His conclusions that predoctoral education should emphasize general practice and avoid early specialization have remained largely in place, and his support for hospital internships and a broad array of graduate specialty programs has been influential.

In many respects, the impacts of the Flexner and Gies reports were similar, but in one respect the impacts differed. Dental schools did not have the added impetus toward restructuring that was afforded medical schools after Flexner moved to the General Education Board and began directing funds to medical education. Thus, the advance of medical research was due not to government but to philanthropic funding. The Gies report provided inspiration for university-based dental research, but historians credit his founding in 1918 of the *Journal for Dental Research* as being a more powerful stimulus. The Gies report would be one of the forces leading to the dental fellowship program, founded in 1929 at the School of Medicine and Dentistry of the University of Rochester.

The School of Medicine and Dentistry (SMD) was established on the premise that there would be a school of dentistry in Rochester offering a DDS degree. George Eastman in particular felt that the establishment of a dental school at the university was necessary to further the success of the dispensary.

"The initial plan [of 1920]," George Whipple wrote in 1955, " . . . was that there be about fifty students in medicine and about twenty-five in dentistry going on together during the first two years and then one group going into the hospital for medical training and the other going into the dispensary for dentistry training."[14] Whipple insisted that the dental students should first get a broad biological background; second, work for PhD and master's degrees but not for MD degrees; and third, immerse themselves in research.

The original admission requirements for both medical and dental students were a minimum of three years of college, including courses in biology, chemistry, and physics, so that the students could work together and proceed with the same speed along their basic science training. This was the plan agreed upon by Flexner, Eastman, and Rhees. But, it didn't work. No dental students applied. "Not a single adequately trained candidate appeared,"[15] Whipple recalled in 1955. By 1928, plans for the dental component of the SMD had been abandoned, with plans to develop the University of Rochester Dental Research Fellowship Program taking its place.

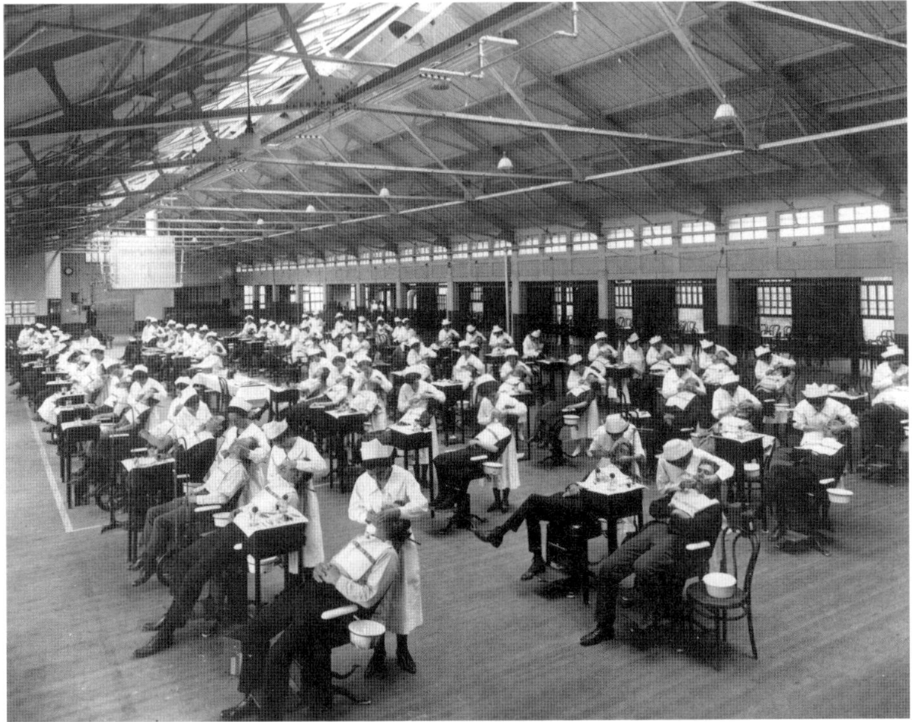

All of Kodak Park gets its teeth cleaned, 1927. (Author's collection)

Why did no "adequately prepared" dental students apply? If you wanted to be a dentist, the path was easier elsewhere. Most dental schools of the time had lower admission standards than did the School of Medicine and Dentistry. Because medicine paid better and was held by some in higher esteem than dentistry, students who met the high qualifications standards for admission to the school might be tempted to switch midstream to medicine.

According to recollections of some early students, George Whipple interviewed not only prospective faculty but also prospective students. When prospective dental students were interviewed, these sources say, they were told that they could not start out as dental students and then switch after two years to medicine. As a result, some prospective dental students switched to medicine before matriculating; this was the one reason there were no candidates for dentistry. Whipple himself explained it this way in 1955:

The Rockefeller Foundation gave generously to support experiments in three schools of medicine, this one and two others. Dental graduates were to be taken in and given further training. This school felt that the training should be in research and teaching leading to the degree of Doctor of Philosophy but not to the degree of Doctor of Medicine. The other two schools decided that the dental candidates could work for their medical degrees. As a result, all of the individuals who went through medical training got their M.D. in addition to their dentistry degree *and they practiced medicine*. The group here . . . received graduate training, attained distinction, liked teaching because they participated in the teaching in the department in which they chose to work. This development could not have been predicted but might have been hoped for.

In this way, the failure of the undergraduate dental program to materialize led to the important transformations to the fellowship and research programs that did emerge at the School of Medicine and Dentistry. Whipple explained, "They had to make a change because no one applied to become a dentist, so they took graduate dentists and turned them into teachers, deans, associate deans, research directors, department heads, etc."

UNIVERSITY OF ROCHESTER DENTAL RESEARCH FELLOWSHIP PROGRAM

In 1929, the University of Rochester Dental Research Fellowship Program was formed under the auspices of the Department of Medicine, receiving an initial five-year grant from the Rockefeller Foundation to provide fellowships supporting dental research and training in the fundamental biological background underlying dental health problems. Further contributions and support from the Carnegie Corporation, the Markel Foundation, the Eastman Dental Dispensary, and the National Foundation of Dental Research helped this curriculum become a unique and outstanding success with national and international recognition. The program evolved into the Department of Dental Research and the foundation of the current Center for Oral Biology at the university. It was set up so that the training in research and teaching would lead to a PhD degree and a career in academia. By contrast, Yale let dental candidates work for a medical degree in addition to their dentistry degree, and as a result, they all practiced medicine.

UNE 22, 1920.

THE ROCHESTER HERALD, TUESDA[Y]

WORK AT MEDICAL AND DENTAL SCHOOLS IN ROCHESTER TO BE ENTIRELY IN LINE OF PREVENTION AS A MEANS OF HEALTH

Dr. Harvey J. Burkhart Tells Members of Kiwanis Club How Dental School Will Be Formed—Medical and Dental Men To Receive Same Training the First Two Years.

That the new Rochester medical school, hospital, dental school and the Rochester Dental Dispensary will do work of almost entirely a preventative nature was the statement made by Dr. Harvey J. Burkhart of the Rochester Dental Dispensary at a meeting of the Kiwanis Club yesterday noon. Dr. Burkhart discussed the new schools and hospital in an informal manner, with the idea of giving as much information as possible, to as many people as possible.

He began by explaining the difference between the Rockefeller Foundation and the General Education Board, the latter having the distribution of the immense sums of money Mr. Rockefeller gives for education, and stated that, as time goes on, all will hear more of the work of each. He then spoke as follows:

"The donation by the General Education Board for the medical and dental schools and the hospital here was made on a 50-50 basis. The board never gives above that basis. The $5,000,000 given to Rochester is to match the $1,000,000 of the Rochester Dental Dispensary and the $4,000,000 given by George Eastman. The dispensary and its equipment cost $500,000, but the Education Board never matches equipment in existence; hence George Eastman has given more than the $4,000,000.

Fertile Field in Rochester.

"The primary reason for the gift was because there was not previously a medical or dental school here. When the new institutions are established, they will be of the highest type that can be gotten together. In the newer institutions they bring men from the older institutions who have received the proper training. Johns-Hopkins Hospital is not a hospital of the ordinary rescue and relief kind, but a clinical hospital. The obscure and unusual cases come there and receive the best attention and observation. The new hospital will be similar.

"The dental school will be along the same lines. There are now many dental and medical schools in the country that have no university connection. Such schools have not had a very good effect on medicine and dentistry and a good many of them are going out of business because they cannot give the best teaching. Now that there is a medical school in prospect for Rochester, I feel that we can establish the best dental school in the world here. We will have connection with a fine university and the benefit of connection with the medical school for teaching medical dentistry. And we will also have the hospital. In the same way the medical school will have unusual advantages.

"The new school will teach dentists the same as the medical men are taught to-day. The first two years the dental men will receive the same instruction as the medical men, then will come the specialization, and, when the dentist has been graduated, he will have the advantage of a training in general pathology. It will uplift dentistry, as it will put dentists on a higher educational plane than they are to-day.

No Competition with Others.

"We will not be in competition with the medical and dental schools that are now in existence to get men. But we are going to get the highest class of men for the professions and have them developed to the greatest proficiency. They will not be big schools, but their product will be the best in the world.

"We are not going to have money to burn for fancy salaries or for a whole lot of buildings. We have enough to start in a comfortable way and we will have the assistance of the Rockefeller Foundation and the General Education Board, Johns-Hopkins and other similar institutions, so that we are off to a fine start. The people here will have to assist when calls for money come; but we will show our goods and prove by our works that we are entitled to more and get assistance when needed.

"The object of the whole proposition is to arrange the teaching and contributions so as to meet the end of preventive dentistry and medicine. Our main hope in the betterment of the race is producing means to the end of prevention. Hence our work with the children, first of all, to educate them to take care of themselves physically. When the dental college is established, we will do adult work to give instruction to dental students. It is a case of work for the future, rather than for the present, and in our dental work it has already gotten to the stage where we can see results."

Rochester's first dental fellows did research on oral and dental topics, an entirely new idea in the 1920s. Basil Bibby, who followed Burkhart as dispensary director, was one of those original fellows. "Up to that point," Beatrice Bibby said in 2004, "they didn't realize there was so much overlap between teeth and other parts of the body. The fellows attached themselves to various departments. The [medical men] accepted the dentists and encouraged them and made life easy. [Even though the dentists] were working in separate departments, they were also creating a unit among themselves as a dental research group."[16]

Instead of the academically sound but clinically oriented dental school envisioned by Eastman, Burkhart, and Flexner, the fellowship program initiated by Whipple provided advanced education for academic and research-oriented dentists. Whipple believed that the development of the fellowship program "was very fortunate, infinitely more so in my opinion than the original program." The men who came "wanted to do something different . . . learn something about basic science and teaching."[17] Whipple thought that the early fellows were "brave young men," because no one knew if dental schools wanted men trained in research on their faculties. He warned them that it might take years to build up demand: "This is not a five year plan but a 25 or 50-year plan."

George Washington Corner, MD, was the original chair of anatomy at the nascent School of Medicine and Dentistry, 1924–40. He is known chiefly as the discoverer of progesterone, which to led to the development of the birth-control pill. Corner was also the Whipple biographer who wrote that the early dental fellows "own success as investigators and showed that a medical degree is not the only passport to research in the medical life-sciences." The program prepared fellows for leadership roles, Corner wrote in the Whipple biography.

The dental fellows organized a weekly seminar to moderate any sense of isolation from their own profession. Candidates for the program came from many states, Europe, and Asia. Each of the basic science departments received fellows as temporary members. Whipple's own department, pathology, trained nineteen, more than any other.

By 1955, the dental fellows program had fifty-eight alumni. They had come from thirty-three different dental schools, twenty-two in the United States and eleven in foreign countries. Of the fifty-eight, thirty-three had received one or more university advanced degrees—eighteen received masters, eigh-teen received PhDs, and three of these received both. All basic science departments—anatomy, bacteriology, biochemistry, pathology, pharmacology, physiology, vital economics, and radiology—contributed to the training of the fellows. Most impressive were the men's postfellowship careers: five became deans of dental schools, three associate deans, one director of a dental institute, three directors of dental research, one director of medical research, twenty-three professors, thirteen associate professors, assistant professors, instructors, or research associates, two army officers, five public health officers, and ten in private practice.

These appointments represented fourteen U.S. and three foreign dental schools. The former fellows estimated that they gave 24 percent of their time to teaching, 34 percent to research, 16 percent to administration, 24 percent to practice, and 2 percent to professional activities. Nearly all continued to carry on research, producing more than 1,000 papers in twenty-five years. In announcing these statistics, Dean Donald Anderson, who succeeded Whipple, noted, "Very few efforts in education have ever paid off so handsomely."[18]

Later, Basil Bibby estimated that between 1930 and 1988, up to 100 of the University of Rochester dental fellows had been appointed to teaching or research positions in dental schools throughout the world.[19] Some cases in point illustrate this global influence:

George W. Burnett, DDS, PhD, established that proteolysis of the dentine could not take place prior to decalcification. He was the first to purify and establish the chemical structure of the mucopolysaccharides in saliva. Burnett went on to become chief of the Department of Dental Research, American Medical Service Graduate School, Washington, DC.

S. Wah Leung, DDS, PhD, established bicarbonate as the principal buffer of saliva. Leung became professor of physiology at the University of Pittsburgh.

Kanwar L. Shourie, PMID, John W. Hein, DMD, PhD, Leung, and Norman S. Simmons, DMD, PhD, devised a Puerto Rican dental survey in 1948–49 that was the most comprehensive ever conducted up to that time. It set the standards for clinical dental research for a long period.[20] Shourie became dean and professor of dentistry in Bombay, India. Hein, who also demonstrated the powerful caries prevention effect of copper ions (1952–54), became dental director for the Colgate Palmolive Company. Simmons, who later joined the Harvard faculty, was also the first to purify and establish the chemical structure of the mucopolysaccharides in saliva.

Erling Johansen, DMD, PhD, was the first to develop a method of following the progressive development of caries and periodontal disease in small un-anaesthetized animals.

HAROLD HODGE:
EARLY FLUORIDE RESEARCHER

Harold Hodge, PhD, professor of pharmacology and toxicology (1931–71) at the university, published a paper entitled "Fluoride Metabolism and Safety of Water Fluoridation" that considered two questions: (1) Does it work? and (2) Is it safe?

Hodge then answered his own questions: "The evidence now available of the effectiveness of water-borne fluorides (whether naturally or artificially present at a concentration of about 1p per-million) in reducing dental decay is overwhelmingly convincing. Safety is also established with reasonable surety."

Hodge spent the remainder of the paper explaining that last sentence. He concluded: "When the metabolic evidence is put together with that from studies of the known toxic effects of fluoride, it is concluded that water fluoridation provides adequate factors of safety. At present, the evidence does not justify the postponement of water fluoridation."

Whereas most of the early fellows were trained as dentists, Hodge, a chemist, early became interested in the structure of teeth, and with colleagues from radiology, he participated in developing a technique for the quantitative analysis of tooth structure. He then quickly produced a paper on the structure and metabolism of tooth and bone—reprinted by the University of Arizona Press as a "classic in radiology." Hodge would present his work on tooth hardness to students using a special diamond-tipped scribe.

Hodge also made chemical analyses of dental enamel and dentine and observed the effects of fluorine in preventing dental caries.[21] He also headed a research group that tested sodium monofluorophosphate as a hardener of tooth enamel. His work attracted wide attention and he was asked to contribute the definitive chapter on fluorine in a multi-volume work on mineral metabolism.[22]

Hodge was chosen as the first president of the newly formed Society of Toxicology in 1961. He served as president of the International Association of Dental Research in 1947, and in 1966 he was named president of the American Society of Pharmacology and Experimental Therapeutics. He was the recipient of numerous awards, and his publication record encompasses 286 papers and five books.[23]

ENTER FLUORIDE . . . AND CONTROVERSY

Dental fellows Dr. Harold Hodge, Dr. Kanwar L. Shourie, and Dr. John Hein were among the first to demonstrate the ability of complex fluorides to prevent decay. The year was 1934, twenty years before the fluoride wars heated up nationally. These researchers showed that topical applications of fluoride protected teeth against caries. Basil Bibby and Harold Hodge began the initial work on the use of the topical application of fluoride as a caries preventive agent, work that continued from 1939 to 1941. Hodge and Dr. Joseph F. Volker established the mechanisms by which fluorine could decrease the solubility of tooth structure. Volker went on to become dean and director of dentistry and medical research and subsequently president at the University of Alabama.

Burkhart reluctantly gave Bibby permission to test the effects of fluoride applications on the teeth of the school children under the care of the Rochester Dental Dispensary, a test that lapsed after Bibby left Rochester in 1940. At that time, most researchers believed that fluorine strengthened teeth through the bloodstream and thus worked by being ingested. However, the research fellows' findings were that applying fluoride mixtures to the exterior of the teeth would prevent dental decay. After these findings were reported in the newspapers, Burkhart and the American Dental Association criticized the School of Medicine and Dentistry for "unethical action in making unjustified claims that would be harmful to dentistry." To reinforce this disapproval, the *Journal of the American Dental Association* was required for a number of years to refuse publication of research papers from the Rochester dental research fellows.

In 1936, a follow-up study was done in Brockton, MA, that vindicated the laboratory research done by the Rochester dental research fellows. The study indicated that dental caries could be prevented by making applications of fluoride solutions to the exterior of the teeth. "As a result [of the fluoride

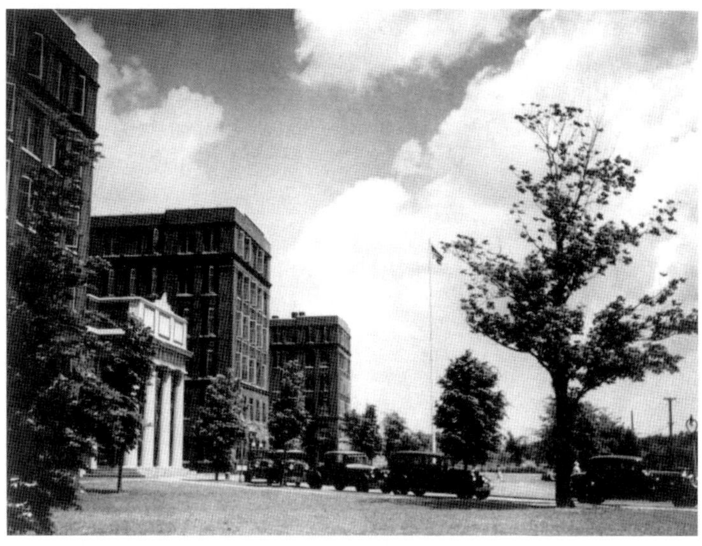

*Original entrance to Strong Memorial Hospital,
now the School of Medicine and Dentistry*

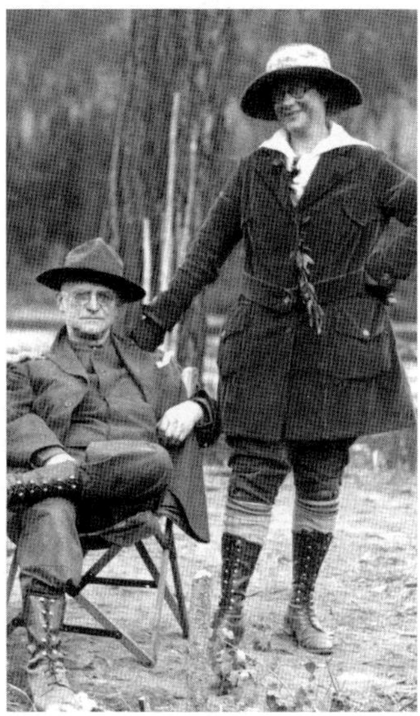

*George Eastman and Katharine Whipple
(Courtesy George Eastman House)*

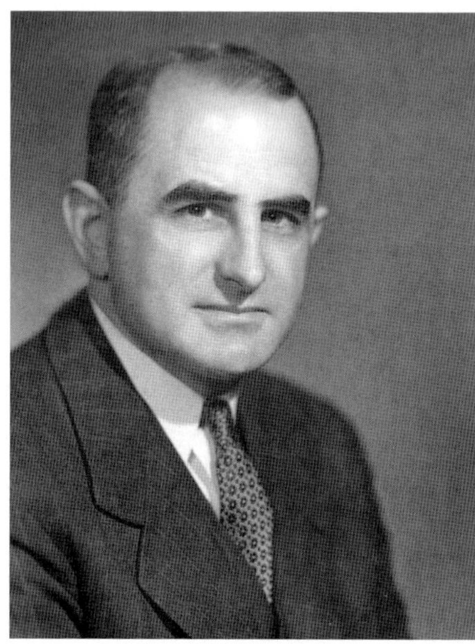

Basil Bibby

applications]," Bibby wrote later, "dental decay throughout the Western World has been reduced by about 60 percent." Considering that dental decay is the world's most prevalent disease, more common than asthma, this constituted a significant breakthrough.

The controversy over fluoride demonstrates that despite Eastman's patronage and influence, his vision for a school of medicine *and* dentistry was never really accepted by the physicians and administrators who designed and ran the School of Medicine and Dentistry. Notwithstanding Eastman's hopes and intention, the funding that was partially set aside for training young dentists who would serve the community (as well as providing dental care for indigent children and training hygienists who would take the program into the schools) was never used for that purpose. Instead, the graduate program in oral biology and the dental fellowship program became an alternative to a real dental school. While many positive connections developed between the dental center and university basic science departments, including collaborative research projects, echoes of that early dissatisfaction lingered.

FORESHADOWING THE FUTURE

Basil G. Bibby, who received his dental degree from Otago University of the University of New Zealand in 1927, graduated first in the initial dental fellows class. Dr. Bibby was practicing in New Zealand when he saw an advertisement in a dental journal about the research program for graduate dentists that Dr. George Whipple was starting at the University of Rochester School of Medicine and Dentistry. Bibby was accepted into the fellowship program and would serve as an assistant professor in SMD's Department of Bacteriology for ten years.

In New Zealand, Bibby had observed how the teeth of the native Maoris deteriorated after they started eating a European diet following the arrival of the English and Dutch colonials, and he became interested in caries prevention. While in Rochester in the 1930s, Bibby and the other fellows conducted considerable research into the uses of fluorides—salts of the gas fluorine—in checking tooth decay. He wrote or collaborated on about sixty publications, principally on oral bacteriology. He received a doctorate in bacteriology in 1935 at the University of Rochester and a doctorate in dental medicine in 1939 from Tufts University. The next year he was recruited to become dean of the Tufts University School of Dentistry.

Whipple, a research man through and through, assumed that George Eastman's promise to do "something else for dentistry" meant that he would provide funds to establish a dental research institute. Whipple believed that the Dental Research Fellowship Program, financed for five years by the Rockefeller Foundation, would serve as forerunner for this institute. Whipple told Basil Bibby to hold on just a little longer as a fellow, leading Bibby to believe he might become head of the institute that Whipple envisioned. This would prove to be a dead end. Funds failed to materialize and Bibby moved on.

* * *

The following essay by Dr. William Bowen, of the Center for Oral Biology is included in this chapter rather than in chapter 9 where the other histories of the departments and divisions of the Eastman Department of Dentistry are placed. The department that is the subject of this essay, now the Center for Oral Biology, had its beginnings in the fellowship program established at the University of Rochester (UR) School of Medicine and Dentistry (SMD)

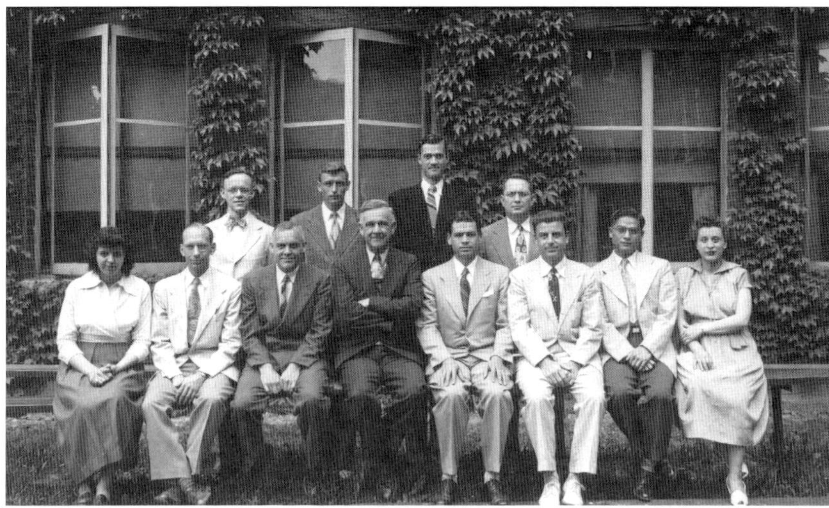

George Whipple (sixth from left) and some of the early fellows

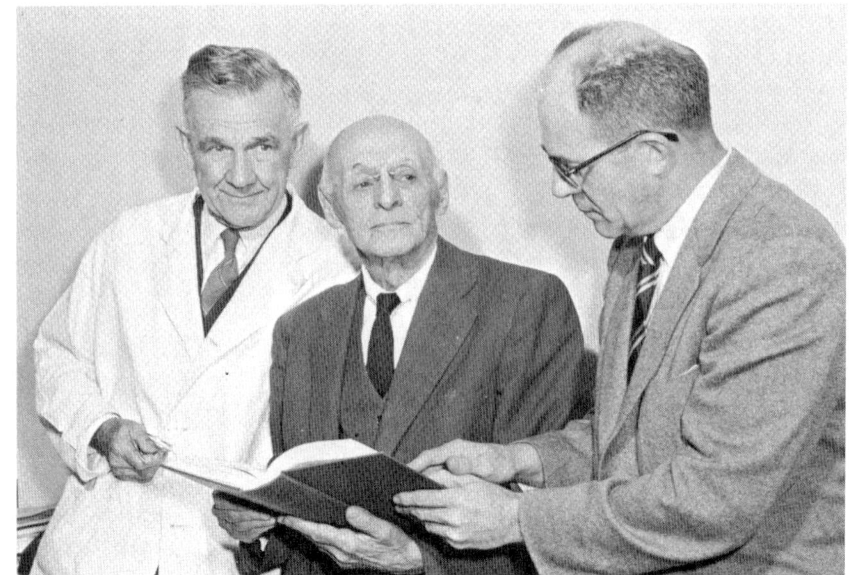

George Hoyt Whipple, Abraham Flexner, and Donald Grigg Anderson (from left to right) on the occasion of Mr. Flexner's return visit to Rochester in 1954. He died in 1959 at the age of 92.

in 1929 during the time period described in this chapter. This foundation led to the creation in 1947 of the UR Dental Research Division under Dr. John Hein, which become in 1955 the Department of Dentistry and Dental Research under Dr. Erling Johansen. In 1972, the department was renamed the Department of Dental Research (still under Johansen), and a new Department of Clinical Dentistry under Dr. Fred Emmings was created. This chronology of name changes is reflected in the remainder of this book.

BRIEF HISTORY OF THE DEPARTMENT OF DENTAL RESEARCH— CENTER FOR ORAL BIOLOGY

William H. Bowen

INTRODUCTION

A plaque hanging outside the Miner Library bears the following inscription: "The School of Medicine and Dentistry was established in the University of Rochester in 1920 by the gifts of George Eastman and the General Education Board founded by John D. Rockefeller and is dedicated to the advancement of knowledge and to instruction in Medicine and Dentistry for the promotion of the Health and Happiness of Mankind."

As described previously, a conventional dental school was never established because of an alleged "lack of qualified candidates." In its stead, with George Eastman's approval and Dean George Whipple's enthusiastic support, the Dental Research Training Program was initiated with additional funds from the Rockefeller Foundation. Whipple promoted the concept that trainees would come to the university with their dental degree, become immersed in the biological sciences, and work toward their PhD degree. This was certainly a revolutionary concept, particularly for a young profession geared at that time toward restoration and replacement of teeth. George Whipple was given the title of "Father of Teachers" by one of the early fellows, Harold Hodge. The program succeeded beyond expectations,

and its graduates have had a profound influence on dental education and research worldwide. The program continues to have the following goal: "To conduct research and to train prospective teachers, investigators and practitioners in the fundamental biological sciences underlying the practice of dentistry."

The history of oral and dental research in the University of Rochester mirrors the evolution of dental science in the United States. The foundation of dental research and training in Rochester ironically was conceived from failure. When George Eastman funded the School of Medicine and Dentistry, he clearly intended to have a dental school. Through a combination of circumstances, not the least of which was a lack of will by the medical school administrations, the dental school languished and died.

With most amazing foresight, George Whipple (Nobel Prize, 1936) saw the need to establish a program for the training of dentists to pursue careers in research and teaching. He obtained financial support from the Rockefeller Foundation and thus was born what must surely be one of the outstanding success stories in the history of the university. Indeed, more than fifty years later an external review team referred to the Department of Dental Research as a gem. There is an abundance of evidence that the program established by Whipple and which continues today has had a profound influence on research and dental education worldwide. George Whipple, speaking on the occasion of the twenty-fifth anniversary of the program (1955), noted, "We were fortunate in the men who came here—they wanted to do something different. They wanted to learn something about sound basic science and teaching. I think their accomplishments have been quite extraordinary. They were a good bunch."

The early fellows were certainly pioneers. When they entered the program, there was no set curriculum or a "dental faculty." Fellows were encouraged to visit numerous laboratories, find a problem that was attractive to them, and pursue it to a logical conclusion. Philip Jay appears to have been the first fellow, and he had a particular interest in the role of lactobacilli in the etiology of dental caries. Indeed, the first four fellows, including Basil Bibby, focused their research on oral microbiology and the effects of saliva on their growth and laid the foundation for generations to come. However, it would be an error to believe that the fellows had a narrow approach to oral research. At the International Association Annual Meeting in 1934, there were sixteen papers presented by University of Rochester trainees out of a total of ninety presentations. The Rochester presentations included x-ray absorption properties of normal and pathological dentins; form, size, and position of maxillary sinus at various ages; and influence of high-sugar diets upon teeth of white rats. It is of interest to note that there wasn't a single paper on fluoride presented at this meeting.

The arrival of a cyclotron in the university in 1935 provided more opportunities for the dental fellows, and, to their credit, they grasped the significance of the instrument and exploited it fully. They laid the foundation for some core principles that remain valid today, even though they were not universally accepted at the time.

Using P^{32}, Joseph Volker (later president of the University of Alabama) and his colleagues demonstrated that phosphorus in enamel could exchange for phosphorus in saliva, thus providing the basis for the future remineralization studies of early enamel carious lesions described by Koulerouides (MS, 1958). Koulerouides subsequently joined Volker in the University of Alabama Dental School as a member of the faculty.

Perhaps use of the cyclotron provided the earliest indirect demonstration of how fluoride prevents dental caries, that is, through rehardening of demineralized enamel. Furthermore, using some ingenious techniques in rodents, Joseph Volker, Virgil Cheyne, Sidney Finn, Basil Bibby, and Dick Manly demonstrated that the primary mode of protection of fluoride is topical. It is noteworthy that this material was first presented at the American Association for the Advancement of Science (AAAS) annual meeting in Columbus, 1939; this illustrates elegantly one of the guiding principles in the foundation of the dental fellows' program, that dental science is part of the mainstream of scientific endeavor. Much of the data presented ran contrary to the dogma of the time—for example, that fluoride prevented decay solely by being incorporated into enamel. This of course was understandable because of the obvious effects of excessive fluoride on enamel (fluorosis-pitting of enamel). The data presented at the AAAS meeting showed very clearly that fluoride was "taken up" by enamel, and even in sufficient concentrations to affect the growth of bacteria on enamel. They also demonstrated that topical application of fluoride on erupted teeth in rats reduced the incidence of decay by 75 percent. It is significant that the authors discounted the possibility of using fluoride in powders or paste by the general public because they deemed it "unsafe." They advocated topical application by professionals.

The concept of fluoride acting locally on the tooth was so revolutionary that one major dental journal declined to accept any papers on fluoride from the University of Rochester for many years.

Cheyne, who was one of the leaders in developing the hypothesis, took a position in the Indiana Dental School. I suspect he had a strong influence there on Dr. Joe Muhler, who was responsible for the first successful introduction of a fluoridated toothpaste (stannous fluoride—Crest, which contained stannous fluoride, received FDA and ADA approval in 1961).

Following identification of fluoride as an effective method of preventing dental caries, investigators naturally turned their attention to the possible effects of additional trace elements. This research was led by Jack Hein, who completed his PhD in Rochester and who demonstrated the effects of strontium, iron, lead, and other elements. Unfortunately, none proved more or even equally as effective as fluoride. This work led to additional research on mineral content of enamel and to numerous epidemiological studies.

INTERNATIONAL FLAVOR

From its inception, the Dental Research Training Program has attracted overseas graduates of the highest caliber. Basil Bibby, from New Zealand, was one of the earliest fellows. The 1940s saw the arrival of several young researchers from Norway and Latin America. Among these was Reidar Sognnaes, a graduate of the University of Bergen and one of the leaders of the famous Tristan da Cunha expedition, which demonstrated the influence of sugars on prevalence of dental caries. While in Rochester Sognnaes pursued the uptake of phosphorus by enamel and eso-exchange and explored the topical effects of fluoride on dental caries. He subsequently became Dean of the School of Dentistry at the University of California, San Francisco.

Dr. Humberto Grandos was the first fellow from Colombia. He had a particular interest in epidemiology and the effects of nutrition on tooth development. K. L. Schourie arrived in Rochester in 1947 from India and pursued his interest in the nutritional and dietary aspects of dental caries.

Clearly the fame of Rochester was spreading internationally and nationally. As noted earlier, in 1948 the U.S. Public Health Service contracted with

University of Rochester dental group to conduct a survey of dental and oral disease in Puerto Rico. Thus the connection to Puerto Rico goes back more than sixty years.

DIRECTORS AND STRUCTURE

The university decided in 1952 that a formal structure for the dental program was required. Dr. John Hein was appointed as first director of the Department of Dentistry and Dental Research (later the Department of Dental Research). Hein had very ambitious plans for the department, which he laid out in a comprehensive memorandum. Clearly it called for expenditure of significant amounts of money, justified by Hein on the grounds that when the dental school did not materialize after the establishment of the School of Medicine and Dentistry, the funds given by George Eastman went into the coffers of the medical school. It became readily apparent to Hein that he was not going to receive any support so he resigned and became director of dental research at Colgate Palmolive. Dr. Hein later was appointed head of the Forsyth Dental Clinic in Boston and was a leading advocate for federal support for dental research.

Dr. Erling Johansen became director in 1954 shortly after he had completed his fellowship. Dr. Johansen had a particular interest in electron microscopy and used the hamster as a model for dental caries. He also worked closely with colleagues in radiation oncology to prevent caries in persons who had undergone irradiation for head and neck cancer. This was certainly a much-neglected area, and he is to be commended for drawing attention to this problem.

Dr. Johansen was regarded by many as cautious and conservative. Relations between the dental unit and Eastman Dental Center were not strong, and several opportunities for significant joint programs were missed. Johansen later became dean of the dental school at Tufts.

There was a steady flow of well-qualified fellows, most of whom went on to very distinguished careers in government or academic dentistry. The Department of Dentistry and Dental Research, as it was originally named, had been moribund for several years following the departure of Dr. Erling Johansen. Indeed, there was serious consideration given to closing the department permanently.

Having initially turned down the invitation to be chair, I accepted and took office in August of 1982. The task ahead was indeed daunting. The faculty and staff were composed of one technician and myself. The facilities and equipment were outdated and in disrepair. My goals were very clear. I wanted to recapture the essence of what was the core of past success. This could be accomplished, I believed, by collaborating with the extraordinary talent available within the University and in the Eastman Dental Center. My personal research was focused on the etiology, pathogenesis, and prevention of dental caries. Also in the early 1980s, the National Institute of Dental and Craniofacial Research (NIDCR) decided to launch a number of disease-oriented centers. I approached a number of persons in the departments of microbiology, biochemistry, biostatistics, and the Eastman Dental Center and invited them to collaborate. I was overwhelmed by their enthusiastic participation, and the department was awarded the first cariology center in the United States. Dr. Robert Marquis, department of microbiology, was particularly supportive, and his contributions to oral microbiology have been invaluable. He is certainly one of the icons of dental research. His work on acid tolerance in microorganisms is a key in the pathogenesis of dental caries.

It had become apparent that there was a dearth of persons involved in caries research in the United States and that there was a major opportunity to construct a training program for "cariologists." I devised a program, again tapping into the intellectual reservoir of talent in the university and the Eastman Dental Center. The collaborative efforts were exceptional, and once again they were successful. Thus in a short period Rochester had a major center grant and a training grant.

Around the same time, NIDCR noted the relative lack of clinically trained PhDs and decided to develop the Dentist Scientist program. The objective of the program was to recruit dentists into specialty training and a PhD program in a basic science. Rochester was in a particularly strong position, because a somewhat similar program had been jointly supported by the School of Medicine and Dentistry and the Eastman Dental Center. It was one of four successful applicants. Once again, support from colleagues throughout the university was extraordinary. Thus the department was back on track to its roots—research and training. Twenty-five years later it is still among the leaders in craniofacial and dental research and training.

There was of course an urgency to hire faculty, particularly persons who were likely to be successful in the ever-competitive grant arena. I was most fortunate to have attracted some extraordinarily skillful young people who have gone on to internationally acclaimed careers. Because of my interactions with the faculty of the department of microbiology (I had served as acting chair for two years), I had the opportunity to observe a talented postdoctoral trainee, Dr. Rob Quivey, and a predoctoral trainee, Dr. Bob Burne. Both became members of the faculty and now are full professors. Around this time, I met Dr. James Melvin, who was pursuing his PhD with Dr. Bob Hamill in Neurology. Dr. Melvin decided to take a postdoctoral position in NIDCR, and when the occasion arose, he was offered a faculty position at the university, which he accepted.

Shortly after I had arrived in Rochester, I met Dr. Larry Tabak at the University of Buffalo. I attempted to recruit him, but Tabak was unwilling because he had obligations to his mentor which would take a year or so to discharge. A year later I called Tabak. Tabak expressed interest, but after some negotiation he declined. I suggested that he postpone his final decision until the following Monday and he agreed. I then proceeded to call several of Tabak's friends to exert a little persuasion, and Tabak decided to accept the offer.

After serving as chair for thirteen years, I decided the time had come for me to pass the torch. The position was offered to Dr. Tabak, and he became chair of the Department of Dental Research, as the department was now called, in 1995. He brought exceptional scientific and administrative skills to the department. He is regarded as one of the leading experts in glycobiology, in which, coincidentally, the department had been a pioneer. Dr. Tabak introduced the use of transgenic animals into the field and greatly expanded the use of molecular biology and genetics into the study of saliva and salivary glands. Indeed, the first investigations on the use of transgenic animals in caries research were conducted in the department.

Dr. Tabak also developed a short-term training program focused on underserved minorities. The trainees traveled to Rochester at no expense to them and were provided with accommodations and a modest stipend. This is an exceptionally successful program; nearly all of the trainees have gone on to enter full-time programs.

Dr. Tabak was part of the team that developed the inclusion of the Eastman Dental Center into the University of Rochester Medical Center and the evolution of the Eastman Department of Dentistry in 1998. The Department of Dental Research became the Center for Oral Biology (COB) and moved into modern laboratories (a total of 20,000 square feet) in the newly constructed Kornberg Building.

Dr. Tabak's talents were recognized when he was promoted to senior associate dean for research, a position he held when he left the university to become director of NIDCR. He was the second person from Rochester to be director of NIDCR; Dr. David Scott was the first.

Following the departure of Dr. Larry Tabak, Dr. James Melvin was appointed chair of the Center for Oral Biology after a national search. Dr. Melvin received his DDS from Case Western Reserve and his PhD in neurobiology and anatomy from the University of Rochester. He is regarded as a leading researcher in the world on ion transport in salivary glands and has brought the most sophisticated biological tools to bear on his research, including transgenic animals. Dr. Melvin is also a leader in exploring the proteomics of saliva. Anticipated outcomes of this research will almost certainly lead to saliva being used as an aid in diagnosing systemic and oral diseases. Dr. Melvin has been spectacularly successful in obtaining grant support. The recent awarding of a novel training grant illustrates his progressive and forward thinking. Dr. Melvin, among others, has recognized the small number of persons entering academic careers in dentistry. In collaboration with the University of Puerto Rico (see earlier mention of the Puerto Rico survey program) and Marquette University, dental students come to Rochester to complete their final year and commence PhD studies. The program is unique to the University of Rochester and is in the spirit of the very foundations of dentistry at the university, dating back more than eighty years. Thus it is anticipated that Rochester will continue its tradition of providing leaders in research and teaching. Dr. Melvin stepped down in June of 2008, and Dr. Rob Quivey was appointed the chair of the Center for Oral Biology.

SOME NOTEWORTHY FELLOWS

Harold Hodge was one of the earliest fellows and joined the program in 1931. Although the program was designed for dentists, Hodge, a chemist, was welcomed. How fortunate for dentistry! He became one of the "Fathers of Teachers" (so named because most of the fellows went on to be teachers), one of the leading researchers into the action of fluoride on teeth, and contributed enormously to understanding the physiology of fluoride. Dr. Hodge became the director of toxicology for the Manhattan Project in Rochester, which was devoted to exploring the toxicity of beryllium and uranium in the 1940s and 1950s. He maintained his interest and support in dental research throughout his illustrious career. Dr. Hodge was professor of pharmacology from 1938 until 1970. His contributions to dental research were recognized when he became the recipient of the Swedish Patent Fund Prize in 1988. It is perhaps noteworthy that originally he was less than enthusiastic about the introduction of water fluoridation; however, like all great scientists, he allowed the facts to guide him and became an avid supporter.

Paul Keyes was a dental fellow in the early 1950s. He recognized the wonderful animal facilities and superb faculty. He placed animal caries studies, using both rats and hamsters as models, on a solid scientific basis, and also initiated research into determining the effects of topical applications of a variety of fluoride compounds. Keyes subsequently went on with Fitzgerald to demonstrate the infectious and transmissive nature of dental caries and subsequently to identify *Streptococcus mutans* as the prime microbial culprit in the etiology of dental caries. It is rumored that Keyes and Fitzgerald came close to receiving the Nobel Prize for their work.

David Scott was also a fellow in the early 1980s. Scott was one of the pioneers in the use of electron microscopy in dental research. His elegant work on the structures of enamel and dentine still illustrate textbooks today. He also produced wonderful images of cell walls of fusobacteria and spirochaetes, illustrating the complexity and interaction of these microorganisms. Scott eventually became the fourth director of the National Institute of Dental Research.

Dr. Paul Abadom, from Nigeria, became a fellow in 1955 and received his PhD in 1959, under the guidance of Dr. Hodge. He and I were good friends. One evening we were having a beer in a pub on Eastman Street when we noticed that when Paul finished his beer, the barman would break his glass. We ensured that he broke a lot of glasses that evening.

Given the research environment in the university, it is hardly surprising that many innovative approaches to oral health research were introduced here. For example, John Salley, a fellow, introduced the first animal model to study oral cancer by painting a carcinogen on the cheek pouch of hamsters. This model continues to have value.

The critical role that saliva plays in the maintenance of oral health was elegantly demonstrated by Virgil Cheyne. He surgically desalivated animals and observed a devastating increase in the incidence of caries. I have used this model extensively and expanded its use to model oral and esophageal candidiasis.

The unit was the first in the world to use transgenic animals in caries research and thus open a completely new avenue in oral biology.

ORAL BIOLOGY AT URMC

The commitment to excellence by the faculty of Dental Research (later COB) is evidenced by the range of awards received by faculty and students internally and externally. For example, in 1982 there was no federal support in the Department of Dental Research. By 1992, annual grant support was in excess of three million dollars, and the department was ranked six in dental schools receiving grants. The level of external support has continued to grow over the years. In 2001 it exceeded five million dollars and by 2005 it approached six.

The COB continues to be one of the most successful unit at the university based on support per capita and per square foot of space, metrics that are of increasing importance to administrators. An external review group, including a member of the National Academy of Sciences, evaluated the Department of Dental Research and noted, "The effect of the group is clearly more than the sum of the parts. . . . They interact with a large number of faculty in research across the University." They further concluded, "The unit is a model for the way a basic science department should integrate itself into the University as a whole. It is truly a 'small gem' and should be nurtured by the School of Medicine and Dentistry."

The department has excelled in competing for training grants. The success was based in large measure on its ability to demonstrate that their approach to training was broadly based, encompassing all of the basic biological sciences, and certainly was not narrow or parochial; over the years, persons in the department have been awarded PhDs in anatomy, pharmacology, biophysics, microbiology and immunology, biochemistry and neuroscience. The unit has had sustained support for the past twenty-five years and recently was awarded the Training Program in Oral Science (Dr. Melvin is P. I.), which is the largest training grant in the School of Medicine and Dentistry.

The trainees have been recognized for their excellence. Over the past twenty years, eight of its trainees have received the Hatton Prize, which is awarded at the annual meeting of the International Association for Dental Research, an accomplishment unmatched by any other institution.

The faculty, too, have been the recipients of numerous university, national, and international awards. For example, four of the faculty have received university recognition for teaching and mentoring. They have been awarded major international prizes by dental groups worldwide. Two members of the faculty have been elected to the Institute of Medicine of the National Academy of Medicine, an accomplishment achieved by only one other department university-wide, and three of the chairs have received MERIT awards from the National Institutes of Health.

Members of the university dental community have played major roles in the affairs of our national and international research organizations. The unit has influenced the tide of events in education and research far beyond what its size would appear to warrant.

In the early days of the program, there was little continuity in the research emphasis. This apparent lack of continuity could be attributed to an absence of core dental faculty. However, this situation allowed for a most extraordinary exposure to a plethora of research topics in the weekly seminars, and I recall somewhat wistfully that these were so well attended by senior faculty, residents, and students that the classroom was frequently packed. It is difficult to imagine a more scientifically invigorating environment. Nevertheless, as fellows took up positions in other universities, they brought their specific expertise and knowledge acquired in Rochester with them, and thus Rochester's influence on a huge range of diverse scientific challenges is displayed in government, industry, and academics.

The expansion of the faculty, which occurred in the 1980s and later, certainly allowed for consistent themes of research to be pursued vigorously. Current faculty are recognized internationally for their expertise in microbial physiology, craniofacial development, and salivary gland physiology. They attract graduate students from across the university. The future indeed continues to glow with success.

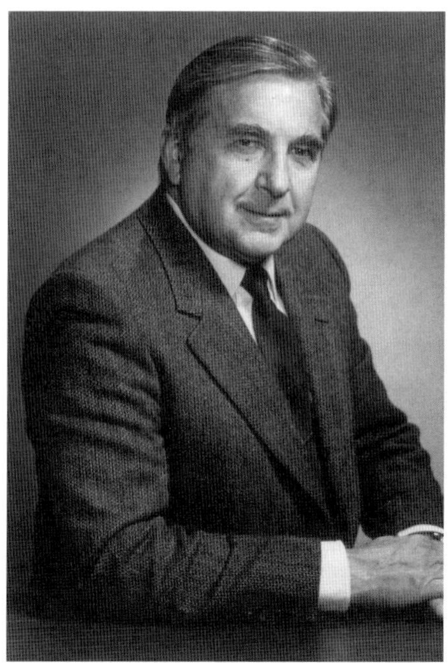

Erling Johansen

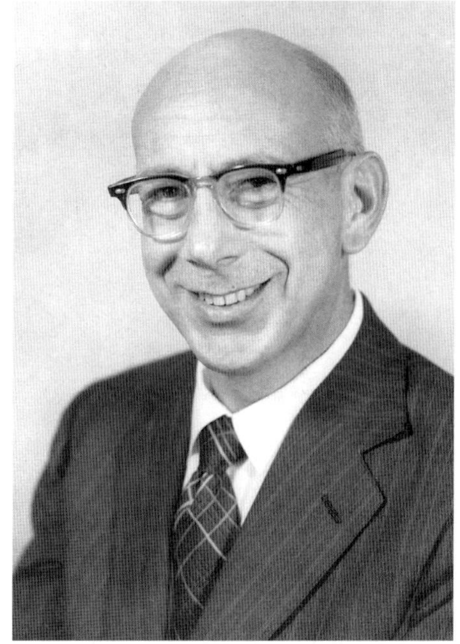

Jack Hein

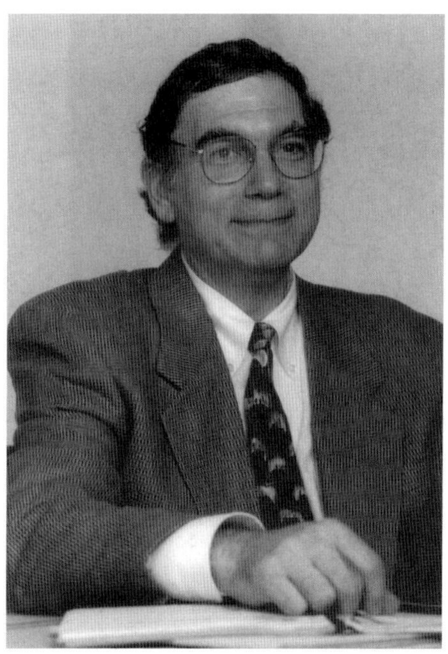

Larry Tabak

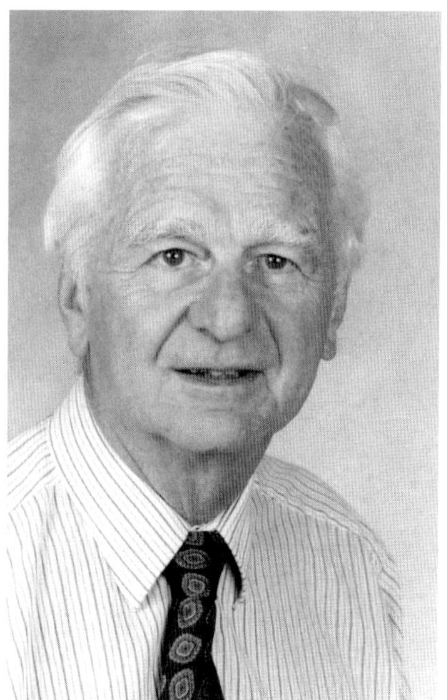

William Bowen

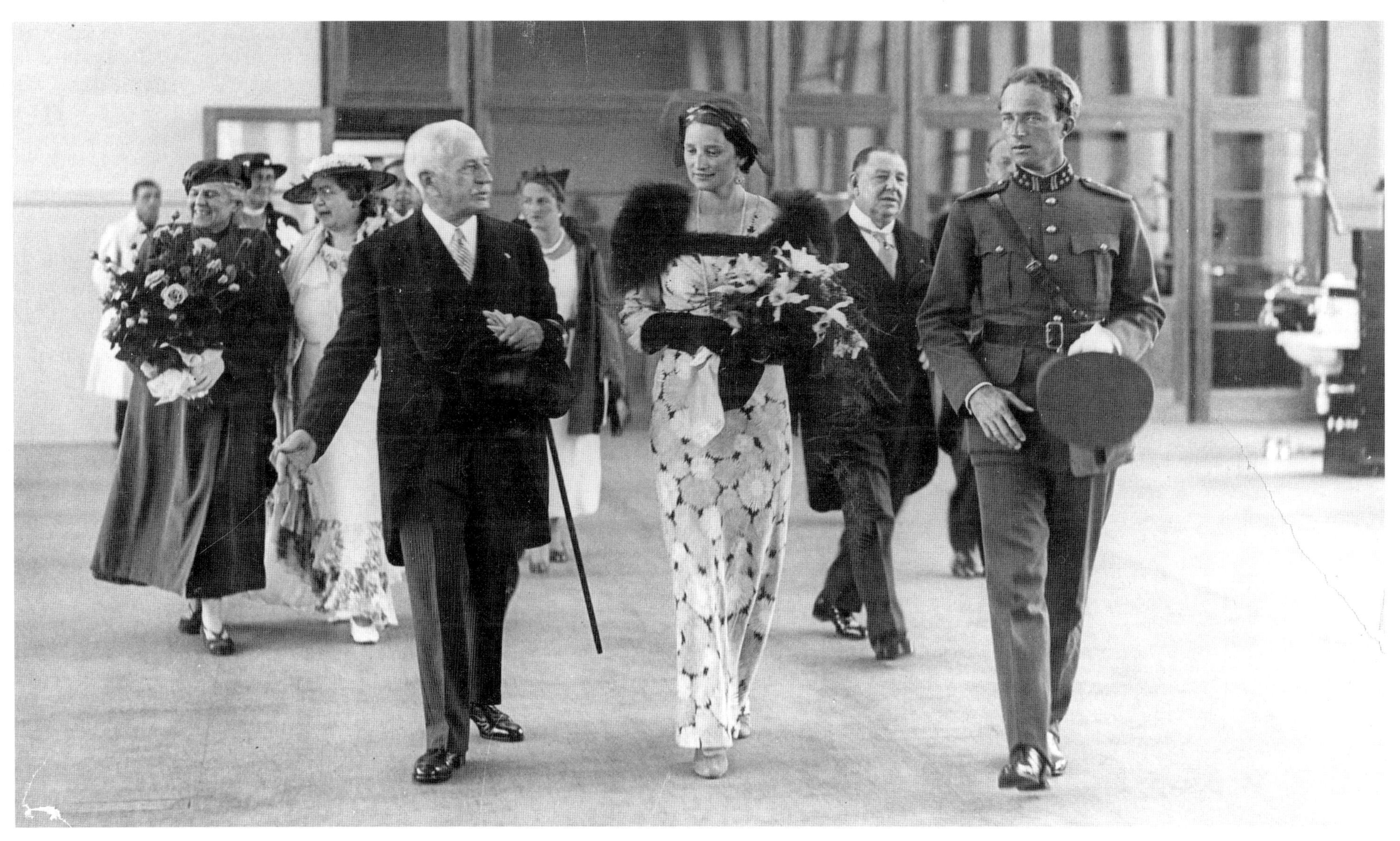

Dr. and Mrs. Burkhart whoosh into Brussels with rock stars King Leopold III and Queen Astrid to dedicate the Eastman Dental Clinic there.

Chapter Three

THE INTERNATIONAL CLINICS

"KODAK MAN TO BE WORLD'S DENTIST"

Even in the dark days of the German occupation, these buildings stood as reminders of Rochester philanthropy,
a symbol of the ministrations of peace that conquer the ravages of war.

Rochester newspaper on the fiftieth anniversary of the
opening of the Eastman Dental Center, 1967

EASTMAN DENTAL CLINIC, LONDON, 1930

GEORGE EASTMAN'S ENDURING MEMORY OF THE BRITISH HE KNEW SO WELL in the 1890s was that they all seemed to have bad teeth. "On his numerous visits," Harvey Burkhart wrote, "Mr. Eastman became concerned with the necessity for improving the condition of the mouths and the teeth of adults and children."[1] It was about 1925 when Eastman first expressed an interest in supporting a dental demonstration project in London, a city in which he had spent almost as much time, especially in the 1880s and 90s, as he had in Rochester. Indeed, London, the photographic and financial capital of the world in the nineteenth century, was, in 1879, the scene of Eastman's first triumph in photography and, in 1898, his biggest financial success. London became the seat of the corporate headquarters of Kodak from 1898 to 1901. Only the taxation of foreign corporations brought on by the Boer War led Eastman to move the corporate headquarters from London to New Jersey in 1901. So why should London not be the initial European site for the latest Eastman enthusiasm—dental dispensaries?

In 1926, Lord Riddell, chairman of the board of the Royal Free Hospital, approached George Eastman to fund a dental clinic in London. Eastman agreed to give £200,000, which was matched by £50,000 ($250,000) each from Lord Riddell and Sir Albert Levy, the honorary treasurer Royal Free Hospital. The clinic would serve four of the most needy districts of London.

During the Christmas holidays of 1927, while en route to Africa, Eastman spent several weeks in London firming up plans for the London clinic and beginning discussions about a clinic for Rome. Eastman authorized Burkhart to offer "a dental dispensary on the lines of the one in Rochester" equipped with its full complement of chairs and other equipment, ready to begin operation "providing Lord Riddell and his friends will arrange permanently for its running expenses."[2] Riddell had already suggested that the building should be constructed on the grounds of the Royal Free Hospital. "My idea would be to have this dispensary . . . cover a definite territory and be limited if possible to an area containing . . . five or six hundred thousand people," Eastman wrote. "This would enable the clinic to make a complete job of taking care of the teeth of the children in that territory."[3] Of all the European clinics, the facade (increased to seven arches) and plan (reversed to take advantage of natural light on Gray's Inn Road) of the Eastman Dental Clinic in London most resembled the facade of the Rochester Dental Dispensary. In London, the children's waiting room was enlarged and other improvements made to reflect the thirteen years of experience of the Rochester dispensary.

Burkhart went to London in 1929 to negotiate, and his letters to Eastman chronicle a melodrama of clashing egos in the attempt to get the London clinic off the ground. Yet soon Eastman could write that his offer had been accepted, adding, "If there is any place in the world that they need dental propaganda it is in London."[4] Then "that highwayman" Abraham Flexner got wind of the project and tried to charm Eastman out of another medical school, this one connected to the proposed London clinic. This time the industrialist resisted, noting "I have sent Burkhart over to London to cough up the necessary to build a dental dispensary there . . . Lord Riddell is the Abraham Flexner of the picture."[5]

"Our institution in Rochester has been so successful," Eastman wrote to Murry Guggenheim, a Sears Roebuck executive whose foundation would fund dental clinics in New York City and Chicago, "that I have been encouraged to build a duplicate in London to demonstrate, in probably the best place that exists, what can be done for children's teeth. . . . We have selected four parishes, St. Pancreas, Holburn, Finsbury, and Islington, and are building the Clinic on Gray's Inn Road under the aegis of the Royal Free Hospital. The number of poor inhabitants in the territory (about 1,000,000) is just sufficient to be covered in an institution of the size that is being built and it is proposed to clean up this territory just as we have in Rochester, affording a better demonstration than to 'spatter' our work over a larger territory."[6]

London dentists were skeptical, but according to Eastman, the opposition was already melting away. When the London cornerstone was laid on April 30, 1929, Eastman was characteristically 4,000 miles away at Oak Lodge, his North Carolina retreat. Dr. Burkhart and Frank B. Kellogg, former secretary of state, represented him, and a Kodak film, a very early example of a "talkie," recorded the occasion. The Prince of Wales (later Edward VIII) and Prime Minister Baldwin came equipped with long speeches and bad jokes at which the crowd of 3,000 laughed and cheered appreciatively. "Upon teeth rests digestion and upon digestion rests the temper," explained Prime Minister Baldwin, "and if all people had perfect teeth there would be great deal less rot talked, and a great deal less of those gloomy tomfool letters to the press about England and America and a half a dozen other subjects [Laughter and cheers]." Therefore, Baldwin went on to more laughter, he was all in favor of good teeth; they did not matter so much to a woman, who only held a cigarette in her mouth, but to a man who smoked a pipe, teeth were important.[7]

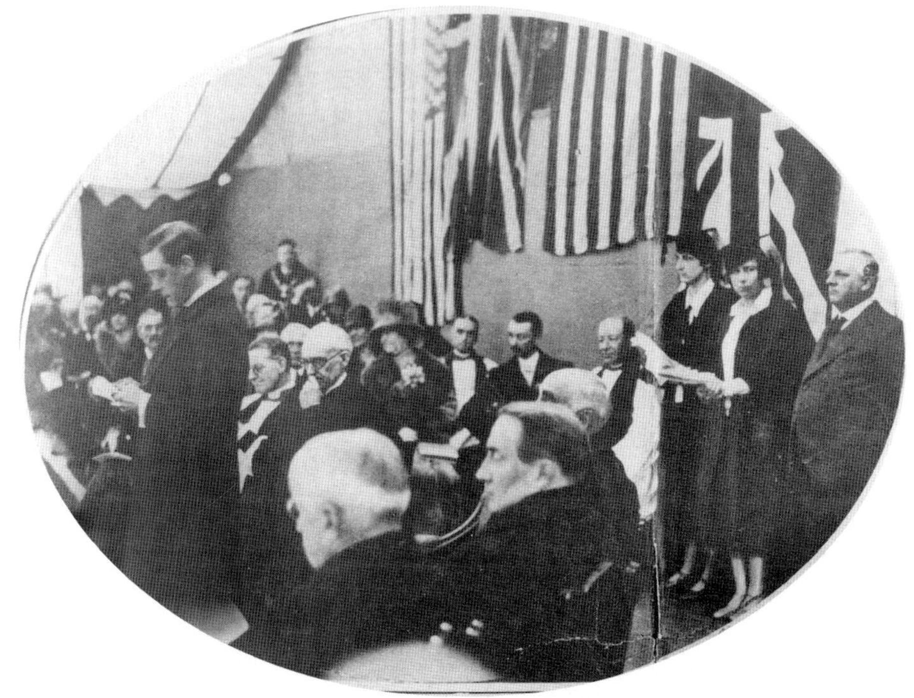

The opening ceremony was presided over by the Prince of Wales, later King Edward VIII. (© Reproduced with the kind permission of the Eastman Dental Hospital)

The London clinic was dedicated and opened in November 1930, with the United States ambassador, Charles G. Dawes, making the principal address in the presence of Sir Neville Chamberlain, then the minister of health, and a crowd of hundreds, many of them Americans. The Crown Prince of Sweden was present, foreshadowing that Sweden was also on the list for an Eastman dental clinic. The presence of the Duke of York (later King George VI), who would succeed Lord Riddell as chairman of the clinic board, numerous members of the royal family and the nobility, and various maharajahs and their retinues indicate that the sun had not yet set on the British Empire.[8] The European clinics (except in Rome) were private institutions at their founding and not yet part of a national health service.

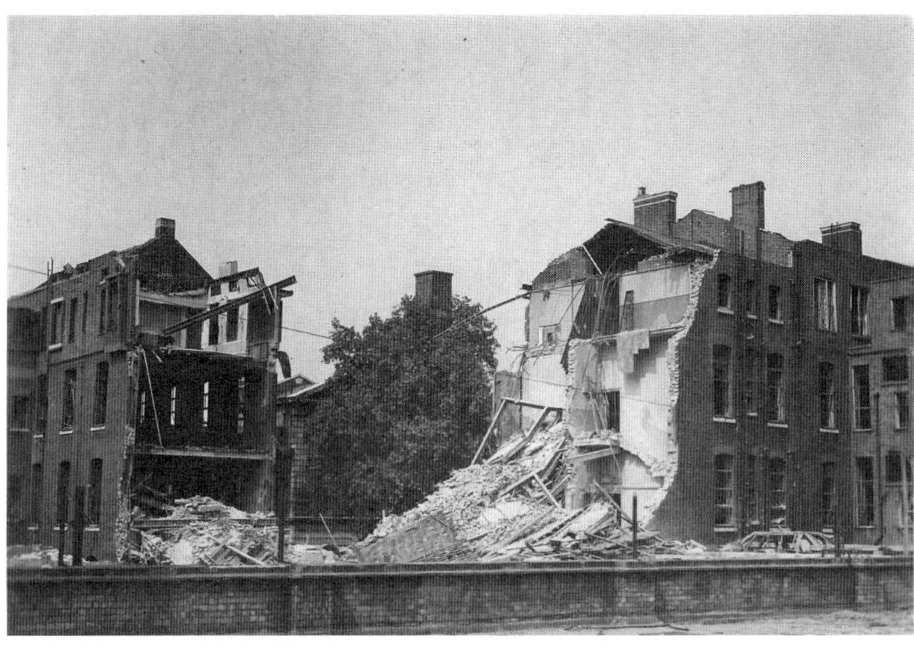

Wartime damage (© Reproduced with the kind permission of the Eastman Dental Hospital)

In the 1930s, the Ministry of Health under Neville Chamberlain approved the organization of the first school for the education of dental hygienists in Europe. The graduates not only would do prophylactic work on children but also would serve as "lecturers and advisers to parents and children in matters relating to oral hygiene and the benefits to be derived from early attention to the teeth."[9] Soon after community/clinical dentistry began, an educational component was added, and as in Rochester, research would come later. In England, research would become the most important component. From the beginning, unlike the situation in Rochester, the dental clinic building was totally integrated into the Royal Free Hospital. It included three wards, for oral, ear, nose, and throat, and cleft lip and palate surgery, and it was dedicated to providing dental care for children from the poor districts of central London. Soon 500 treatments a week were being performed.[10]

During World War II, the London clinic was spared total demolition from a German robot bomb that landed nearby. Because the dental clinic building was constructed of steel, brick, and stone (just as George Eastman House and the buildings of Kodak Park were), it survived so much better than the rest of the hospital. Thus 185 general hospital beds were moved into the dental clinic for the duration of the Blitz. Because the Royal Air Force wanted hygienists, the clinic continued to train them.

EASTMAN DENTAL INSTITUTE, LONDON, 1948–1998[11]

Moving beyond preventive measures and the dental needs of the poor and untreated (the original purpose of all Eastman clinics) to advanced training and education, a new umbrella organization named the Eastman Dental Institute, incorporating the postgraduate Eastman Dental Clinic and Institute of Dental Surgery, was established in London in 1947. Although the first directors of the Eastman Dental Clinic and others had argued for a multidisciplinary teaching clinic, it was not achieved until 1947–48 when the Eastman became independent of the Royal Free Hospital and was established as the postgraduate dental institute of the Postgraduate Medical Federation. The objects of the institute were the following:

- To train consultants, specialists, and teachers in various branches of dentistry

- To provide facilities for and encourage research by members of staff and students

- To provide clinical and laboratory facilities and instruction for candidates working for higher degrees or diplomas

- To provide short courses for general practitioners, in so far as it is possible to do so without interfering with the main objects as set out above

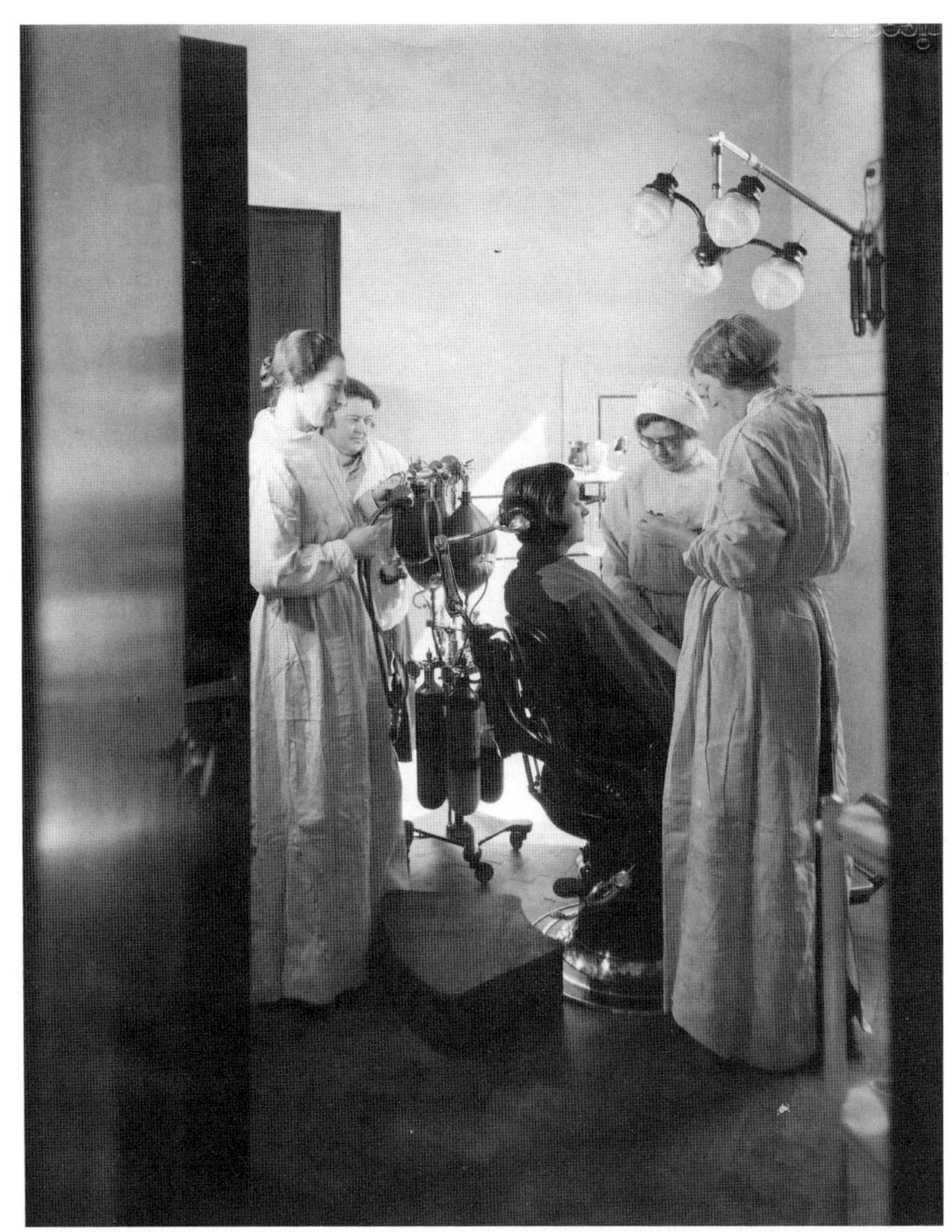

(© Reproduced with the kind permission of the Eastman Dental Hospital)

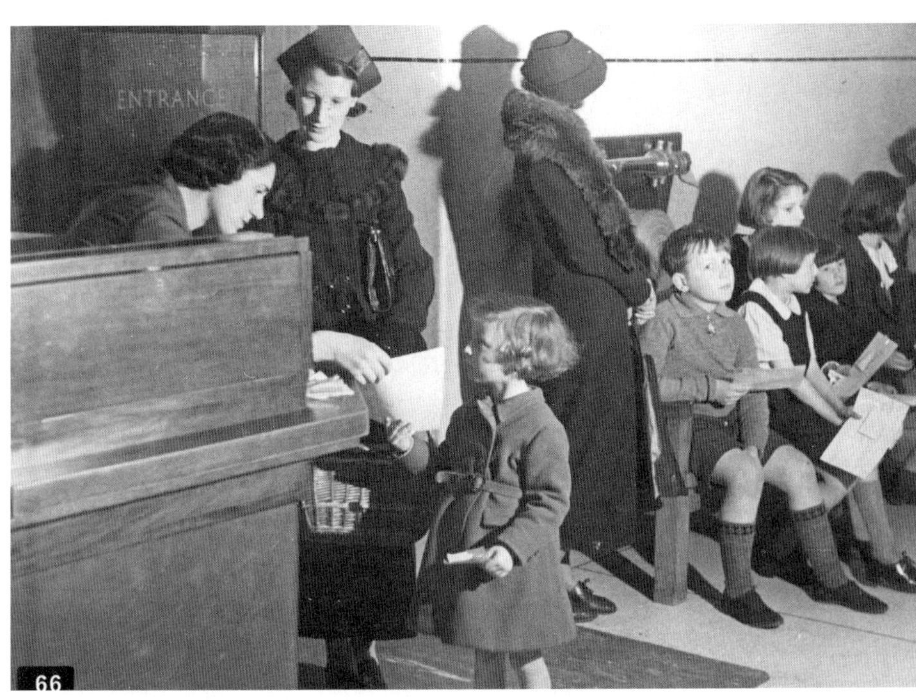

Checking into the London clinic
(© Reproduced with the kind permission of the Eastman Dental Hospital)

The clinical service, education, and research themes that evolved in the postwar London clinic narrative prefigure the unfolding Rochester story of conflicts between the Eastman Dental Center and the School of Medicine and Dentistry and their ultimate merger in the 1990s. By 1948, there were four London departments: periodontology, preventive dentistry, conservation, and orthodontics. In 1949, a department of pathology and microbiology was created. In 1950, free primary dental care became available throughout the United Kingdom and the Eastman clinic ceased to provide routine treatment apart from retaining a casualty service; its name was then changed to the Eastman Dental Hospital. During the next nine years, a full range of departments, including children's, oral surgery, and prosthetics, was established.

During this period, "the Eastman"—as it is invariably referred to in London—became an international center of excellence for education. A new director consolidated the international role of the Eastman as a postgraduate school and created a department of oral medicine. In 1967, plans were made to rebuild the Eastman elsewhere. Kodak gave £100,000 to help establish new research laboratories. In order to overcome the shortage of space, an oral surgery research laboratory was set up in the former orthopedic plaster room in a derelict wing of the Royal Free Hospital. A modest group of four squatters created the first of the future Eastman Research Laboratories. By 1988, the refurbishment of the Eastman building was complete and opened by Princess Anne. The organization changed its name to the Eastman Dental Institute in 1992.

Eastman Dental Hospital is now part of the large Eastman Dental Institute complex of medical and surgical excellence, which is geographically right for clinicians, managers, students, and patients. The institute and its hospital are part of a stimulating university hospital complex, together with a unique group of postgraduate institutes constituting a faculty in its own right. This has facilitated the creation of an Eastman Head and Neck Pathology Unit serving both the University College Hospitals and Royal Free Trusts.

Since 1999 (when it merged with University College London Hospitals [UCL]), the name of what opened as the Eastman Dental Clinic in 1930 has been Eastman Dental Institute for Oral Health Care Sciences, University of London. Although "the Eastman," as this conglomerate of clinic, postgraduate school, hospital, and research laboratories is still called, almost moved to the London suburbs in 1967, it remains at its original address, 256 Gray's Inn Road, London.

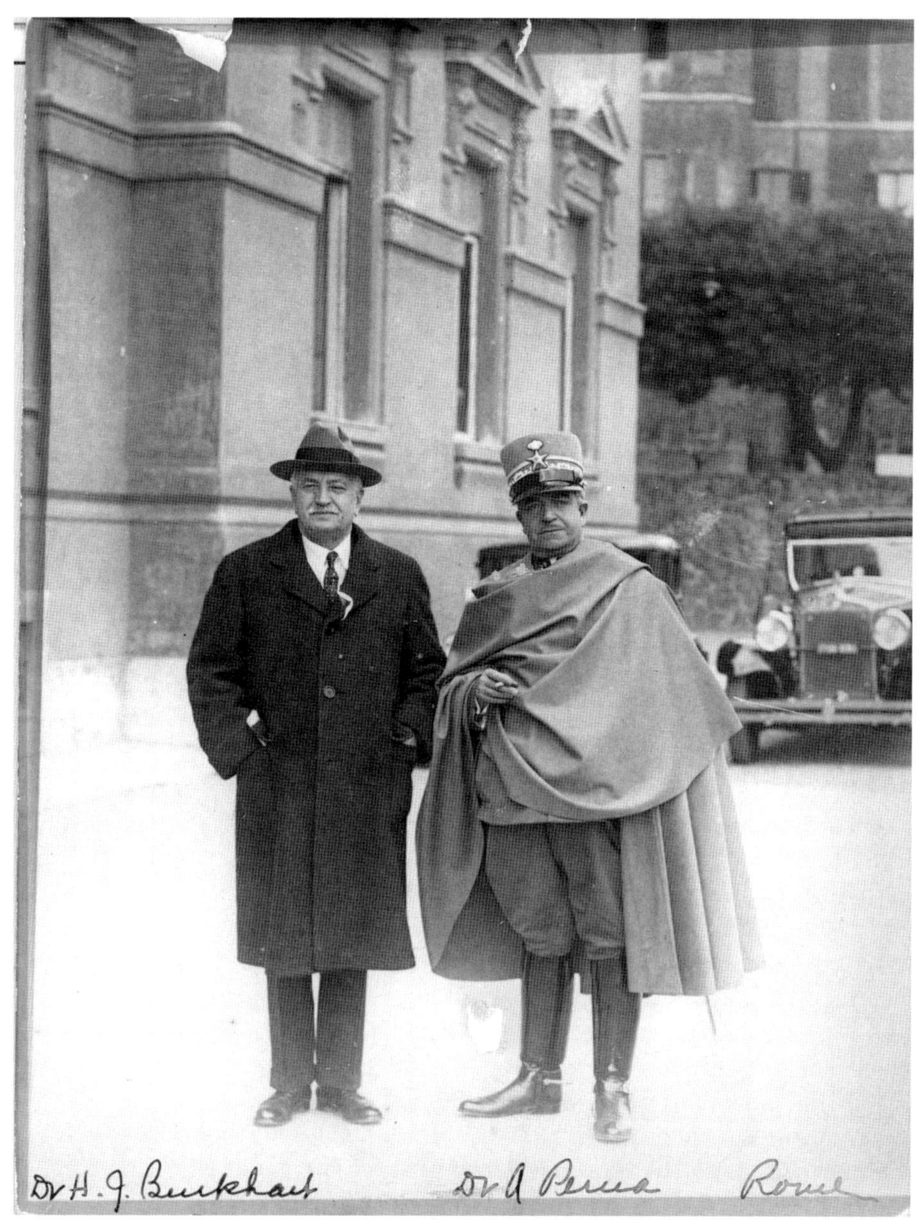

Drs. Harvey Burkhart and Amedio Perna

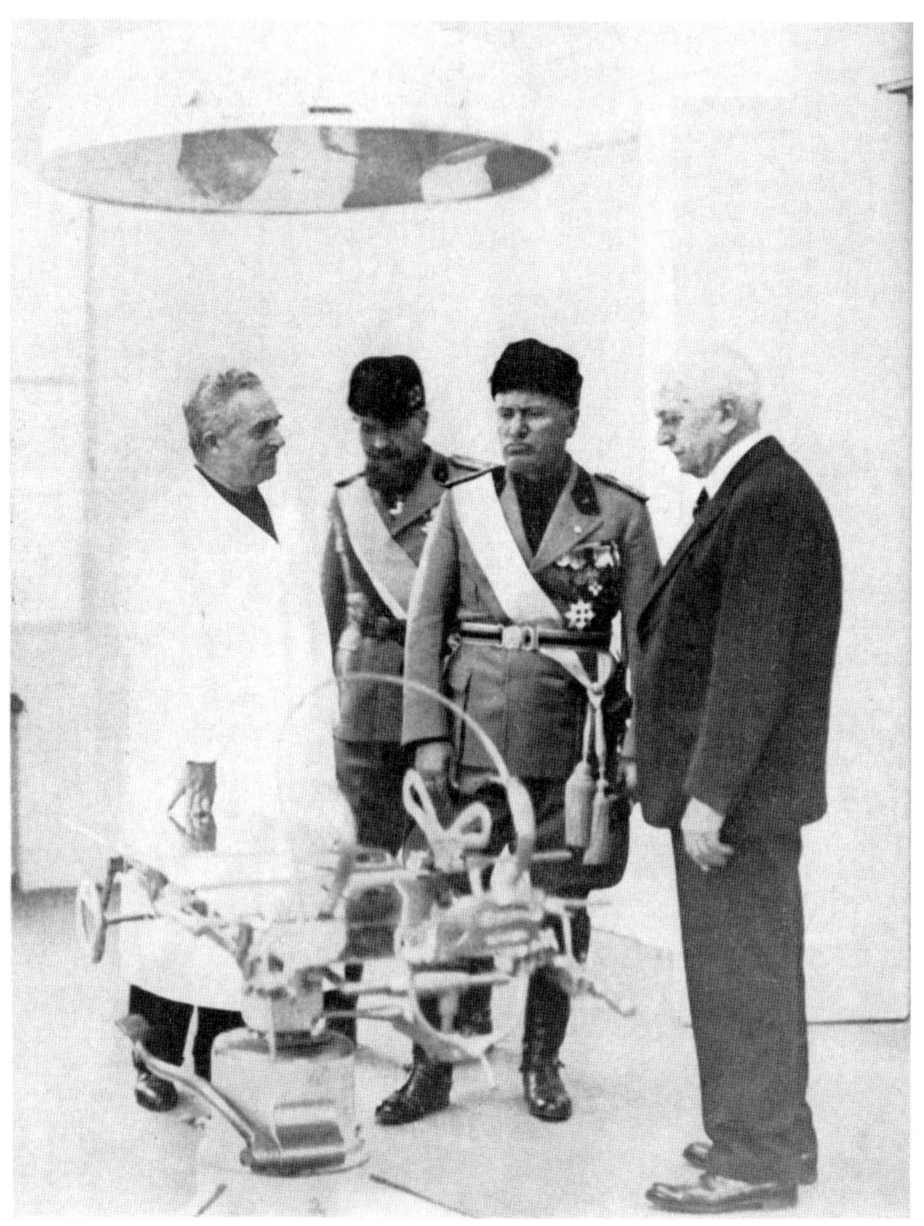

Drs. Perna and Burkhart examine equipment with Benito Mussolini

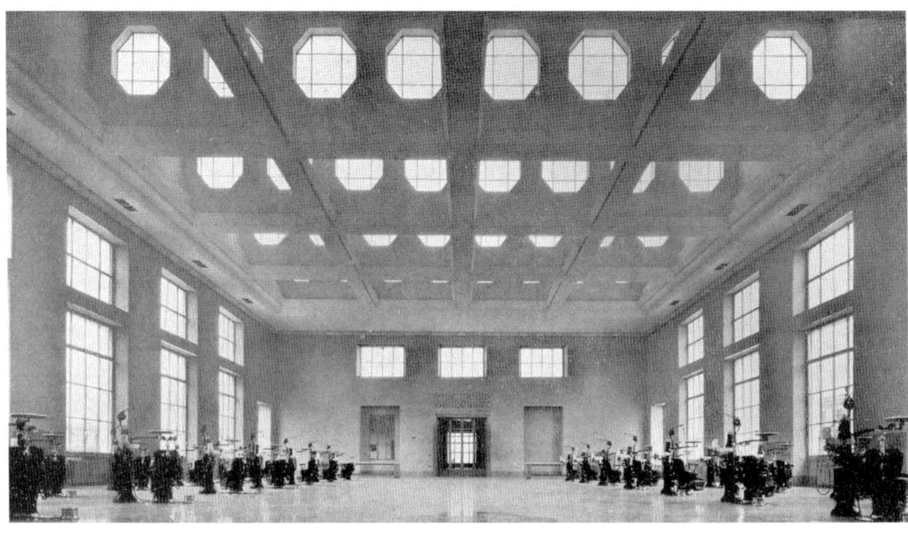

Even the operatory is architecturally brutal.

The man who, as surrogate for George Eastman, founded the Eastman Dental Clinic was honored when the Burkhart Dental Therapists School was built. This school strengthens the educational spectrum of both hospital and institute. The International Centre for Excellence in Dentistry at 123 Grays Inn Road has been established to relate the highest quality private practice with teaching and education and clinical research. In 2002, the Eastman Institute entered and won the Queen's Anniversary Prize for Higher and Further Education. A summary of the winning entry follows:

> The Eastman Dental Institute for Oral Health Care Sciences, together with its associated hospital, is a leading centre of expertise for postgraduate teaching, advanced research and patient care. . . . Scientists work with clinicians in key areas including causes of oral and craniofacial disease, clinical service delivery and materials science. This approach concentrates efforts on areas having optimum effects on quality of life, whether through prevention or cure. Specialisms include the use of novel materials for tooth repair, bone and gum regeneration, and implants, as well as the early detection of oral cancer and advanced and minimally invasive treatments when the disease is already present, infection control and treatment, and special needs treatment including HIV and other disabilities.

The institute has had the largest concentration of dental graduate students in Europe and was designated the first World Health Organization Collaborating Centre in orofacial health, disability, and culture.

ISTITUTO SUPERIORE DI ODONTOIATRIA GEORGE EASTMAN DI ROMA

George Eastman was an opera fan. As a member of the board of directors of the Metropolitan Opera, he regularly wore out younger friends by taking them to New York for an exhausting week of two operas a day. When the Eastman Theatre opened, he made sure Italian opera was well represented. From this grew a friendship with Cesare Sconfietti, Italian consul in Rochester, and an expressed fondness for "the Italian people." When the fascist Benito Mussolini became the dictator of Italy in 1922, Eastman, along with many others, expressed admiration for his "experiment" in bringing efficiency to Italy. Eastman was primed for Sconfietti's overture concerning the next European dental clinic.

On June 4, 1929, following conversations with Sconfietti, George Eastman offered to build a dental clinic in Rome. The government, he insisted, must provide maintenance. Benito Mussolini at once sent Senatore Amedio Perna, a member of parliament, to Rochester with the Italian ambassador. In August 1929 the contract was signed and work began about a year later.[12] In 1930 Burkhart wrote, "The maintenance and support of the Rome clinic is different from that of the London clinic . . . [which] is guaranteed by Lord Riddell, Sir Albert Levy and the Royal Free hospital, while in Rome the Federal Government guarantees its maintenance and upkeep." Eastman agreed to "furnish the Italian Government the equivalent of $1 million to build and equip on a suitable piece of ground in Rome, to be furnished by the Italian Government (to be approved by myself or my collaborator, Dr. Harvey J. Burkhart), a dental dispensary on the lines of the one in Rochester."

> My object . . . is to establish in Rome a demonstration center which will be competent to care for, and as far as possible rectify, the teeth of all the indigent children in the city of Rome up to the age of 16 years . . . [as long as] there are a sufficient number of physicians who can be employed to serve as dental specialists. . . .

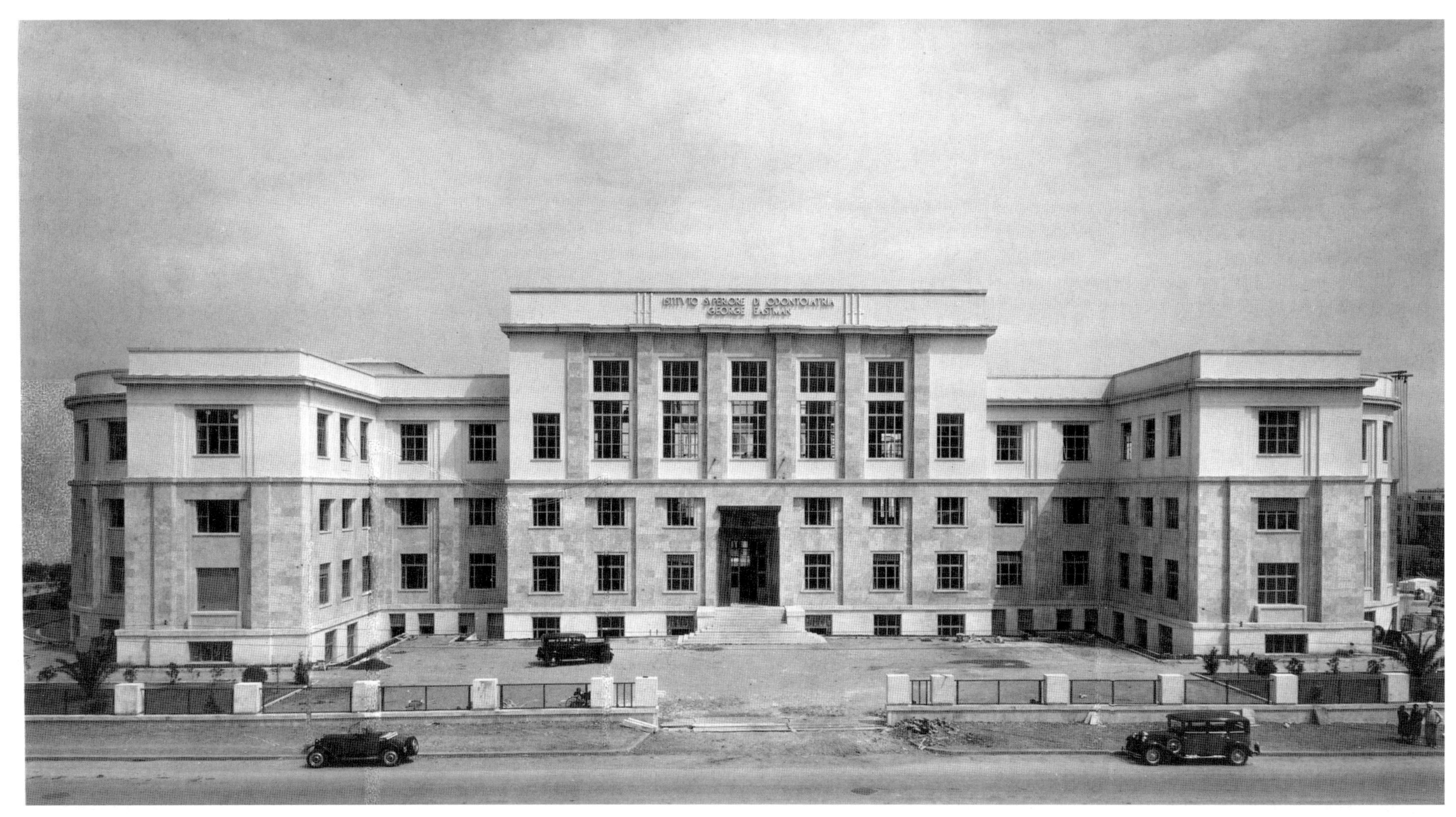

The Rome clinic

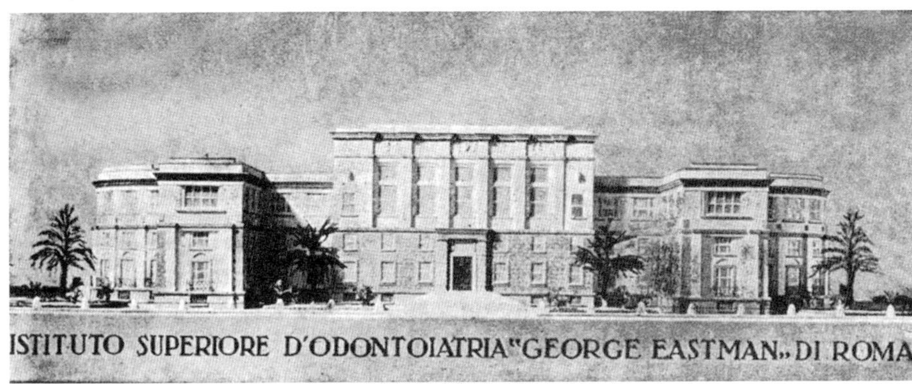

The selection of an architect to be subject to my approval as also the plans of the institution, which in general should follow the lines of the Rochester Dental Dispensary.[13]

In general the architecture did follow the lines of the Rochester clinic, although of all the European clinics, the architecture of Rome's most qualifies for the "Mussolini Modern" label. As such, it blended with the brutal new government buildings in its immediate vicinity. Professor Arnaldo Foschini, considered one of the outstanding architects of Italy, was chosen as architect. Professor Dr. Amedio Perna, director and president of the governing board, had a great deal of input on the details.[14] Eastman and Burkhart would select the equipment, and the Italian government would send the director to Rochester for two months for orientation. Funds remaining after building and equipping the general dental clinic would go toward an orthodontia department.

Eastman's cousin, Mary Eastman Southwick, worried about his schmoozing with Italy's dictator. Cousin George reassured her: "As to Mussolini, on the way back I hope to have an interview with him. I think he is a very interesting person and certainly will be glad to meet him. I do not expect he will eat me up."[15] But six months later, he confessed to Cousin Mary: "I did not get to see Mussolini as he was not in Rome when I was there. Would like to have met him. He is no doubt one of the ablest men in Europe. Whether his dictator scheme will work in Italy is doubtful, but it is certainly a most interesting experiment."[16]

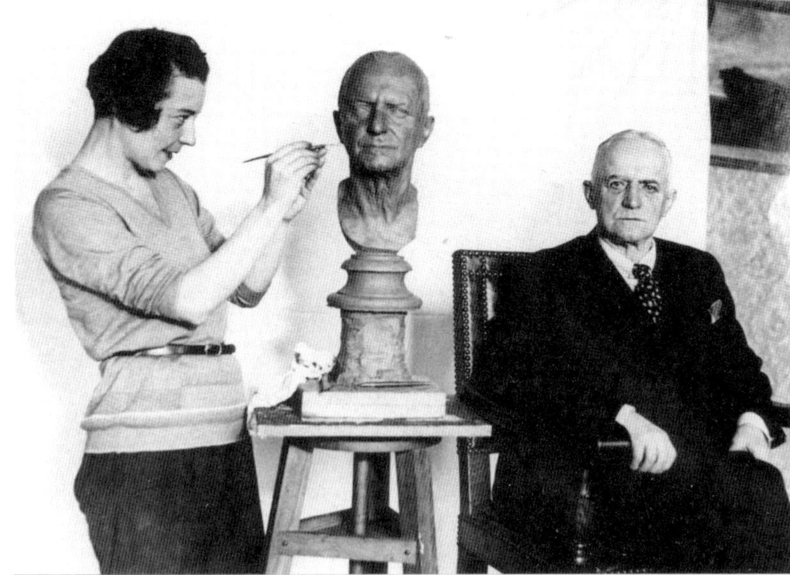

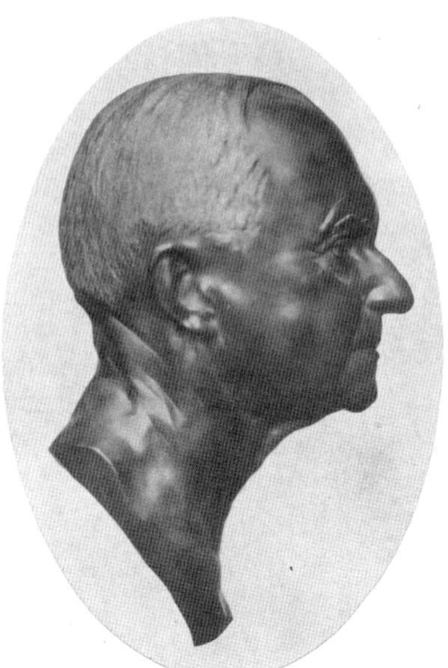

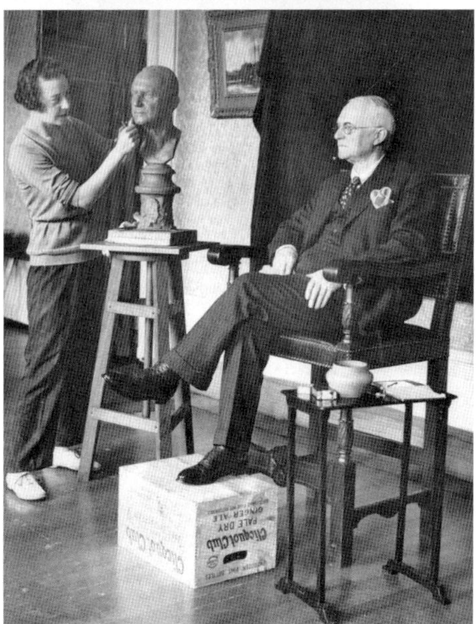

Fausta Menageri sculpted George Eastman in Rochester for the Rome clinic

In April 1930, Harvey Burkhart swept into Rome with his wife, step-daughter Dorothy, a Kodak interpreter, and Eastman's closest relative, his niece Ellen Dryden. They were taken to meet the minister of education, "who could talk very little English but made a good crack at it," then the minister of construction, then the minister of foreign affairs, then the American ambassador, and finally "another one [minister] who has charge of making the law for the King[17] to sign. He showed it to me & as soon as I file the letters you gave me & have confirmation the money is deposited the king will sign the thing."[18] The Burkhart group also went to see "the Polytechnic dental school & the place selected for our clinic. It is a fine location, much better than I expected. . . . The building will look fine in the setting they have picked out. . . . I didn't have any trouble making them see the wisdom of changes in the plans, much different from the London bunch."[19] Burkhart reported back to his boss while zeroing in on one of differences between London and all of the other clinics—the others didn't speak English. However, Burkhart said his "ears are getting tuned to the [Italian] language, no doubt due to your musicale educational efforts in my behalf."[20] The Italians "sent many messages . . . complimentary & appreciative of what you are doing here. All of the big wigs asked for photos of their benefactor." Eventually, the Rome clinic would get a bronze bust of Eastman by the Italian sculptor Fausta Menageri. Burkhart did get that interview with Mussolini in his palace and found the Italians, unlike the English, ready to acquiesce to anything to get the million dollars:

> We were not sure the ladies would be received. We were escorted through numerous corridors & rooms & finally to one that had a lot of old armor, swords, shields etc. . . . Finally we got the high sign. . . . Mussolini was behind a table in the corner of a big fine room, nothing in it but his desk & a couple or three chairs. He got up and greeted me very cordially, inquired about your health etc. I presented the book [Carl Ackerman's biography of Eastman, published 1930], he immediately looked it over with much interest and & seemed very pleased you sent it. . . . It made a hit with him. . . . The minister asked if he would receive the ladies & he told him to bring them along—they say its very unusual. . . . They got some kick you bet. . . .
>
> I told Mussolini how sorry you were not to see him two years ago, & he said he was too. I was with him fifteen or twenty minutes, & really was a very satisfactory interview—on my side anyway. He walked to the door with us & was very

cordial in saying goodbye. He is some fellow all right. Speaks pretty good English & much more friendly than I expected to find him. He is very democratic [!], dressing in ordinary uniform—no decoration. His face & manner indicate a very strong personality. I didn't wear the dam [*sic*] topper I lugged along to show off in, because it wasn't expected. I guess I'll save trouble carrying it back by giving it to some hack driver, of which they have many here.[21]

Before moving on to London, the Burkhart party finished its six-day Roman visit with a papal audience. "You should have seen me at eight in the morning in full dress, some sight I can tell you."[22] The only bad part of the Rome visit was that "Perna insisted on kissing me goodbye. I hoped he would do all of that just to the ladies."[23]

Eastman kept track of the goings-on in Rome to the very end of his life. Eighteen days before he ended his own life, he saw fit to lecture Mussolini about how the Rome clinic was being set up by the Ministry of Education. Not only was the gift to be used exclusively for preventive dentistry for children and not postgraduate education in a university setting, but also Eastman clearly made Burkhart his surrogate.

> February 23, 1932
> His Excellency Benito Mussolini,
> Rome, Italy.
>
> Your Excellency;
>
> I have the honor to acknowledge your reply, through diplomatic channels by Mr. Ceasare [*sic*] Sconfietti, Italian Consul in Rochester, to my letter of interpretation with reference to the establishment of the Eastman Children's Dental Clinic in Rome.
>
> It is quite evident that considerable misunderstanding exists relative to my purposes in making the contribution for the benefit of the children of Rome and the manner in which the institution should be conducted so that the best results may be obtained. My experience in other countries has convinced me that connection with teaching institutions or universities or control by them in any manner or form is not conducive to obtaining of the desired results.
>
> While I am aware of the value of postgraduate and educational work, there is no place for it in an institution such as I have proposed to found. . . . I realize that

in the inauguration and establishment of a new enterprise that misunderstandings may arise due to a lack of appreciation of the efficient and modern plan of managing and conducting a children's dental clinic. I regret to inform you that the reply to my letter of interpretation is not satisfactory to me because I am convinced from past experience that the plan proposed by the Ministry of Education will not accomplish the objects which we are seeking. . . . My collaborator, Dr. Harvey J. Burkhart of Rochester . . . is authorized to represent and act for me in all matters connected with the building and establishment of the Eastman Children's Dental Clinic in Rome Italy, also all matter pertaining to the carrying out of my ideas and plans in the future management of the institution.

Permit me to express to Your Excellency my appreciation of your splendid interest and cooperation in this project. With best wishes and high regard, believe me,

Sincerely yours,
George Eastman

It is not known today whether Eastman knew when he wrote this letter to Mussolini that he would end his own life in mid-March while Burkhart was in Rome. Eastman had promised Burkhart when the dental school part of the School of Medicine and Dentistry in Rochester failed to materialize that he would do "something more for dentistry." Whether this meant the $1 million bequest that Eastman left the Rochester Dental Dispensary or the $1 million gifts each to the clinics in five European capitals or both, Burkhart assumed the latter and spent the remaining fourteen years of his life protecting the dispensary endowment and closely supervising the beginnings of the European clinics. He would die with his boots on.

The formal dedication exercises at Istituto Superiore di Odontoiatria George Eastman di Roma were held on the evening of April 21, 1933, presided over by the minister of education. The American ambassador read a message from President Roosevelt that thanked Eastman while expressing a hope of strengthening the bonds uniting the people of the United States and Italy. Burkhart, on behalf of the executors of Eastman's will, formally presented the institution to the board. Earlier that day, Mussolini and staff had visited every part of the clinic; Il Duce ("the leader") was particularly interested in the units and chairs provided by the Ritter Manufacturing Co. and the sterilizers by the Wilmot Castle Co., both of Rochester.[24]

Dr. Perna lost no time organizing the various departments. The government provided three beautiful new busses to transport children to the clinic. Difficulties did arise because the Romans began to treat adults as well as children (probably to the detriment of the children), and fascism soon began taking its toll. But before that happened, the clinic became so busy with clinical and educational activities that it was considered congested. To relieve congestion in the institute, an elementary school was built nearby that utilized the resources of the institute.

In 1935, using machine guns against Haile Selassie's bows and arrows, Mussolini invaded and conquered Ethiopia. The next year he entered the Spanish Civil War on the side of Franco and in 1940 invaded southern France. By then it was common knowledge that Mussolini controlled through murder, exile, and prison camps. Yet the Rome clinic was considered to be functioning satisfactorily up until World War II.

In 1939, Burkhart made his last prewar visit to Rome. The director at that time was a member of the fascist Blackshirt paramilitary group and was appointed by Mussolini. News from the Rome clinic was meager throughout the war.[25] It was January 1945 before Burkhart received the first detailed news in three years from Rome. Dr. Alton D. Brashear, who served an internship at the Rochester dispensary in 1935 and was stationed with a general hospital unit in Italy, wrote to Dr. Burkhart, "On Christmas morning [1944] while I was walking about the streets of Rome, I happened upon the Via Regina Margherita and the Eastman clinic. . . . The clinic is still existing and somewhat in operation although closed on this particular day [Christmas]."

Though the clinic was closed for the day, Brashear learned that the building had been damaged in air raids and many of the windows broken. Professional operations had been seriously hampered by a lack of supplies. The British had operated it for some time, although some work was also being done for civilians. A special clinic for refugees and the homeless had been organized in December 1944 and a branch opened for plastic surgery. A clipping from a Rome newspaper stated that the clinic was employing forty dentists, whereas there had been only eight the previous June, and that 350 patients were being treated daily. Branch clinics were being organized near the largest suburban elementary school to provide free dental care to the poor who, because of lack of transportation, were unable to attend the central institution.[26]

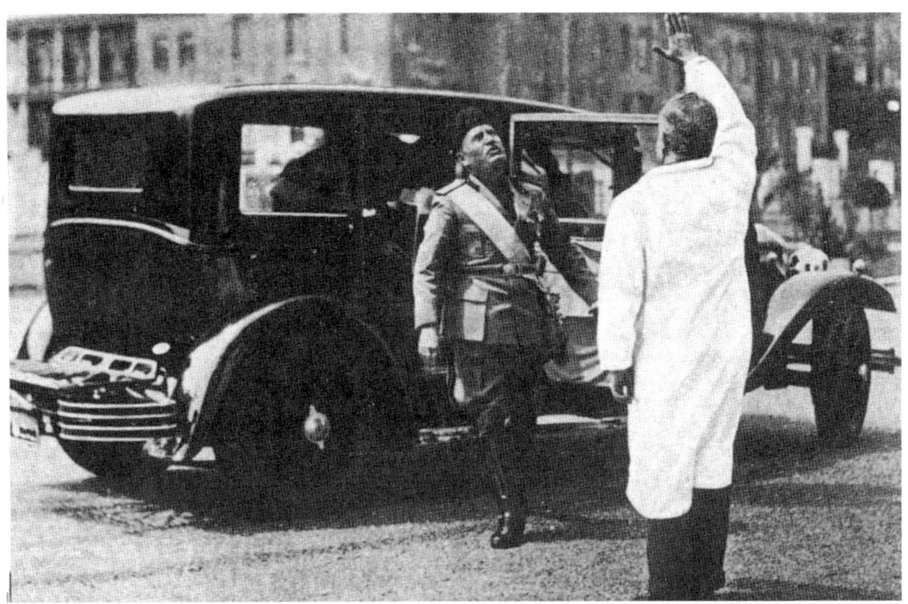
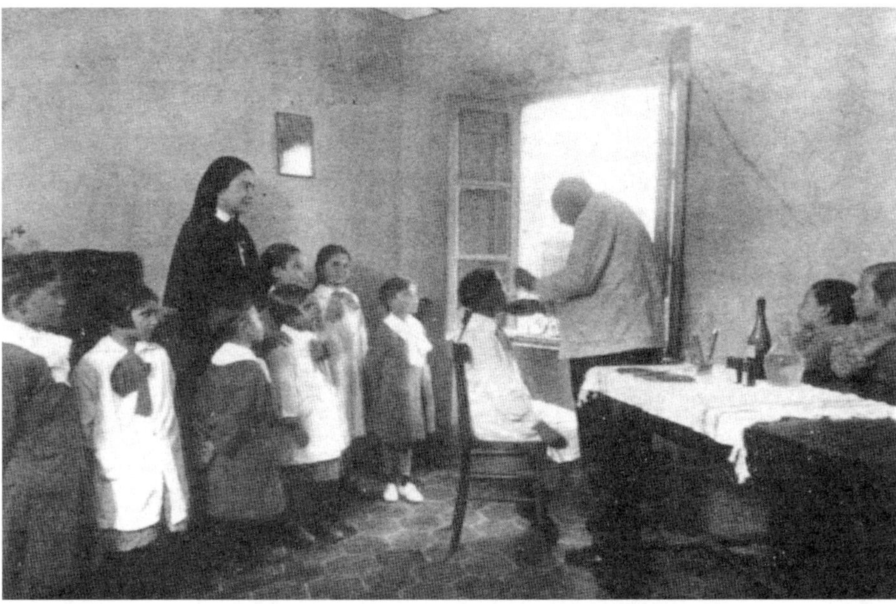
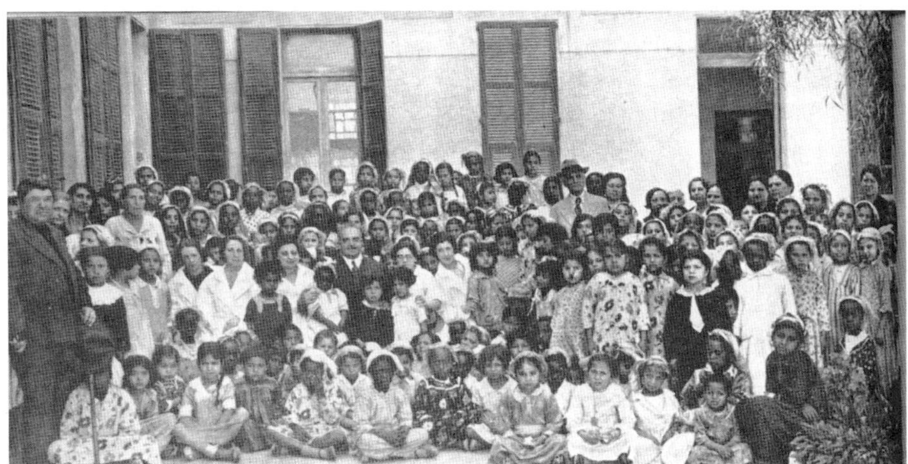
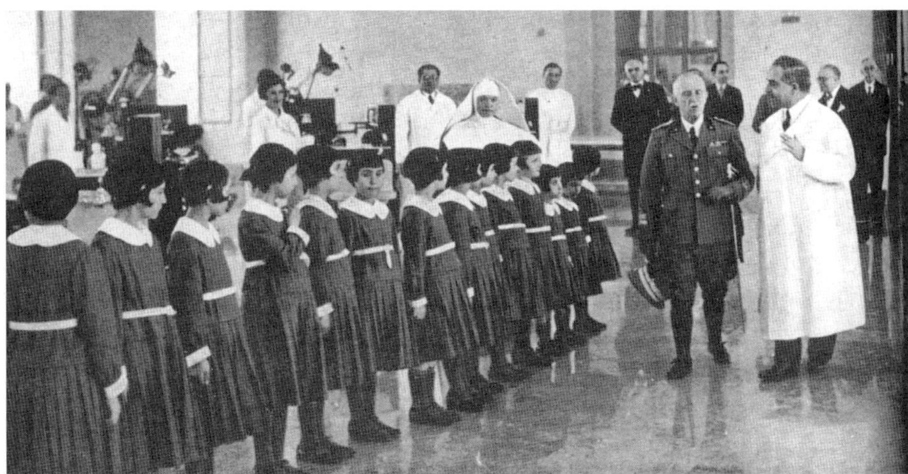

Scenes from the early years of the Rome clinic

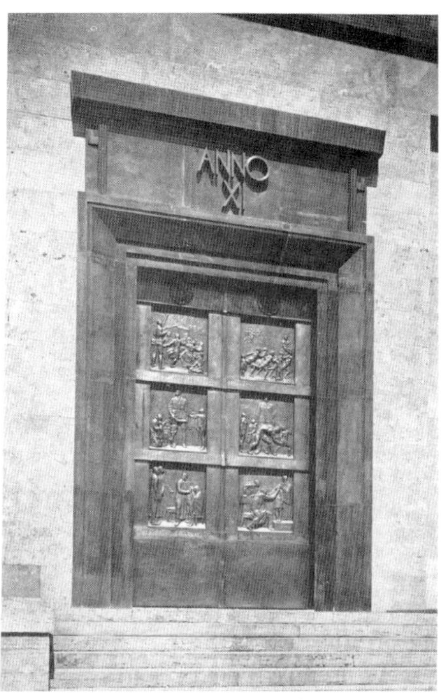

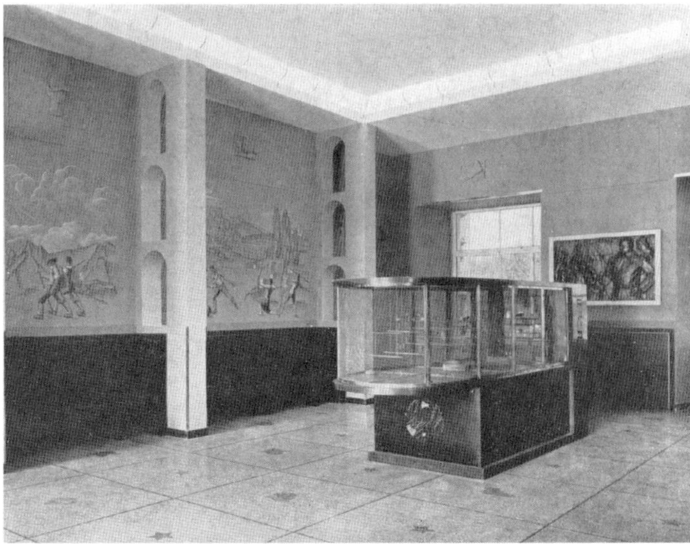

Clinic door and birdcage

The clinic declined during the war, but Professor Beniamino de Vecchis, Perna's successor as director in 1948, and Professor A. Benagiano, who became director in 1951, renewed it with reorganization, improvements, expansions, and ultimately the opening of new schools. As one sign of its postwar growth, the clinic saw 8,830 patients between 1942 and 1946 and 16,672 in 1947–48. According to the clinic's history publication, "Clinical practice and research boomed" as did the "international outreach of scholarship."[27] The art featured on the relief panels of a door to the clinic, obviously derived from the famous doors of the Baptistery in Florence, featured Mussolini leading a crew of Italian youth. Later, this and all fascist symbols were removed.

The Rome clinic went through a period of ossification and decline, much as the Rochester clinic did in the latter Burkhart years. Visitors in the 1980s, including Dr. William McHugh, director of the Eastman Dental Center in Rochester, found the Rome clinic outdated, in poor repair, and somewhat depressing. Since then, the Rome clinic has undergone a major transformation, and visitors in 2007 and then again in 2009, including Cyril Meyerowitz, director of the Eastman Dental Center in Rochester, found that it is still very much in operation in a modernized and renovated facility. In addition it has added mobile units called Odonto-ambulances and Odonto-vans that provide services to underserved and special needs patients in the Rome area.

INSTITUTE D'HYGIÈNE DENTAIRE ET DE STOMATOLOGIE DE LA VILLE DE PARIS, FONDATION GEORGE EASTMAN

In 1930, applications for Eastman-funded dental clinics were received from Paris and Stockholm. Brussels applied in 1931. The Paris application of October 1930 was approved by Eastman days before his death, and the cornerstone was laid in July 1935. The original site selected off Avenue Clichy was not to Burkhart's liking, so he lobbied mightily with "Officers of the Municipality" until a location he approved was chosen. The site was at the far end of a large new park and playground at 11 de la rue George Eastman near the place where it intersected with Avenue Edison. Because the change of location necessitated the redrawing of plans, considerable time was lost. The clinic was eventually dedicated in October 1937 in the presence of

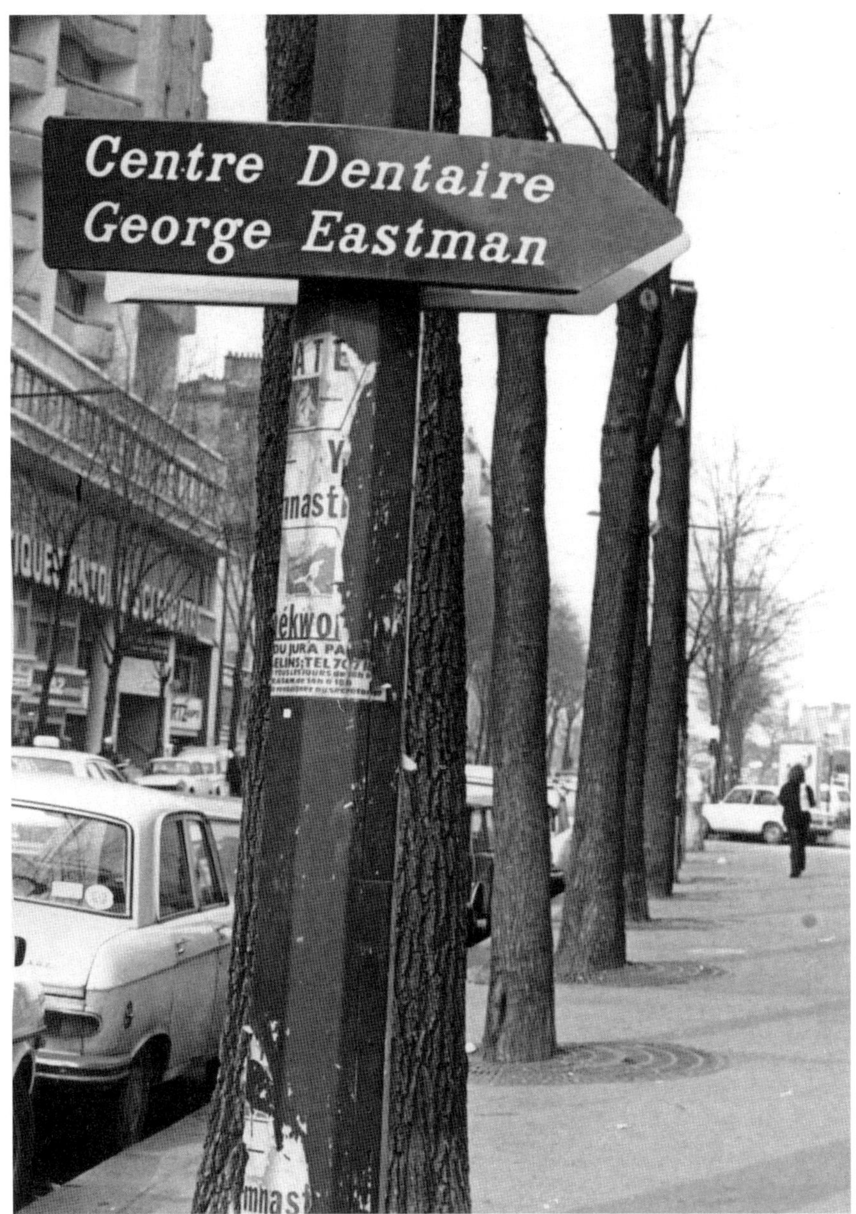

Street sign indicates clinic location

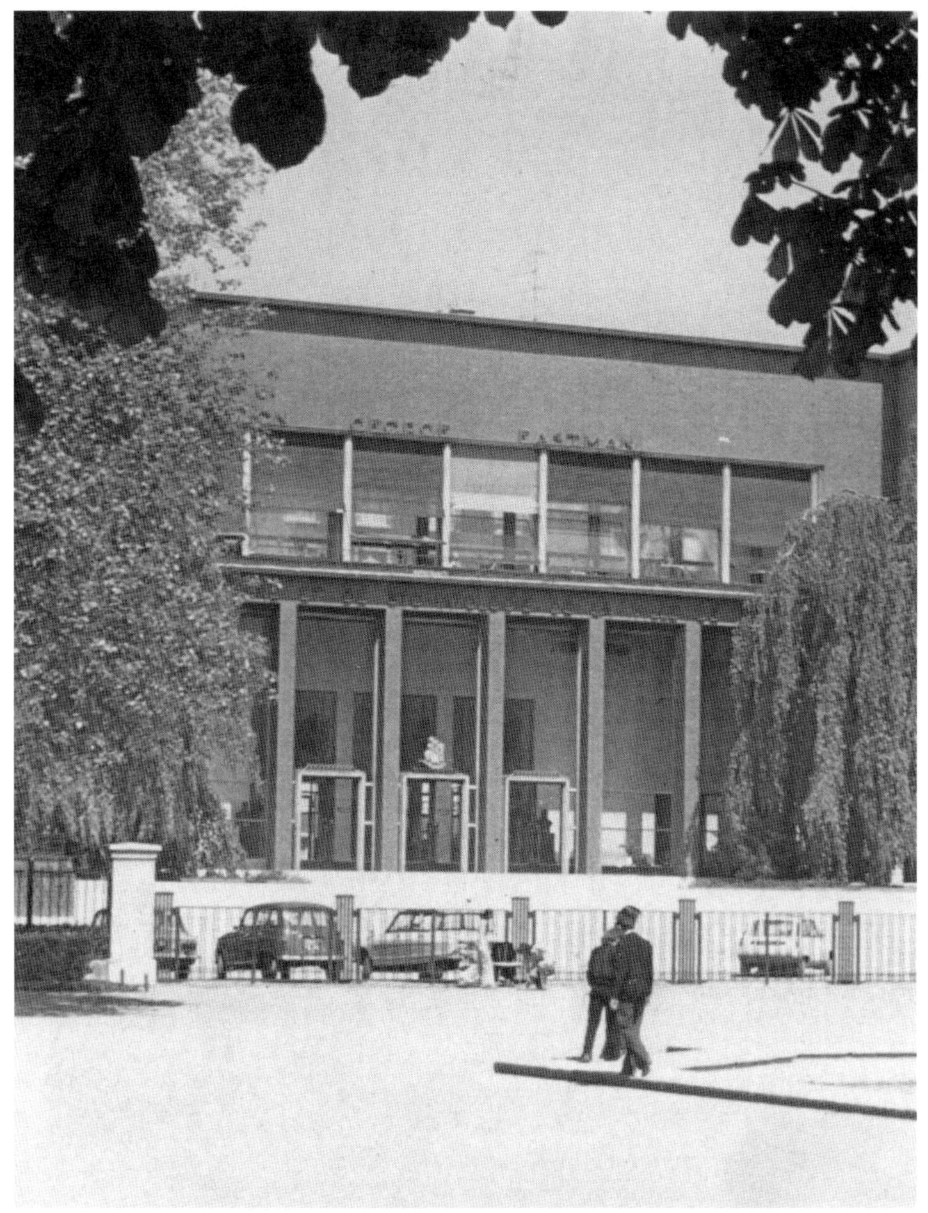

*Institut d'Hygiène Dentaire et de Stomatologie de la
Ville de Paris, Fondation George Eastman*

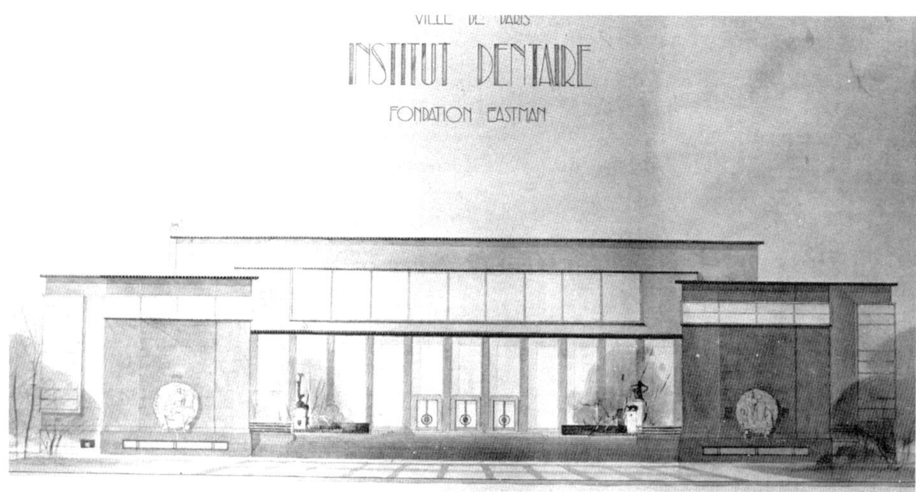

Rendering of Paris clinic

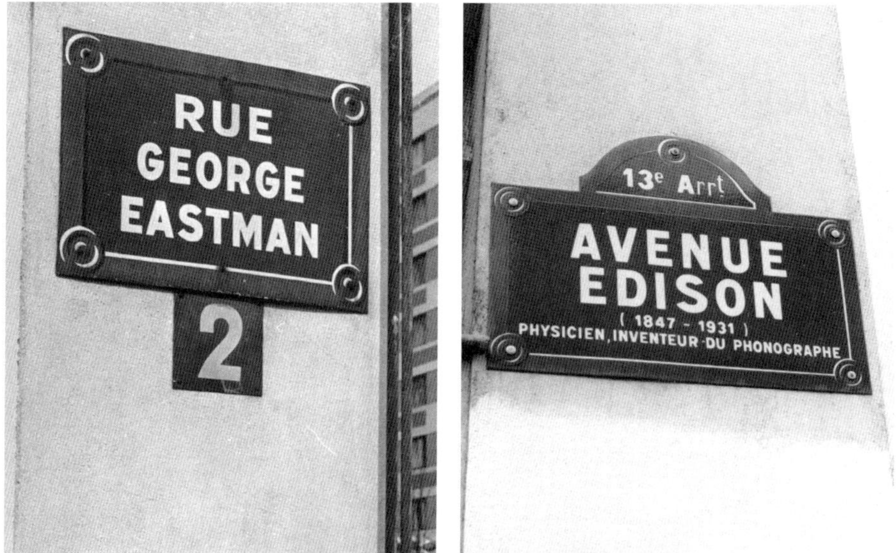

representatives of the French government, the Municipality of Paris, the United States government, members of French and American dental societies, and many friends of George Eastman. The clinic only had a short time to begin operations, because as Burkhart reported in 1939, "At the beginning of hostilities practically all of the male and female professional staff of the institution, and also those connected with the business management were immediately called to the colors. At the same time the children in the immediate neighborhood were sent into the country, so activities ceased at once.[28]

"Eastman Clinics, Seized By Foe, Aid Nazis" read a headline of March 16, 1943. The United Press dispatch continued, "The fortunes of war have cast the philanthropies of the late George Eastman in a strange light. In war-ravaged Europe are three . . . million-dollar dental clinics established by Eastman as demonstration centers to care for the teeth of indigent children. But today those clinics—in Rome, Paris, and Brussels—are rendering service to the armed forces of our nation's enemies. . . . Instead of protecting the teeth of growing children, the clinics now perform surgical work on the heads and jaws of injured soldiers, including skin grafting."

Although the German army occupied the Paris clinic, Burkhart reported that "the director, Dr. Pol Nespoulous, before and since the occupation has been rendering devoted and loyal service." At first the only clients were

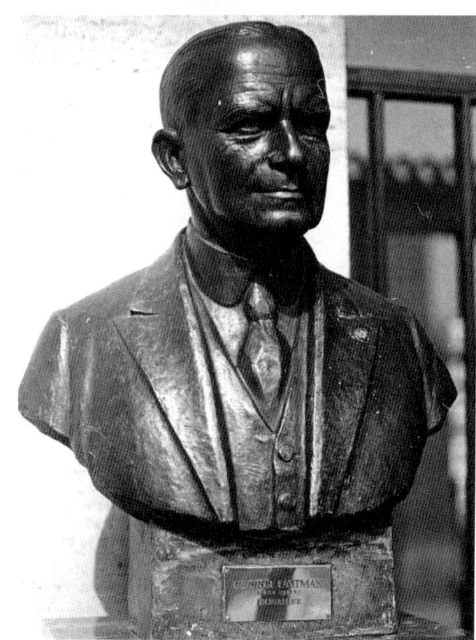

The bust is of George Eastman. The clinic stood at the intersection of Rue George Eastman and Avenue Edison.

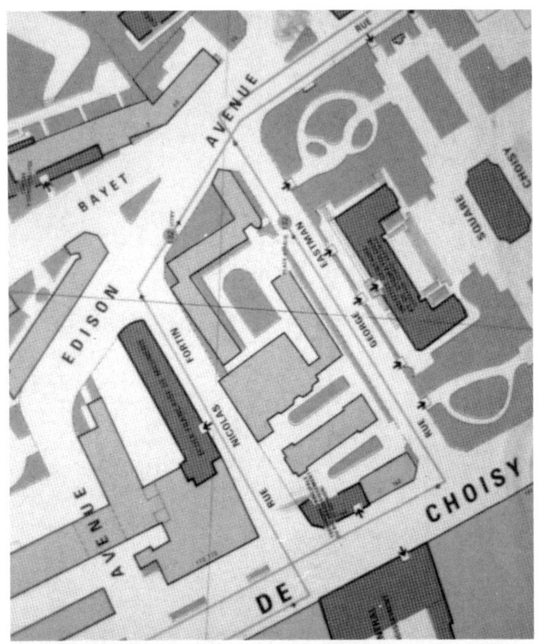

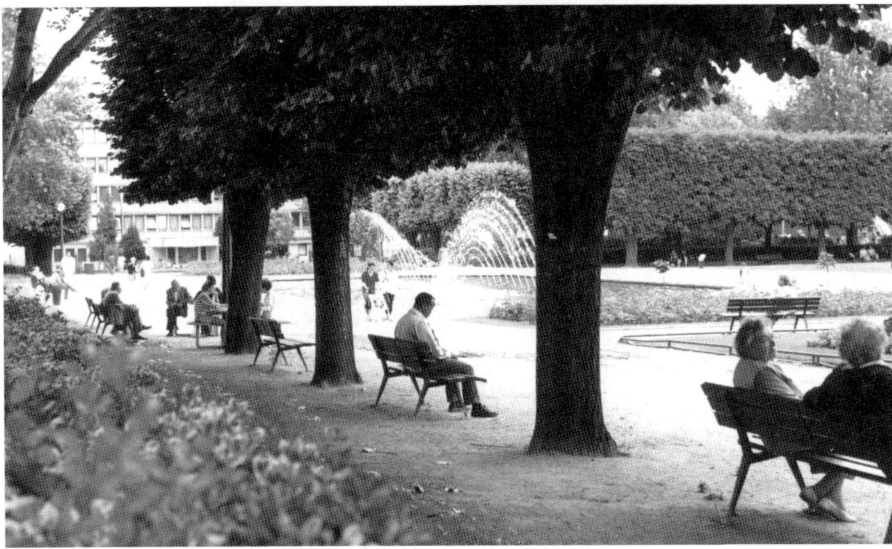

*The subway map pointed patients to the Paris clinic,
located on the edge of a verdant park.*

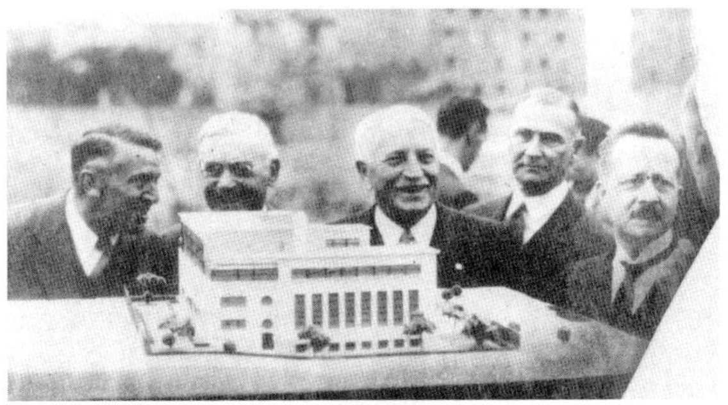

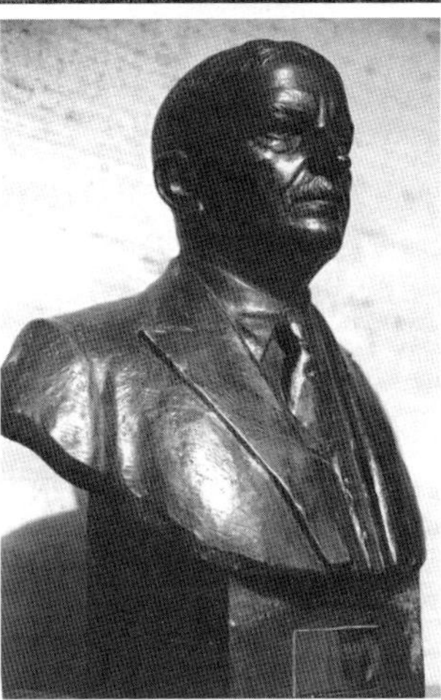

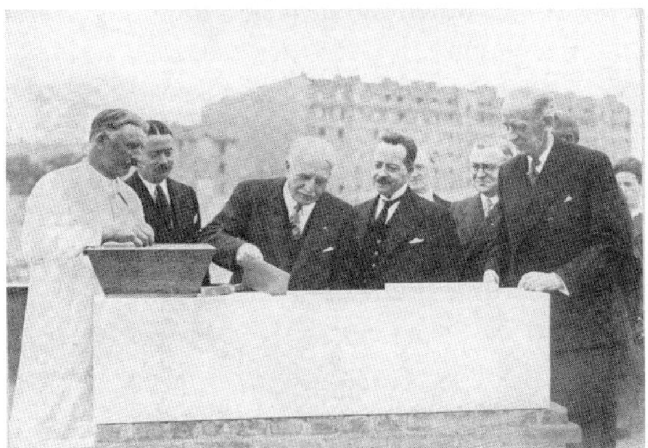

*Burkhart (center) inspects the model (top) and
lays the foundation of the Paris clinic (bottom).*

members of the adult population who had nowhere else to go; but then many children drifted back to Paris and began to receive treatment by a staff composed largely of young women dental operators. Although occupied by German troops, the Paris clinic fared better than the London or Brussels clinics.

Information about the clinics came to Rochester via the grapevine, since the war had severed normal communication lines. One source was Burkhart's nephew, a Parisian dentist who relayed news until he was "invited" by the Nazis to leave France. Still another was the former head of dental service in Germany, a member with Burkhart of the International Dental Federation. Fortunately, the Paris clinic fell into the hands of this man, who knew the original purpose of the clinic. He got word to Burkhart that as far as army regulations would permit, he would try not to interfere with its operation. Many French dentists were prisoners in Germany, and there were hardly enough left to care for the emergency adult work, let alone perform repair and preventive dentistry for children.

Lt. Col. William B. Ryder Jr., an American dental surgeon in the Seine Section during the war, visited Paris and supplied Burkhart with the first detailed information regarding the fate of the clinic. He wrote that the American army was using about 80 percent of the space for military purposes by occupying the second and third floors of the east wing. In 1945, the whole question of dentistry in France was rather confused according to Burkhart. In addition to the prewar division between the dentist and the stomatologist, a specialist in diseases of the mouth, there was further division between the supporters of the Vichy government and those who were working for the resistance. Burkhart prophesized that there were difficult days ahead for the professions in France, especially in regard to teaching and professional standards.

In 1952, an Eastman Dental Dispensary hygienist and historian, Mildred Skinner, visited the Paris clinic and found that all of the dental interns were women, as were the French dental students at the time. Skinner also reported "an excellent bust of Dr. Burkhart in the main corridor seemed to welcome us to the clinic and I could imagine him saying he was glad that I had the opportunity to see the results of his efforts to carry out the objectives of Mr. Eastman. I feel quite sure that Mr. Eastman would have been pleased to hear the shouts of happy French children in the adjoining playgrounds."[29]

The situation was basically the same when the author visited the Paris clinic thirty years after Skinner. The clinic was fully delineated on Metro maps as located at the edge of a park at 11 de la rue George Eastman at the corner of Avenue Edison, and signs pointing to it were highly visible when one emerged from the subway. In the early 1980s, the busts of Eastman and Burkhart greeted the visitor, the clinics were humming, the waiting room full of a multiracial group of children and their parents, the aviary chirping, and the playground full of the same shouts of "happy French children." Although he spoke and read not a word of French, George Eastman had announced the gift of the Paris clinic in idiomatic French—no doubt through the good offices of a translator at Kodak-Pathé.

A June 1979 article in *Kodéco,* magazine of Kodak-Pathé, entitled "100,000 consultations par an," noted that it was the 125th anniversary of Eastman's birth. The article stated that employment conditions at the clinic reflected the Kodak King's interest in preventive dentistry for children: "Dans la lettre du fondateur, on lit aussi, au chapitre du choix du Directeur de l'Etablissement: 'Les conditions spéciales exigées, outre une instruction et une expérience complète de l'art dentaire, étant la comprehension des enfants et une profonde sympathie pour eux.'" ("'The special required conditions, other than a complete experience with the dental arts, are an understanding of children and a profound sympathy for them.'")

* * *

In 1986, Eastman Dental Center director William McHugh received a letter from Professor René Ackerman, director of the Medical de l'Institut Eastman, Fondation George Eastman, notifying him and asking advice about "the very real possibility that the Institut Georges Eastman in Paris may be closed." The fundamental issue, apparently, was the move by the French government to "privatize institutions which had been funded by the government but need not be. Philosophically, I am in favor of such a policy," McHugh wrote, "and while I can well understand the immediate problems it will cause you and the Institut, I believe that the long-term benefits can be substantial." McHugh continued:

> If you look upon this 'privatization' policy as an opportunity rather than a threat, you can move to establish a new set of goals and objectives for the Institut and then to establish an adequate economic base for its operation. With the dramatic fall in caries prevalence among children and the increase in the number of dentists in France, the need for a clinic to provide care for children is difficult to justify. This then means that you can set new and entirely different objectives in light of today's needs and opportunities. Some of the possibilities that you might consider are the following:

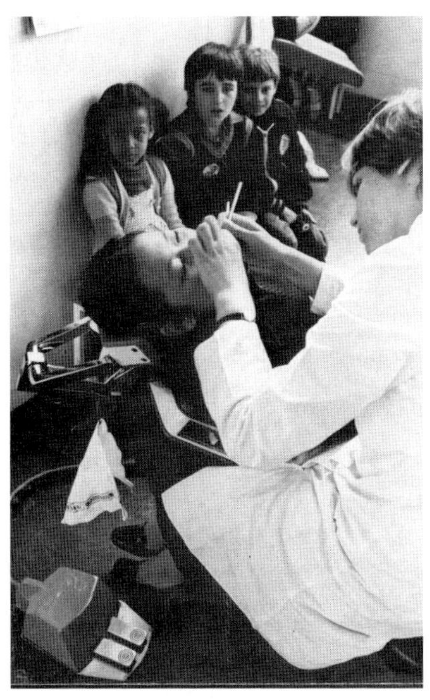

(Author's collection)

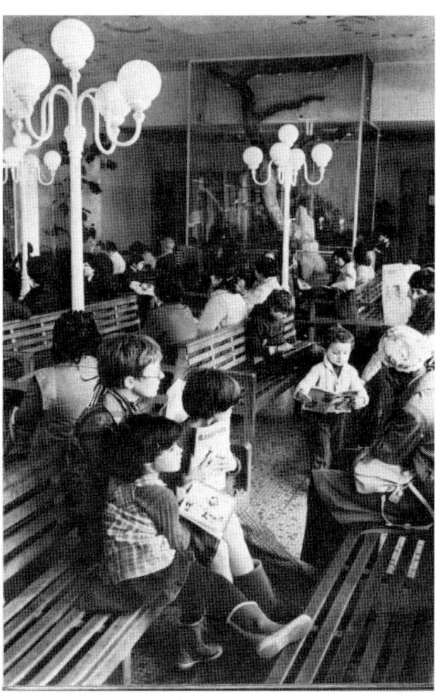

Note birdcage in background (Author's collection)

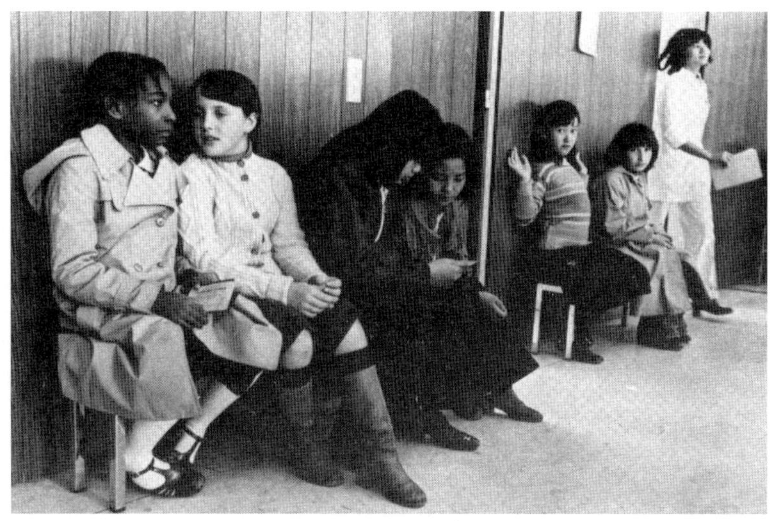

(Author's collection)

1. Education

    a) Dental Schools

You already have a collaborative arrangement with the Dental Schools in Paris and you might develop this by providing clinical experiences or courses that the Schools do not or cannot provide. Presumably the Universities would reimburse the Institut for these services.

    b) Specialty Education

I believe that programs in the dental specialties are developing in France as they have in the United States. You could consider providing selected courses (e.g. Orthodontics, Periodontics, etc.), along the lines we follow in Rochester, in accordance with demand for such courses and the Institut's ability to provide them. Presumably the students would pay fees which would cover the costs of these programs.

    c) Continuing Education

There is a demand from dentists in private practice for continuing education courses and you could try to develop the Institut as a Center for such courses. The courses can be given by you and members of your staff but you can also invite distinguished colleagues from other parts of France and from other countries, including the U.S.A. (Members of our faculty in Rochester have already been invited to present courses in France.) Fees from those attending these courses will cover all costs and often generate a modest profit.

2. Research

Another option to be considered is development as a research center. To do this, you must first assemble a nucleus of talented staff and then seek support from government and industry for specific research projects. I know that the French Government supports a number of research centers in different disciplines and, as you negotiate with ministers, you might explore this possibility in exchange for your current type of funding.

3. Patient Care

Assuming that the need and demand for care by children is diminishing, you might try to determine what are the current demands for treatment in the Paris area. This may involve specific types of diseases/conditions or particular groups within the community. For instance, you might contract to provide dental services to all employees of a company or organization in return for guaranteed annual payments. The key step here is to determine what is needed and wanted, how you can provide that at the Institut, and then how equitable financing can be arranged.

You must realize of course that I know little of the local circumstances in the Paris area and can thus make only general suggestions. While some may not be feasible, I hope you will accept this as an effort to make constructive suggestions that you might find useful.

Thus, the advice from Rochester to Paris was: follow the course of Rochester and London and expand the clinic's mission to include not only preventive clinical dentistry for indigent children, but also education and research. Unfortunately, the dentists of Paris felt otherwise; they saw the Eastman clinic as a threat. Eventually, the Eastman clinic had to leave its beautiful building and move to smaller quarters. However, under dedicated leadership it has maintained the provision of specialized services to underserved populations and, at the time the book was going to press, is considering an expansion of its services.

INSTITUT DENTAIRE FONDATION GEORGES EASTMAN, BRUXELLES

"The choice of Brussels is a sentimental one," Eastman said. That sentiment went back to the early days of World War I when several Belgian women employees bravely and secretly kept Kodak company books and records out of German hands. King Albert (1875–1934), heroic military leader during World War I and wise statesman during reconstruction, and Queen Elizabeth, a Bavarian duchess whose courage under fire matched her husband's, appealed to Eastman for help. Many Rochesterians joined Herbert Hoover's efforts to bring food and aid to destitute and starving Belgians despite the German blockade from 1914 to 1917.

A request for a dental clinic in Brussels came from Dr. Albert Joachin in the summer of 1931. Joachin appealed to Eastman through Prince der Linge, Belgian ambassador to the United States. In October the contract was signed, with Queen Elizabeth serving as honorary president of the clinic committee.

There was considerable delay in starting the professional activities of the Brussels clinic, perhaps a harbinger of things to come. King Albert, Eastman's

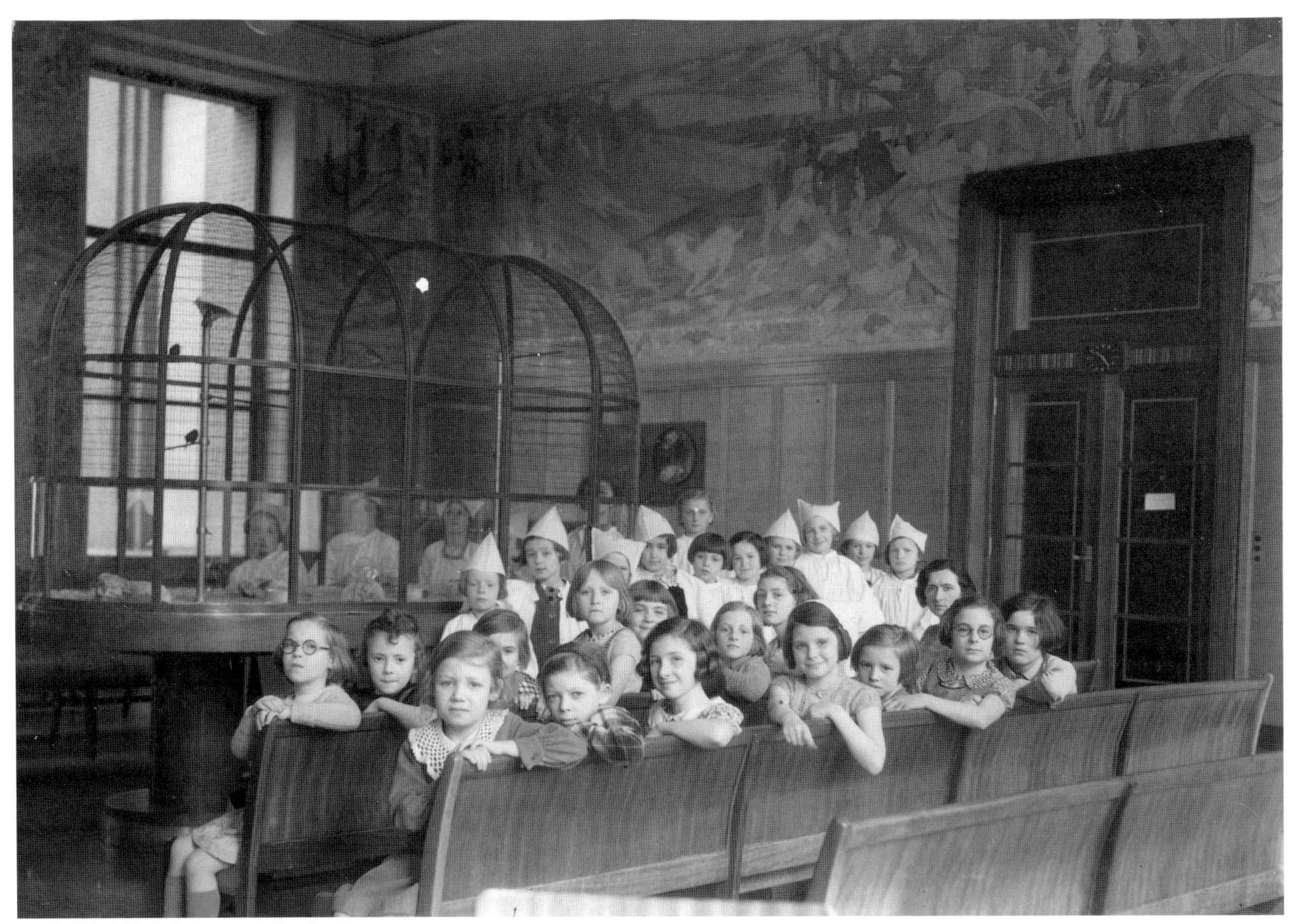

Brussels girls next to birdcage

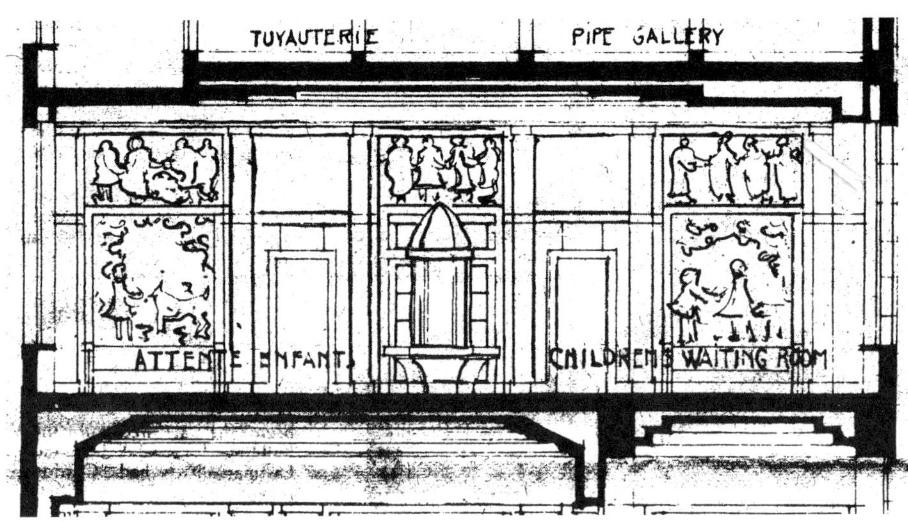

Architect's elevations showing planned birdcage

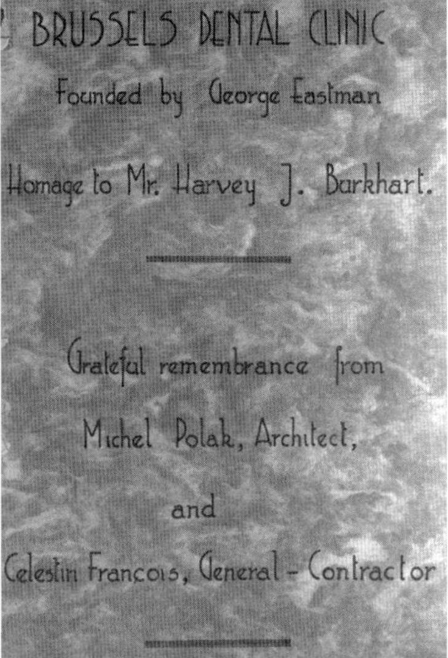

Burkhart's scrapbook

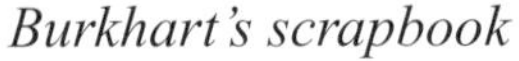

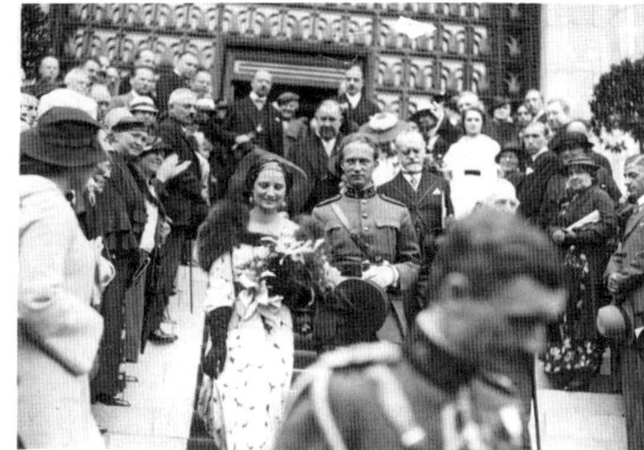
Belgian royalty

original contact whose enthusiasm had propelled clinic plans, died in 1934 and was succeeded by his son, Leopold III. Burgomaster Max picked out one location but then in April 1932 changed his mind and the location.[30] The plans had to be changed then too. Because the Eastman gift covered only the building and equipment, considerable funds had to be raised to provide for operating expenses. The resignation of the American ambassador, who served as head of the Eastman Dental Committee of Brussels, came at an inopportune time. The clinic was located near the communes that it was intended to serve, but the contributions needed for its operation had to be secured from wealthier, more distant communes.

The cornerstone of the Brussels clinic was laid on October 20, 1933, and the clinic was dedicated on July 31, 1934 by the new king, Elizabeth's son, Leopold III. The dedication was the last public function attended by the beautiful and popular Queen Astrid before she was tragically killed in an auto accident in Switzerland. The new director, Dr. Watry, escorted Their Majesties through the clinic. Dr. Burkhart represented the executors of Eastman's will in presenting the clinic to the Municipality of Brussels. Burgomaster Max accepted the gift. The American ambassador and a contingent of Eastman friends from Rochester delivered addresses, and the king decorated Dr. Burkhart with the Order of Leopold II. The dedication coincided with

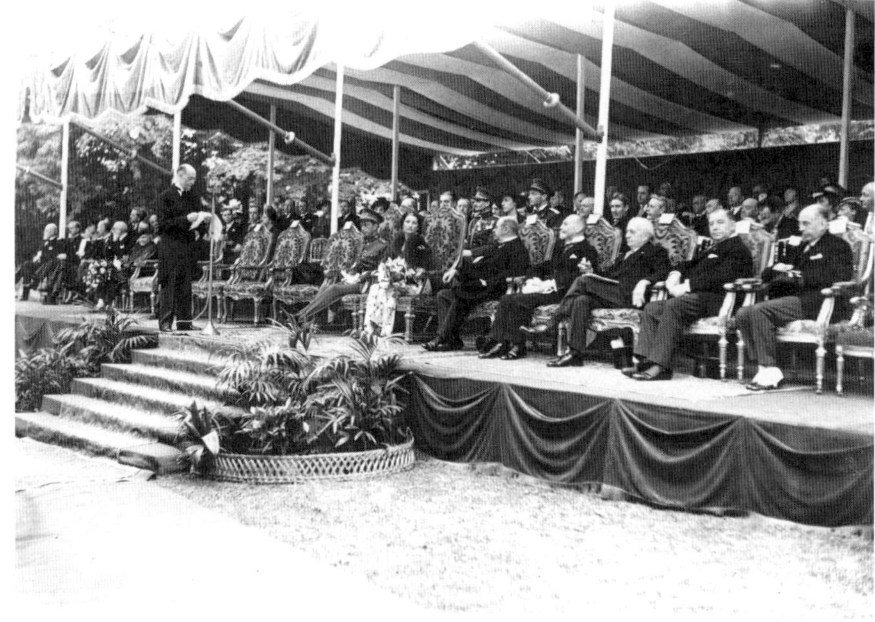
Dedication ceremonies

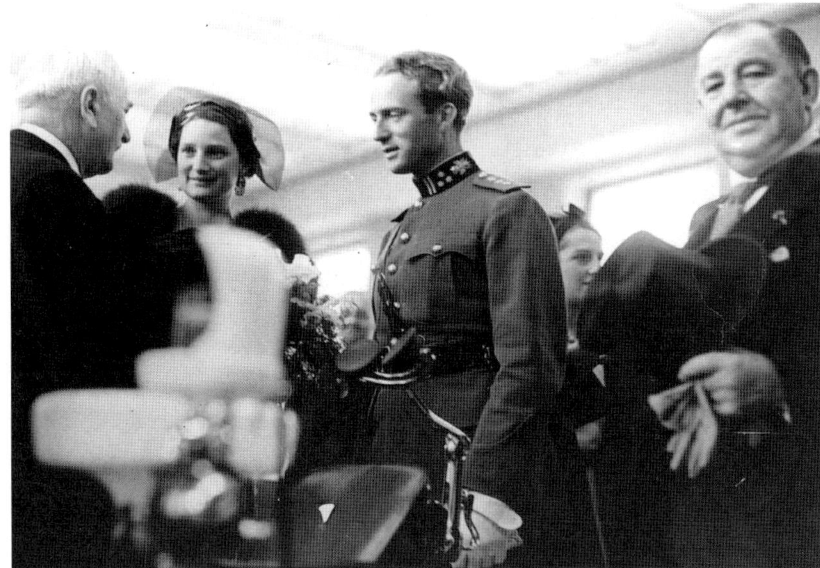

Their majesties

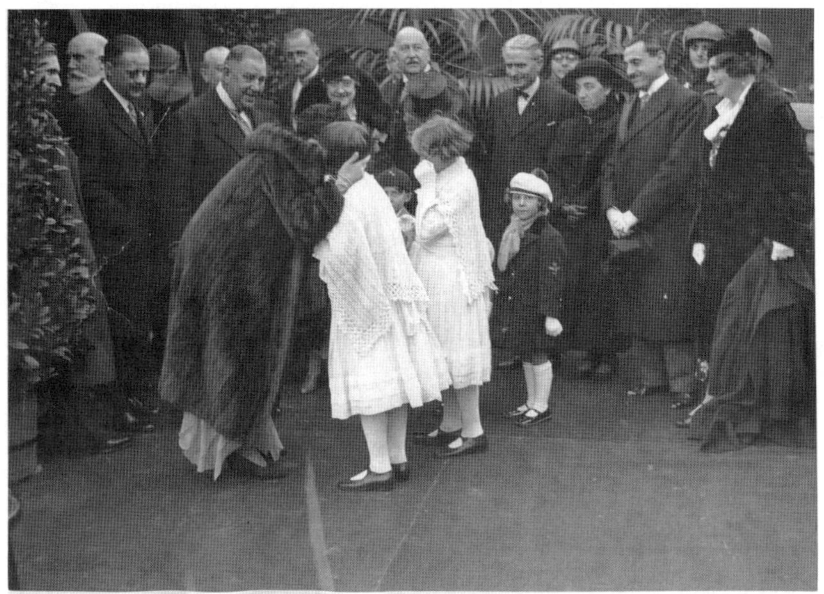

More guests at dedication

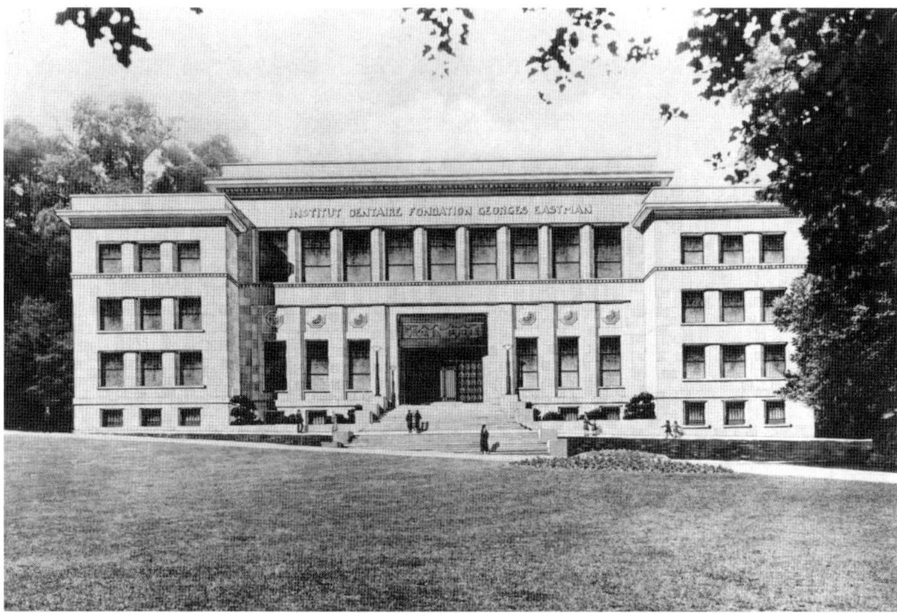

The Brussels clinic

the 1935 session of the International Dental Federation in Brussels; a bumper crop of European dentists attended as well as the presidents and major officers of the American Dental Association, past and present.

During World War II, German authorities requisitioned the Brussels clinic in 1940, using it to perform head, jaw, and facial surgery on their troops. With the permission of the German chief of the hospital, the clinic was plundered of its instruments and its dental, surgical, food, and hospital supplies. Considerable damage was done to the interior when the main clinic room was converted into sleeping quarters. The room was stripped of units and chairs—six of the thirty-eight original units having been sent to other hospitals in the war zone—and walls and linoleum floors were destroyed and cabinets rendered unusable. While some dental work for children and adults was still being done in Rome and Paris during the war, the Nazis operated the Brussels clinic entirely for their wounded. By January 1945, Belgium had been liberated, but the clinic was "merely giving token service to civilians"[31] although arrangements were being made to allow the United States Army to use part of the building for a dental clinic.

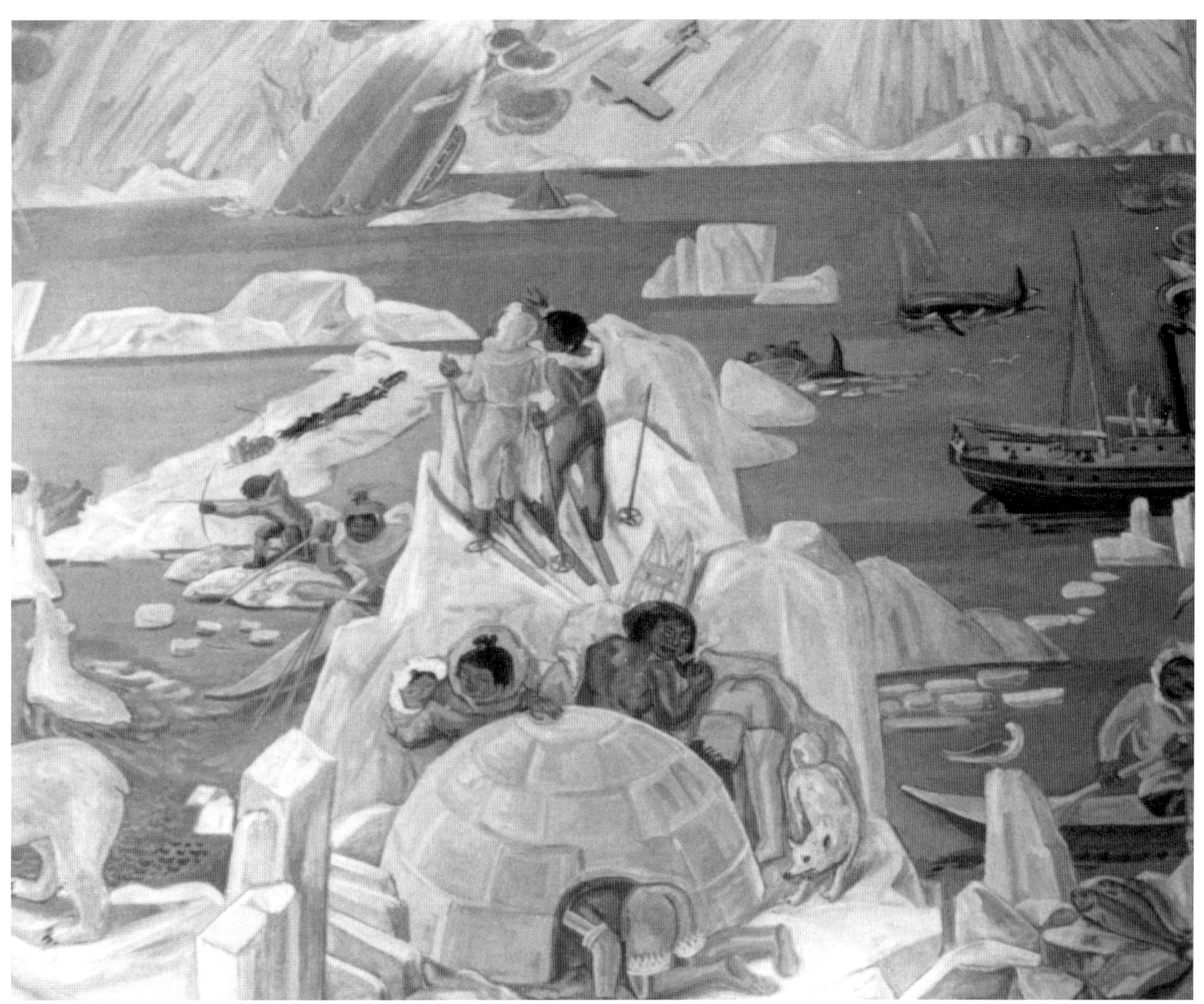

A Stockholm mural

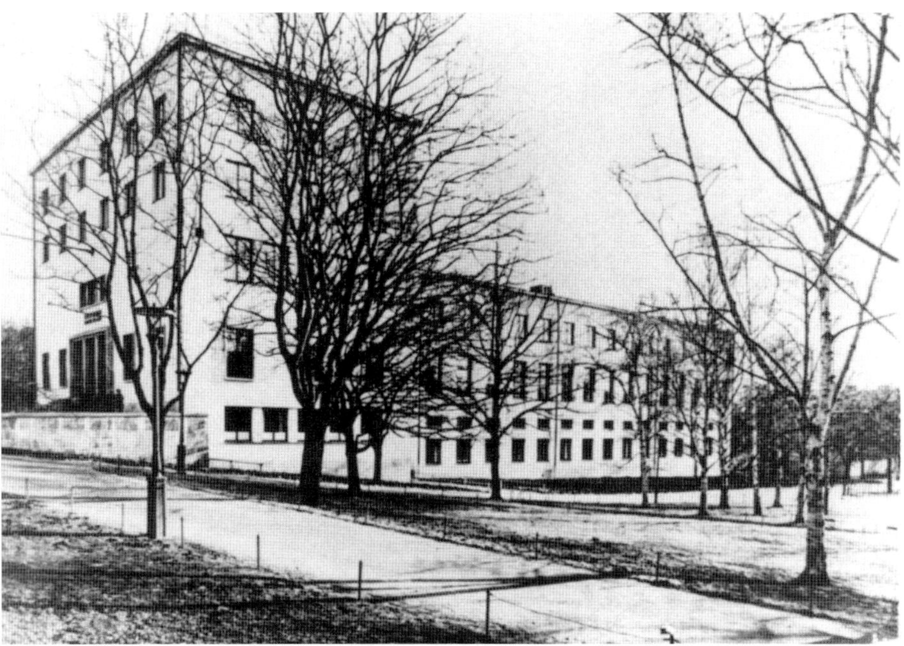

The Stockholm clinic

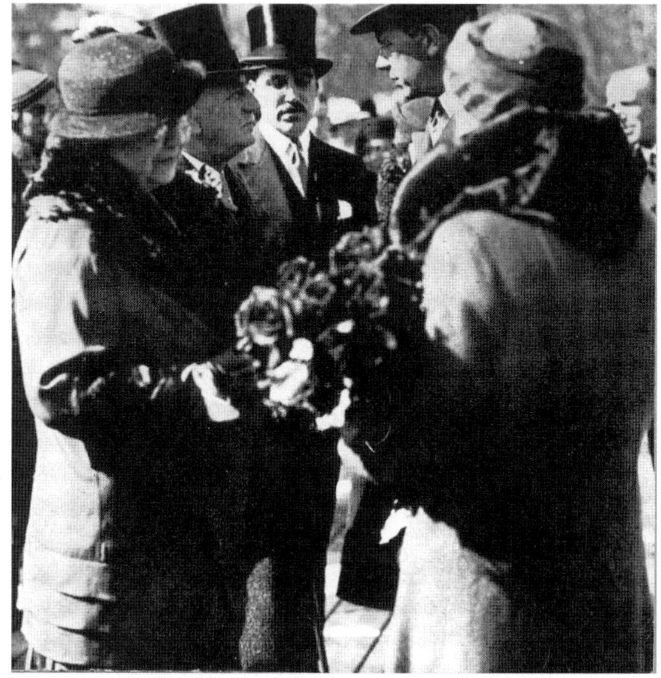

Burkhart's omnipresent top hat in Stockholm

After the war, service was resumed and the number of children's visits was maintained at two-thirds the prewar average. Hobnail boot marks were still evident on the floors. The Eastman Brussels clinic never fully recovered and is the only one that is now moribund.

EASTMANINSTITUTET, STOCKHOLM

The Stockholm clinic was partially the result of Eastman's friendship with Nils Bouveng of Haselblad, the Swedish camera company, and later of Kodak Ltd. (in 1914 Bouveng supplied the rare red dye needed for Kodachrome plates and film, somehow getting it through the German blockade.) When Bouveng died in 1939, Burkhart wrote, "More credit is due to him than to anyone else for the establishment of the Eastman clinic in Stockholm."[32] Eastman's public relations assistant, Colonel Oscar Solbert, another Swede, was also influential. Solbert had connections around the world, including with the Prince of Wales and other European royalty. He would later (1949–58) be the first director of George Eastman House, International Museum of Photography and Film.

Building operations for the Stockholm clinic began in the autumn of 1932. In April 1933, the foundation stone was laid in a ceremony attended by Crown Prince Gustaf Adolf, who gave the dedication speech, Princess Louise, Princess Sibylla, Prince Carl, Princess Ingeborg, Dr. and Mrs. Harvey J. Burkhart, and Dr. Nils B. Forrer of New York, director of the medical department of the new clinic. At the same time as the dedication, Count Folke Bernadotte, nephew of the King of Sweden, placed a wreath on the Eastman memorial at Kodak Park in Rochester. The Stockholm clinic and school for hygienists were dedicated on April 25, 1936.[33]

In a striking similarity to the origins of preventive dentistry for children in Rochester, the first dental clinic in a school in Stockholm had been opened on August 22, 1907.[34] Because of inadequate financial resources, the staff

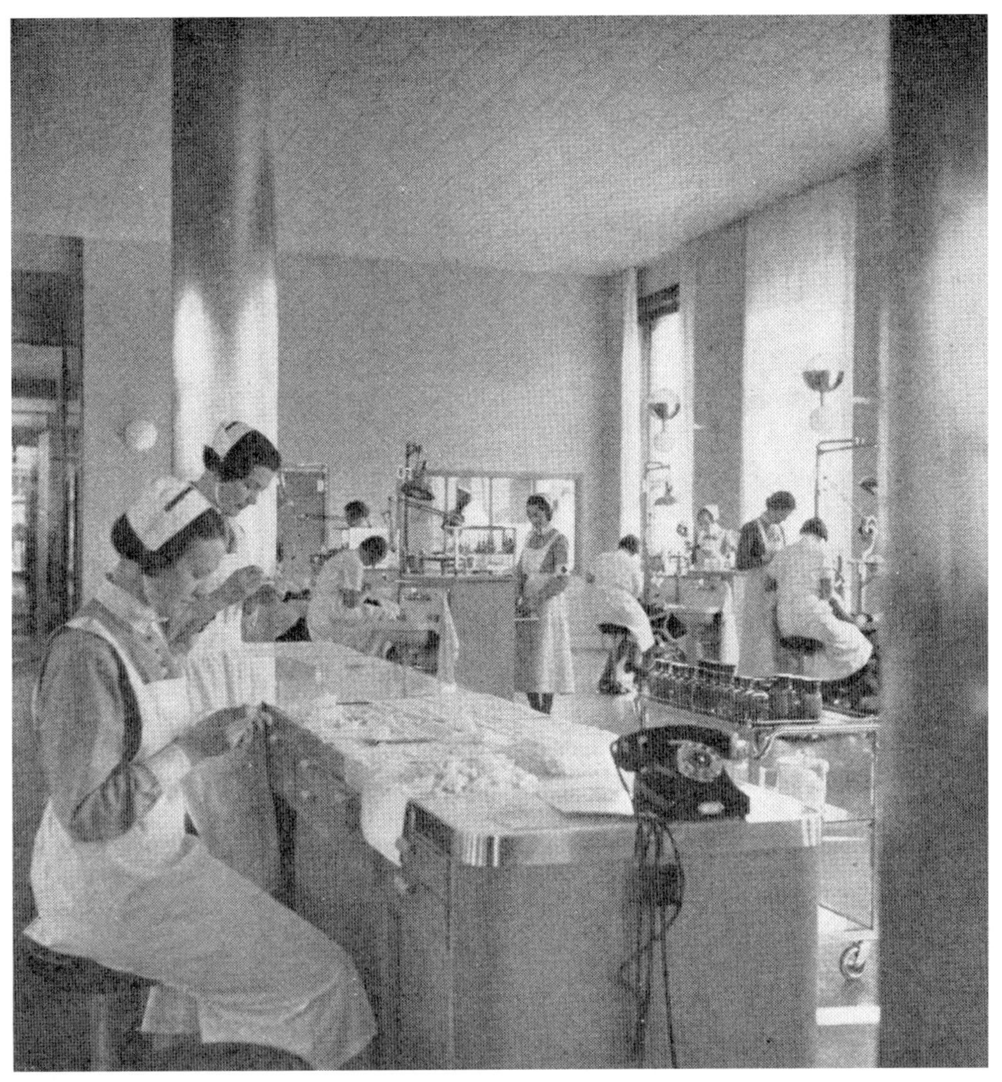

Scene in the Stockholm clinic

consisted of only three dentists and one dental assistant, and work was severely limited. "Experience gained from this first clinic was so promising that in 1911 the city fathers opened an additional clinic. In 1913 it was decided to extend dental care gradually to all children attending the elementary schools of the City. In 1944, secondary and private schools were included."[35]

Stockholm was developing obligatory dental health care for all of its children and teens in the 1930s when the Eastman clinic opened. By then, school clinics were well established. The first generation of dentists employed by the Eastman institute were both Swedish and foreign. The Eastmaninstitutet in Stockholm opened with four dental departments for the treatment of 20,000 children annually:

1. The conservation department

2. The orthodontia department

3. The x-ray and dental surgery department

4. The department for adults

In addition, there was a department for the treatment of diseases of the ear, nose, and throat, which served about 1,000 patients annually and which featured two fully equipped laboratories for scientific research. The institute could accommodate twenty-five patients at a time. It was structured to "provide rational care of both deciduous teeth and permanent teeth" from the time children were three years old onward. Its mission was to stress early dental treatment for children through prophylactic supervision of tooth development.

The specific terms of Eastman's gift included courses for the training of dental hygienists. The eighteen-month course consisted of a six-month theoretical course of lectures and practical demonstrations followed by one year of practical training. For the theoretical course, 300 kronor was charged; during practical training, a small salary was paid to the students. Postgraduate courses for young dentists "desirous of specializing in the dental treatment of children" were arranged for up to fifteen dentists. In other words, the Stockholm clinic was to follow closely the development of the Rochester clinic, with perhaps more emphasis on research.

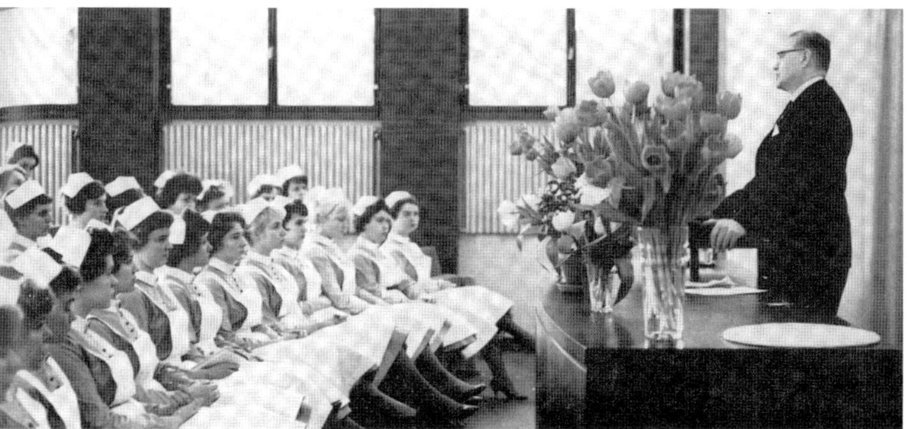

A class of hygienists

As with the London and Rome clinics, the Stockholm clinic was associated with a hospital. "Not only is the arrangement of great importance from a medical point of view, but it also offers certain other advantageous, e.g. food and washing [laundry], which the hospital is well equipped to provide."[36] Standing on the open and beautiful grounds of the Sabbatsberg Hospital, the clinic site was centrally located and easily accessible.

The main feature of all Eastman clinics, and the one most frequently used, was the large hall for general dental treatment. In Rochester, London, and Rome, this large operatory was built on the second or top floor and flooded with natural light via skylights. In Stockholm, it was located on the ground floor and used artificial light.

In his letter of donation, George Eastman stressed that the treatment of malocclusion should also be given at the institute. This was the first time that orthodontics had been officially recognized in Sweden as a necessary item in a dental health program. Through orthodontic treatment it is possible to guide the developing jaw in the right direction, brochures explained, and in the early years it is possible to correct, at least to some degree, the development of malocclusion. "About twenty-five per cent of the children of Northern Europe have such pronounced malocclusion that there is need for corrective measures."[37]

The department of orthodontics was originally equipped for six dentists with only the head and assistant head as qualified specialists and the other

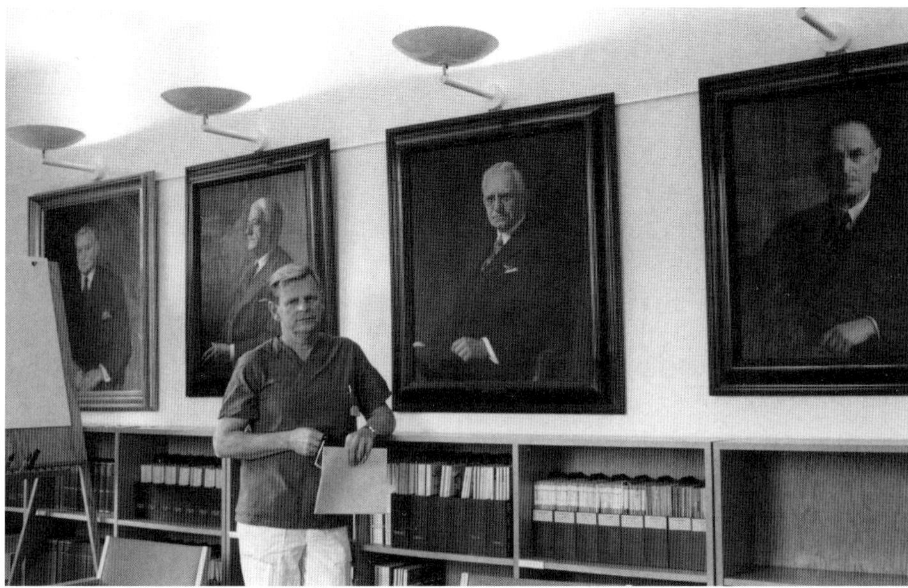

The Stockholm board room in the 1980s featured portraits of Burkhart, Eastman, and Nils Bouveng. (Author's collection)

dentists working as assistants. The number of patients requiring treatment soon exceeded capacity. By giving priority to the children in greatest need of treatment and by applying a means test, it was hoped to keep the number of patients within manageable bounds. However, owing to the large number of cases requiring lengthy, complicated treatment (for example, cleft palate), these measures were inadequate.

The clientele grew considerably. With the abolishment of a means test, the number of children treated tripled. As Sweden moved into a cradle-to-grave system of socialized medicine, the capacity of the departments quickly doubled. A long queue for orthodontic treatment also developed, a report noted, and "the waiting time is now five to six years."

The city of Stockholm took over the institute in 1971. There were some changes in structure as the organization was split into branches of care, education, and clinical trials. "Child dental care in Stockholm enjoys great public confidence," Eastmaninstitutet publications assert, backing up this with figures showing that 98 percent of pupils apply for dental care and 85 percent

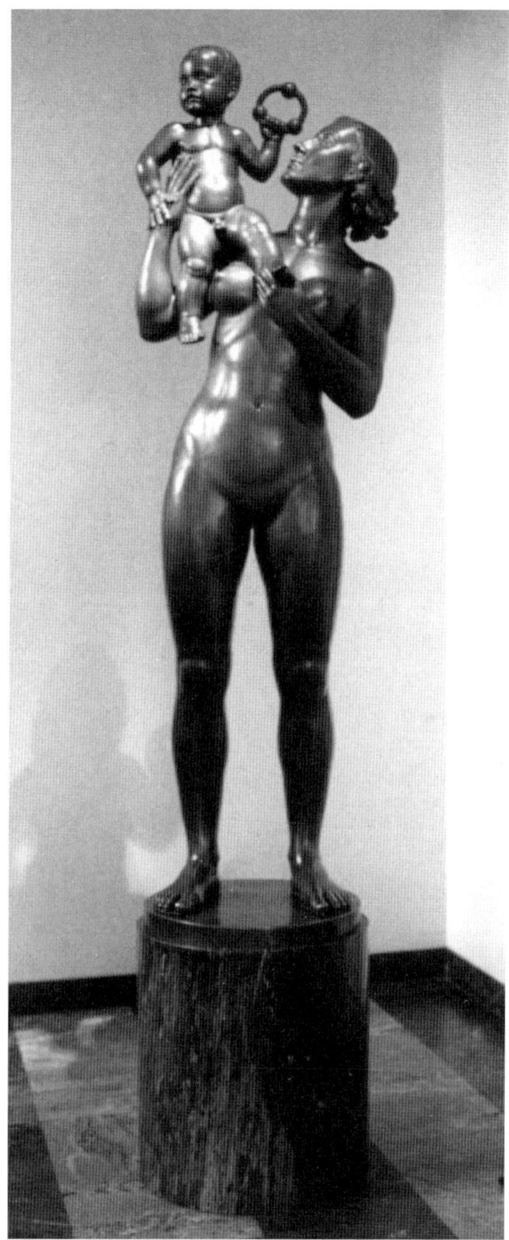

Art abounds in Stockholm

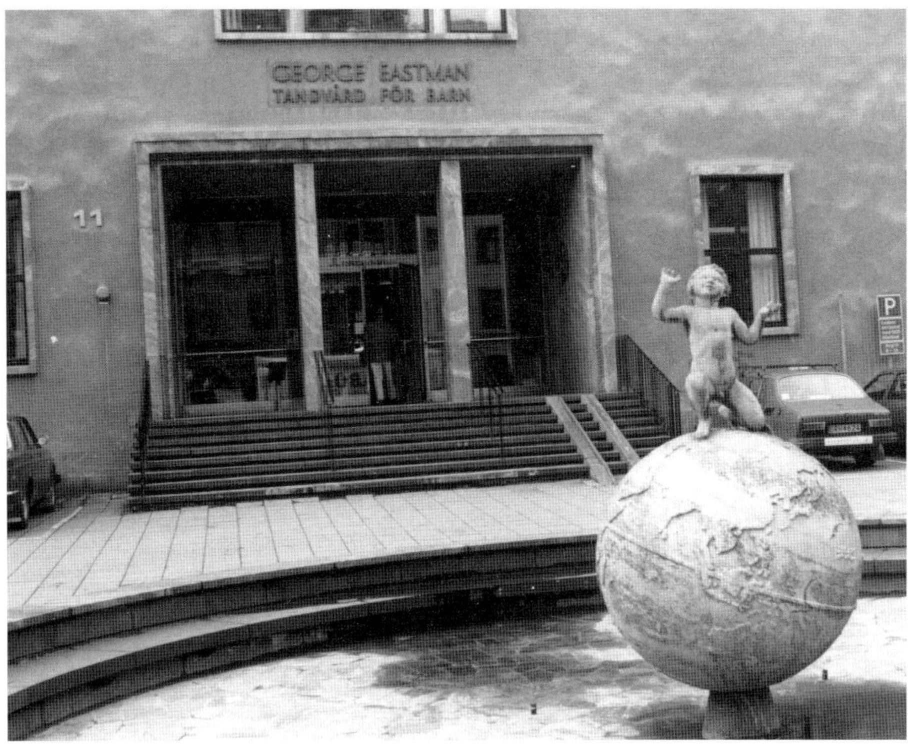

Even the entrance features a sculpture.

administered. The government makes annual grants to each one based on the number of children up to age fifteen receiving complete dental care.[40]

As the only important European capital never to experience a major war, Stockholm has not changed much since the 1930s. Nor has it suffered from urban renewal or "suburban flight." Thus, the clinic site remains centrally located, accessible, and on open grounds.

By its twenty-fifth anniversary in 1961, the Eastmaninstitutet in Stockholm was considered the central dental clinic for the city's Child Dental Health Service. As such, it "assumed great importance not only because dental treatment has been made available to a large number of children of pre-school age, but also because the dental service for children has been provided with a centre where complicated cases and difficult children can be sent in the knowledge that they will be in the hands of well-trained and experienced pedodontists."[41]

Since the early 1950s, the Stockholm Child Dental Health Service has included the topical application of fluorides as part of its program. The fluoride treatment consists for the most part in brushing the teeth with a fluoride solution two or three times a year under the strict supervision of ten specially trained dental assistants. More than 80,000 school children, attending all the elementary schools, come under this scheme.

By 2009 the Stockholm Eastman had added specialty dental services, research, and graduate education to its portfolio and at the time this book was going to press, was in the process of planning a move to a new building.

of preschoolers are enrolled by their parents. At the Eastmaninstitutet, "the demand for treatment far exceeds the capacity."[38] Those accepted are initially examined at age three and receive regular attention until they start school at age seven. An open reception advisory department allows any preschooler and parents to attend and learn; urgent cases are given necessary treatment. The great majority of the cases remitted are children that have sustained injury to teeth and jaws.

The department has been gradually enlarged; single rooms for fractious children have been added, and the number of dentists, both Swedish and foreign, increased. Postgraduate study and training in pedodontics have been added. Signs of the growth of dental service in Sweden include the radical modernization of older clinics, the opening of new clinics, and the increase in annual allocations from 6,200 kronor in 1907 to recent allocations in the millions.[39] Since 1952, all Stockholm dental clinics have been centrally

BERLIN: THE CLINIC THAT NEVER WAS

Until World War II began, the Eastman Kodak Company had a large commercial presence in Berlin, but because of George Eastman's anti-German sentiments during World War I, he did not offer that municipality a children's dental clinic. However, he did influence other philanthropists, such as Julius Rosenwald of Chicago and Murry Guggenheim of New York, to start clinics in their respective cities. Rosenwald in turn offered the municipality of Berlin "a children's dental clinic along the lines of the clinics established by Mr. Eastman in Europe"[42] in June 1931. The offer was gratefully accepted by the city's oberburgermeister, but before it could be effected, Rosenwald died. His children and heirs at first were inclined to carry out the benefaction, but as the years went on and Adolf Hitler rose to power, they changed their minds.

*   *   *

There was some contact with the European clinics during the Bibby years. In his 1954–55 annual report Bibby announced, "Three six month appointments in the overseas Eastman clinics have been offered to dentists who have completed a year's appointment at the Eastman Dental Dispensary in Rochester. The first appointment already has been made and the appointee . . . is now in London."[43] The European clinics, with the exception of the one in London, have generally developed in their own way rather than following the Rochester model as George Eastman intended. In 1967, on the fiftieth anniversary of the opening of the Eastman Dental Center, the directors of all of the European clinics came to Rochester for the occasion.

BIBLE CLASS OBJECTS TO EUROPEAN CLINICS

Gifts of dental clinics to European countries did not sit well with those who believed charity should begin at home. The Men's Bible Class of the First Church of Christ in Grafton, West Virginia, for example, debated the merits of Eastman's gift of the Rome clinic, and a spokesman wrote to Eastman in 1929:

> If you have money to give away why not give it to spreading the Gospel? . . . Why not pay it to your workers in wages? . . . Why not give it to your country where you made same? I told the class you would not answer. Will you?
>
> Yours for America First (P.S. Loan on this church of $8,000).

Remarkably, Eastman did reply, "chiefly because of the economic and social questions that you raise." His response provides a rare glimpse into his thought processes regarding social questions and the role of a philanthropist.

> In the first place, permit me to say that I can understand your present anxiety and the problems that confront you. I had to leave school before I was fourteen years old because I was the only wage earner in the family. When I was a young man I had to work eleven hours a day in a job that I considered drudgery. By the time I reached your age I had large obligations and responsibilities because I felt a personal responsibility for the welfare of thousands of families in this country and Europe who were dependent upon the success of this company for their livelihood and, in a measure perhaps, for their happiness.
>
> Today the employees of this Company are the largest stockholders. They receive more in wages and dividends than I ever received in the course of any one year. In addition the company has provided a pension and insurance plan that practically guarantees that no employee will ever have to face the possibilities of poverty that confronted me.
>
> You state that you have four children. These children face an entirely different situation from that that confronted the children of this country . . . seventy years ago when I was a boy. In those intervening years we have had the telephone, the electric light, the street car, the motion picture, the automobile, free public libraries and the development of the public school, college, and university education that makes it possible for every child to obtain an education. In the meantime, the progress of medical and dental science and the improvement in public health enable every citizen to benefit by the labor and generosity of men and women who have thought more of their fellow citizens than of themselves.
>
> In the building of industry and transportation in this country some men have accumulated great wealth. In most cases these men have given to education, to the church or to some agency serving the public, a far greater proportion of their wealth than they ever used themselves. So that in addition to raising the economic standard of the country, men like John D. Rockefeller, Cleveland Dodge, Jacob Schiff, Julius Rosenwald, Andrew Carnegie and scores of others have improved the social life of our country. What they are doing will most certainly benefit your children.
>
> Because you condemn me for a gift to the people of Italy and because you mention the fact that "your family needs $200 dentist work" I want to acquaint you with a few facts. . . .
>
> About 15 years ago a man by the name of Forsyth in Boston conceived of the idea of establishing a dental infirmary in that city that could obtain expert dental treatment free of charge. The idea appealed to me and I established a dental dispensary in Rochester for all indigent children under age sixteen. Since this dispensary has been open the children of this city have received more than one million treatments free of charge.

Reasons for Founding Dental Clinics Told by Mr. Eastman

Replied to Critic That He and Other Rich Men and Women Were Doing Part of Work That Should Be Done by Government

Explanation in his own words of the reasons for his founding of dental dispensaries in Rochester and foreign capitals was given by George Eastman in a letter made public in February in a speech by Dean Carl W. Ackerman of the Columbia School of Journalism in New York City.

Mr. Ackerman, who is the author of a biography of Mr. Eastman published two years ago, made the letter public in an address before the Men's Class of the Riverside Church at the Commodore Hotel in New York. It was written in response to a letter from a correspondent in West Virginia, who criticized Mr. Eastman for not concentrating his philanthropies on other causes.

West Virginian Asks Questions

"In 1929," said Mr. Ackerman, "Mr. Eastman gave the City of Rome one million dollars for the establishment of a dental clinic for Italian children. It was one of several similar gifts to European communities. The publication of this item in the press of West Virginia caused a debate in the Men's Bible Class of a certain church and the secretary and teacher wrote Mr. Eastman, as follows:

The result of this debate was that men like you and Mr. Blank are the greatest stumbling block to a poor man living a Christian life.

This church is made up of poor working men. I will cite myself as to what poor means. American—42 years old. Family of 6. Work 7 days per week, no vacation. $1,500 mortgage on home. $400 doctor bill. Wife and part of children won't go to church on account of poor clothing. Three children need tonsils removed, no money. Family needs $200 dentist work done, no money. Bills to pay, no money.

The questions I was requested to ask you are as follows:

If you were poor and saw a rich man throwing money away, would it make you doubt God's justice?

Are you a member of any church? (Let God decide the Christian part of it.)

If you have money to give away, why not give it to the spreading of the gospel of Christ?

Why not pay it to your workers in wages?

But if you cannot do either, why give it to a nation like you did? Why not give it to your country where you made same?

I told the class you would not answer. Will you?

Yours for America first
(Signature)
P. S. Loan on this church of $8,000.

Mr. Eastman Replies

"Mr. Eastman," Mr. Ackerman said, "replied to this letter, not because of his own feelings, but because of his sense of social responsibility." His reply follows:

Permit me to say that I can understand your present anxiety and the problems which confront you. I had to leave school before I was 14 years old because I was the only wage earner in the family. When I was a young man I had to work 11 hours a day in a job which I considered drudgery. By the time I reached your age I had large obligations and responsibilities because I felt a personal responsibility for the welfare of thousands of families in this country and Europe who were dependent upon the success of this company for their livelihood and, in a measure perhaps, for their happiness.

You state that you have four children. These children face an entirely different future from that which confronted the children of this country 60 or even 70 years ago when I was a boy. In those intervening years we have had the telephone, the electric light, the street car, the motion picture, the automobile, free public libraries, cheap railroad transportation, excellent daily newspapers and the development of public school, college, and university education which makes it possible for every child to obtain an education. In the meantime, too, the progress of medical and dental science and the improvement in public health enable every citizen to benefit by the labor and the generosity of men and women who have thought more of their fellow citizens than of themselves.

Children Will Benefit

In the building of industry and

Newspaper clipping (Author's collection)

The success of this institution convinced me that there should be similar dispensaries throughout the United States and Europe. I decided to found one in London and one in Rome, because I was convinced that, as the idea spread, other men and women would undertake to build, equip, and endow dispensaries in other cities. Since then Mr. Rosenwald has undertaken the work in Chicago and Mr. and Mrs. Murry Guggenheim in New York City.

Now there should be such an institution in your community in West Virginia and in every city in this country. They should be built and operated by government money, but until that time comes when the government can do the work, men and women of money must carry on the work.

Therefore, instead of denouncing the building of dental dispensaries, I would recommend that your Bible class undertake the more constructive policy of striving for a similar agency in your community.

As to the religious questions in your letter, I would like to call your attention to the Constitution of your country, which guarantees to every American citizen complete freedom, without being accountable to any man or any Bible class for an explanation of his faith.

"Whatever a man soweth, that shall he also reap. . . . Let us not be weary in well doing for in due season we shall reap, if we faint not."

Yours very truly,
George Eastman

In 1998, Malcolm Harris, trustee of the Eastman clinic in London, acknowledged a debt of gratitude on behalf of London and the other European capitals:

At the Eastman [Institute in London], success has been the sum total of the effort and talent of all its teachers, clinicians, scientists and postgraduates. However, Harvey Jacob Burkhart must not to be forgotten. It was his influence that won Eastman's support for dentistry, and his initiative that created a postgraduate school and clinic for children's dentistry and dental hygienists, as part of his visionary concept of public dental health. Without Burkhart's ambitious initiative there would not have been specialist clinics in Stockholm, Brussels, Paris, Rome, and in the Grays Inn Road, London. Tribute must also be paid to George Eastman himself who was industrious and ingenious beyond belief, a man who may not have been above industrial spying, the exploitation of patents and ruthless in his elimination of competitors worldwide. Yet he invested millions of dollars in education, opposed racism in education and the workplace, was concerned about health care, especially dentistry, funded low cost housing, and the urban green environment and supported the arts, especially music. He undoubtedly identified with Kierkegaard; history has to do with results, motives and intentions are the business of ethics.[44]

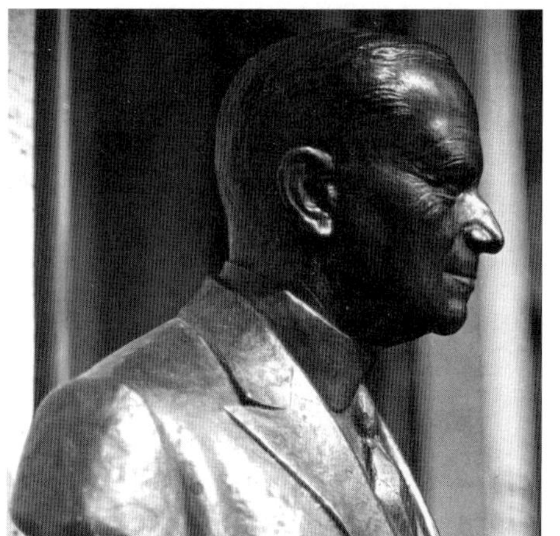

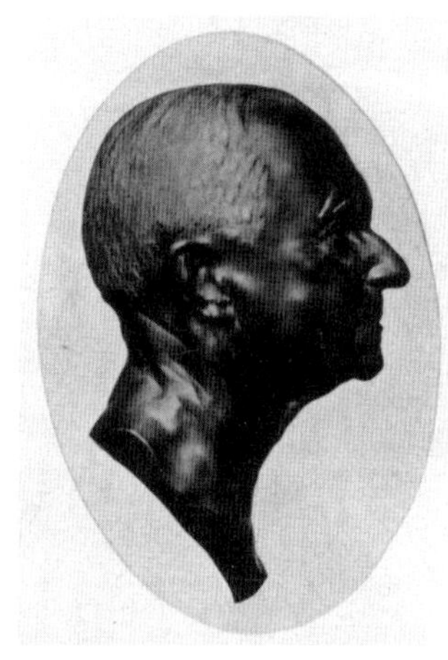

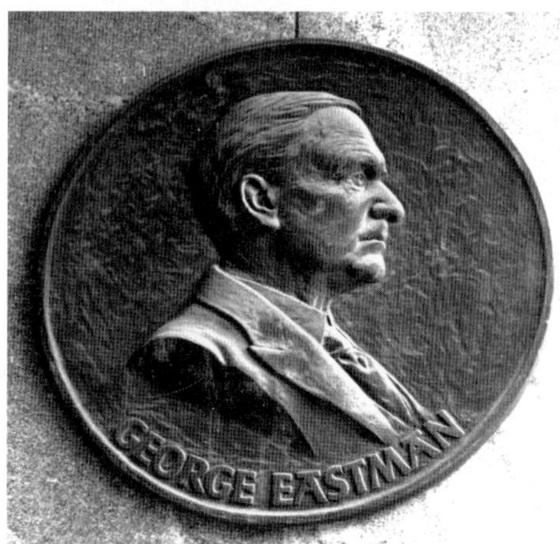

Sculpture and bas reliefs of Eastman varied from country to country. Paris's had a smiling image, Rome's resembled Julius Caesar, and Stockholm featured a crisp businessman. (Author's collection)

Cyril Meyerowitz traveled to Rome in January and February of 2009 to meet with representatives of the Eastman leadership of Rome, Paris, and Stockhold. (London was absent due to snow.) "The time spent with these people was excellent," he reported. We all presented as part of a conference that the Rome Eastman had organized under an organization called SIMO (Societa Italiana Maxillo Odontostomatologica)."

I presented the keynote address, or "lectio magistralis," covering some of the history of the Eastman in Rochester and our achievements in clinical care, community service, education, and research. We decided to talk more about some joint venture in community service and will be discussing this over the next year, meeting again next year in Rome. I was impressed with the ongoing vitality of the international Eastmans and how George Eastman's vision had managed to stay alive and evolve, perhaps differently in the different countries, but in a manner that maintained their relevance. Clearly London and Rochester are the most academic, but the others are moving in that direction, if slower. For example, the Stockholm Eastman has been trying to develop a relationship with the Karolinska Institute. The Rome Eastman has had a thorny relationship with the University Dental School but more recently this is improving.

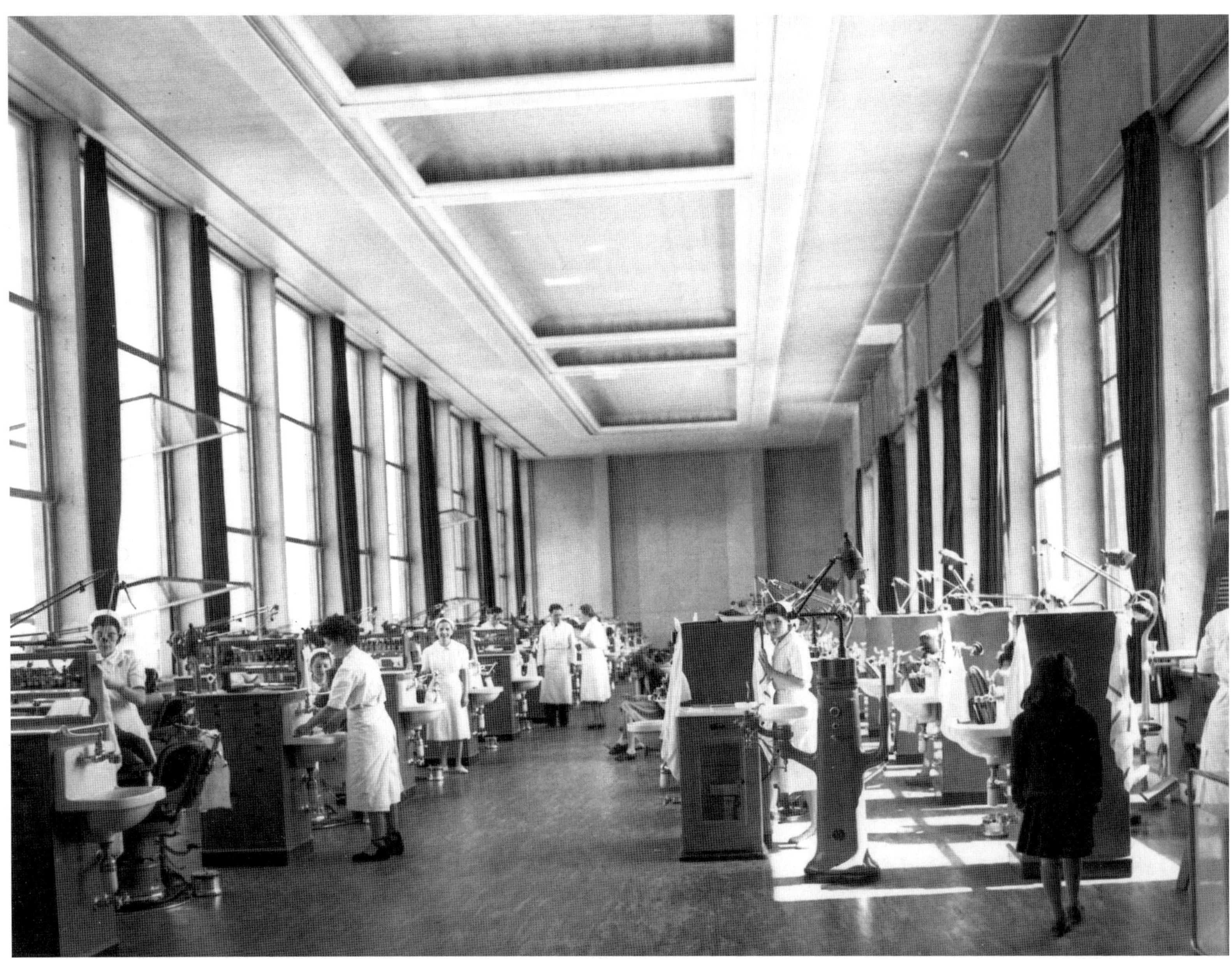

The operatory

HARVEY BURKHART REDUX

"DEAN OF AMERICAN DENTISTRY"

Socialized dentistry will ultimately lead to the "toothlessness" of persons in the United States.
Newspaper headline about Harvey J. Burkhart, DDS, LLD

Uncharacteristically, Eastman insisted on examining in detail each of the separate European contracts. Robinson, who had never had so much as a glimpse of earlier Eastman wills, was asked to read each contract out loud, one clause at a time, as Eastman slowly paced the floor. Then, after another final reading of the five clinic contracts to himself, Eastman discharged the lawyer and his own obligations to the teeth of the world's children with, "Yes, I guess these are right."

At 12:50 P.M. on the fourteenth—not quite the Ides of March—George Eastman lay down on his bed, placed a folded wet towel on his chest to prevent powder burns, and shot himself through the heart. This was the scribbled note he left:

To my friends
My work is done
Why wait?

GE

THREE DAYS BEFORE MARCH 14, 1932, George Eastman called in one of his lawyers, Milton Robinson, to work on a new codicil. Careful provisions had been made for the three European clinics that, as it turned out would be completed after Eastman's death: the clinics in Paris, Brussels, and Stockholm. "Suppose something were to happen to me someday," Eastman posited to the unsuspecting Robinson, "Would there be any hitch? Are these contracts clear as to how that money should be paid in Europe? Are they set up so Burkhart can act?"[1]

The resolution adopted by the board of trustees of the Rochester Dental Dispensary upon Eastman's death noted: "In this institution, founded by him, we have the great honor of carrying on the banner he raised in the interests of children. Pioneer in so many things, he broke new trails in his early recognition of the value of oral hygiene to children."

George Eastman first met Dr. Harvey Jacob Burkhart (1861–1946), mayor of Batavia, New York, and practicing dentist, sometime in 1914; Eastman was wearing a $24 set of ill-fitting dentures, having lost all of his teeth at a

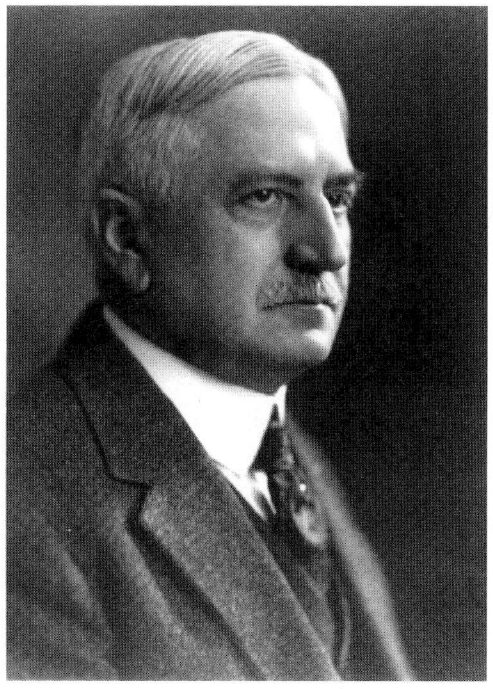

Harvey Jacob Burkhart DDS, LLD

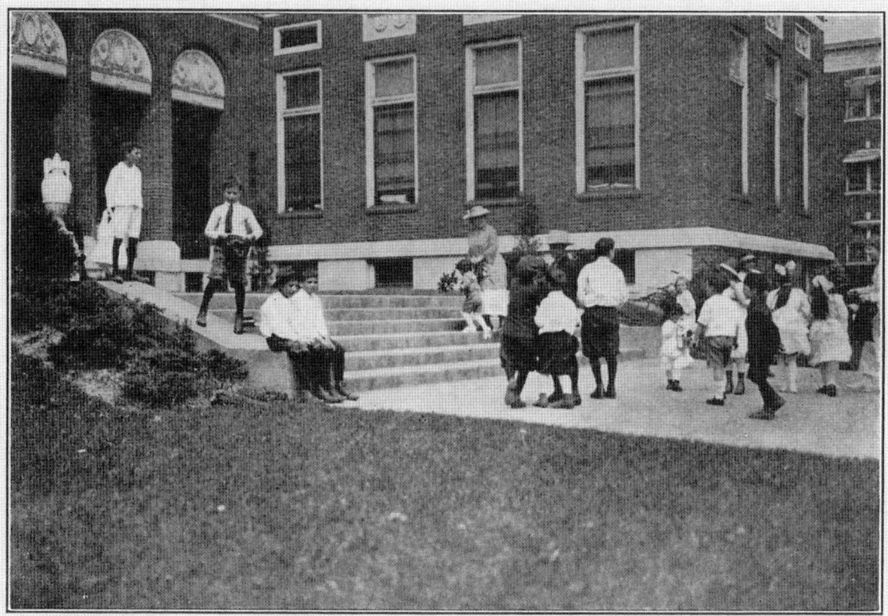

The patients arriving

relatively early age. Burkhart (or his son, Richard Burkhart, a New York City dentist) constructed a more attractive set of dentures that duplicated the original bite and position of the teeth so that Eastman's nose did not meet his chin, as was the case with many countenances of the era. This gave him a fuller, more natural, face. From that time on, the two always called each other "Governor." (By contrast, it took twenty-five years before George Eastman and Rush Rhees, partners in founding the University of Rochester School of Medicine and Dentistry and Eastman Theatre and School of Music, would call each other by their first names.)

Burkhart's personality was often described as "prickly"; probably his dealings with colleagues were less smooth than his dealings with Eastman. Other dentists had expected to have input when the Rochester Dental Dispensary was set up. Eastman and his architects did consult other dentists on the preliminary architectural plans, and even sent one to check out the Forsyth Infirmary. But once the board of directors appointed Burkhart, he ran the operation single-handedly. Other dentists were not allowed any opportunity to participate in the development of the dispensary. Personality difficulties surfaced again between Burkhart and Lord Riddell, chairman of the board of the Royal Free Hospital, when the Eastman Dental Clinic in London was being set up. The most egregious example of the Burkhart prickliness would surface when the School of Medicine and Dentistry was founded and proud Dr. Burkhart learned he was about to be subordinated to a dean thirteen years his junior. Eastman's death meant that Burkhart was henceforth alone in setting policy and tone for the dispensary and its satellites in Europe.

Eastman wanted Harvey Burkhart as the director of the dispensary. He told his biographer, Carl Ackerman, that "the success of the dispensary would depend largely upon the director" and that he had looked upon Burkhart "from the beginning as the ideal head for the institution." He said, however, that he had "declined to exert any influence with the Board of Directors in the selection" and "did not show the directors any of the communications"

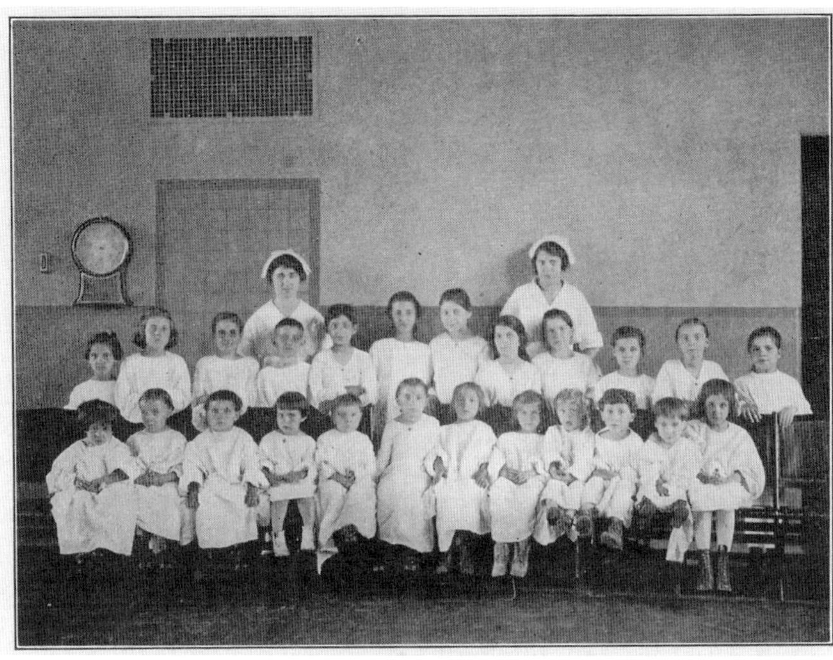

A group of incoming patients

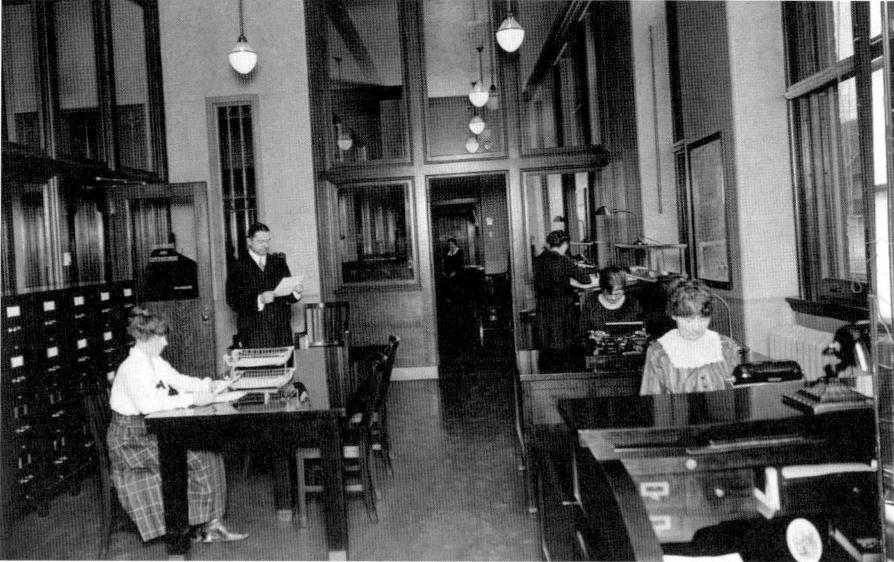

Office of the Eastman Dental Dispensary

he had with Burkhart "throughout the negotiations."[2] So it is not surprising that the search committee of trustees recruited Burkhart—an obvious choice; plus, they had heard of those Eastman dentures—as the first director of the Rochester Dental Dispensary, a post he held for the next thirty-one years. Eastman later told Thomas Forsyth, who visited the building when it was under construction, that "we are fortunate in having a man like Dr. Burkhart as director, as the success of any such institution depends largely upon the personality of the man who is in immediate charge."[3]

Harvey Burkhart was born and grew up in Cleveland. He became interested in dentistry when he moved from Cleveland to Dansville, NY, to live with a brother who was a dentist. Burkhart graduated from the Dansville Seminary and Baltimore College of Dental Surgery in 1890 with the degree of DDS and highest honors. Exactly fifty years later, in May 1940, he received the honorary degree of doctor of science from the University of Maryland, which had absorbed the Baltimore college. In Batavia, NY, where he opened

his first office, Burkhart became interested in the new field of preventive dentistry and soon embarked on the study of orthodontia, or, as he called it, "the remaking and beautifying of faces through the straightening of teeth." Burkhart was mayor of Batavia from 1904 to 1916, served three years as president of the New York State Dental Association, and served a year (1899) as the first president of the new and national American Dental Association (ADA). During World War I, he would be a member of the Committee on Dentistry, Council of National Defense. He would receive many awards and is the namesake for the New York State Dental Association's highest honor, the Jarvie-Burkhart Award. Under his leadership the dispensary became a model for patient care. Burkhart had Eastman's full confidence and once said of his boss: "He was the most sympathetic and loyal friend I ever had."[4]

Clinical dentistry—education and training—not research was what interested Burkhart. Burkhart realized that the School of Medicine and Dentistry had co-opted the research elements. After Eastman was gone, he concentrated on recording and increasing the number of clinical visits to the dispensary and setting up the European clinics. More and more Burkhart was referred to as "the dean of American dentistry." He reveled in the title, and

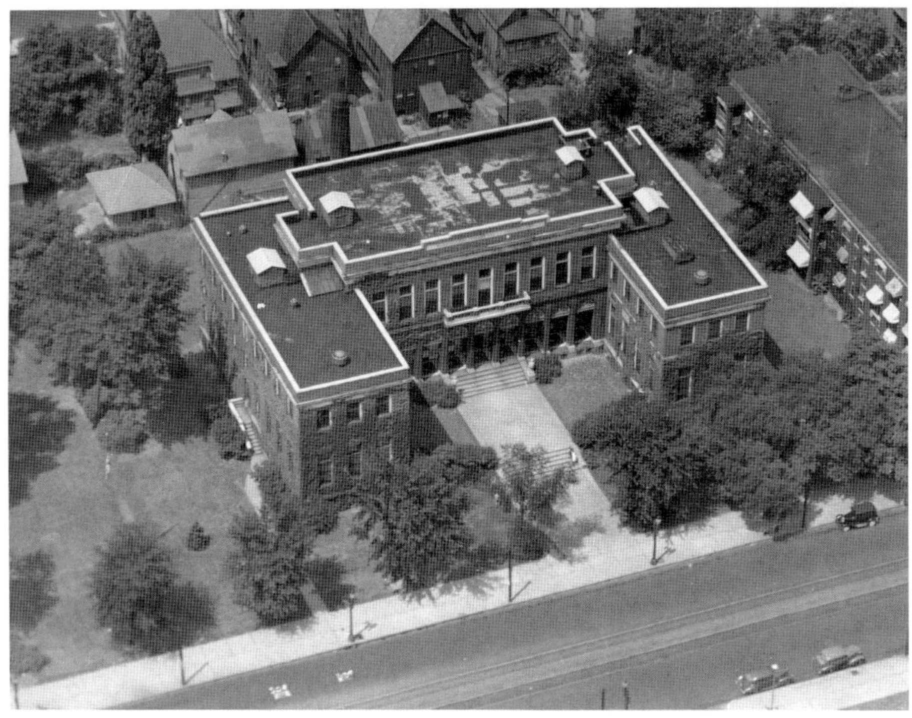

Aerial view of 800 East Main Street, Rochester

and Dentistry of the University of Rochester, to carry on work in dental research." Other 1920s annual reports mention other researchers and the publications they produced.

When he wrote the "Centennial History of Dentistry in Rochester" in 1934, Burkhart said:

> During the last twenty-five years, great strides have been made in appreciation of the value of research work in various directions. This has resulted in dentistry being divided into specialties, with the result that study clubs have been organized in large centers of population. . . . The work of these clubs has been exceedingly valuable, both from the research point of view, and from the opportunity it affords its members for an exchange of ideas and opinions.[5]

In 1938, the Rochester Dental Study Club and 200 dentists nationwide, including the major officers of the ADA, past and present, decided to honor Burkhart. His work for dentistry in five nations was cited and his dental mission described this way:

> If you give children healthy bodies they will be strong—physically and mentally—as adults. Healthy mouths and teeth are of paramount importance to healthy bodies. . . . Two men [Eastman and Burkhart] have been leaders in a movement toward the realization of this platform for youngsters in Rochester, London, Rome, Paris, and Stockholm.[6]

THE EASTMAN BEQUEST

In his will, Eastman bequeathed an additional million dollars to the Rochester Dental Dispensary. Burkhart may have expected more, based on Eastman's promise "to do more for dentistry" when the School of Medicine and Dentistry was founded in 1920. On the other hand, getting the European clinics built and operating occupied much of Burkhart's time during the 1930s, and for that pleasant task he would be his own boss.

Basil Bibby later had a different take on why Eastman never stepped up to the plate to support dental research in the same magnanimous way that he had supported education and clinical care, especially for indigent children. According to Bibby, Burkhart had told Eastman that "we know all we need

when the "dean" arrived in European capitals with his tall silk hat to dedicate yet another Eastman dental clinic, he commanded much respect. One newspaper would say of Burkhart, "His work and hobby was dentistry." Clinical dentistry, that is, since Burkhart's dream of establishing a dental school never materialized.

Burkhart would argue that he was not anti-research. After all, the Rochester Dental Dispensary was founded with a new research lab, and various investigators throughout the 1920s conducted research into the causes of caries. According to the 1928 annual report, in the furnishing and equipment of the research laboratory in memory of her husband, Mrs. Rudolph H. Hofheinz became interested in furthering dental research and "contributed a substantial sum for research work." The 1928 report further notes, "Dr. Philip Jay has been engaged by the School of Medicine

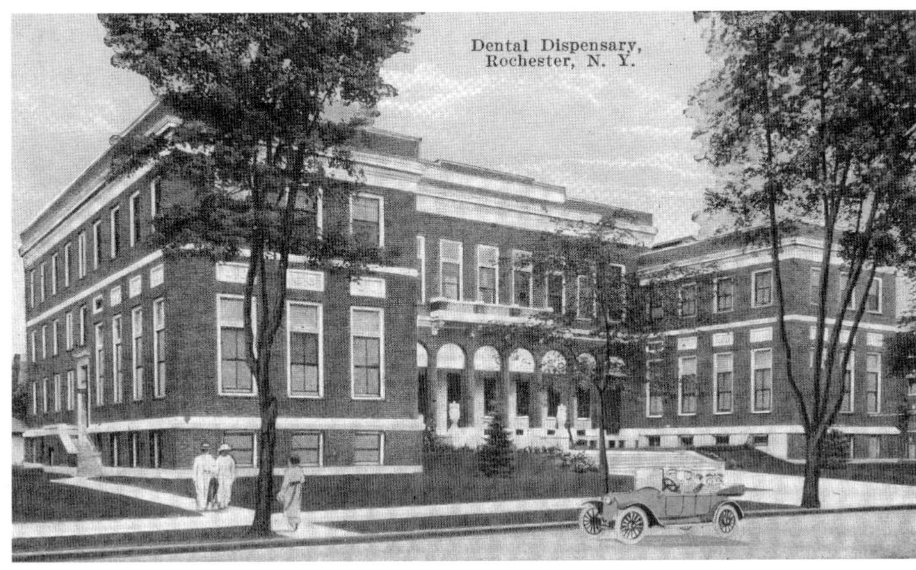

*The Eastman Dental Dispensary became such a
landmark that postcards were made of it.*

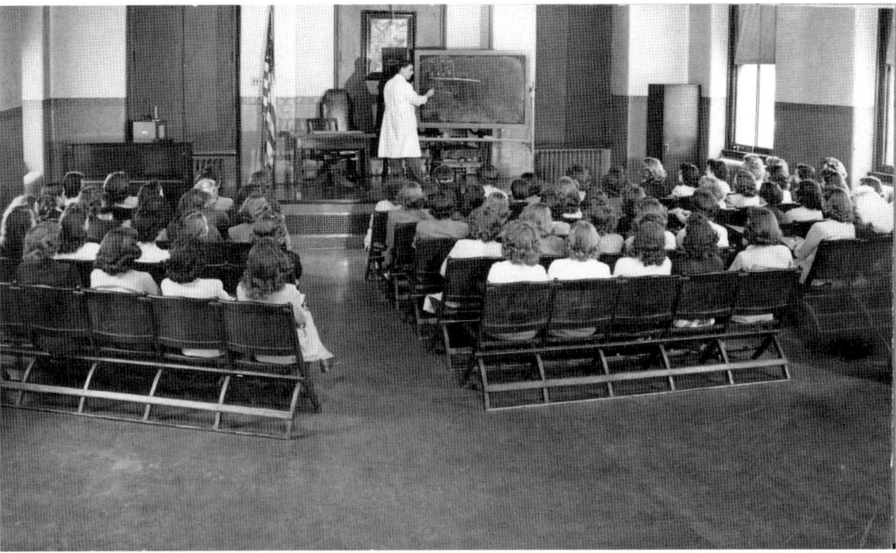

Classroom of the School for Dental Hygienists

Trustees	$16,000
George Eastman	$53,000
Patient fees	$14,000
Interest	$4,000
City of Rochester	$20,000
Hygienist Tuition	$6,000

to know about dentistry," thereby discouraging him from taking the final step of financing a major dental research program before his death.

Clearly, Eastman was not opposed to research. In 1886, he established the first industrial laboratory devoted solely to photographic emulsion research under the aegis of a University of Rochester undergraduate chemist. In 1912, in order to keep up with the photographic research done by 800 scientists employed by the Bayer Company in Germany, Eastman imported Dr. Charles Edward Kenneth Mees from London to start the most modern photographic chemical research laboratory in the world. He supported Flexner and Rhees in the hiring of George Whipple, a research man through and through.

Financially, the operating pattern for the Rochester Dental Dispensary/Eastman Dental Dispensary had changed very little during the years when Burkhart was in charge: In 1920, the dispensary's income of $114,000 was received approximately as follows:

The budget did not change appreciably throughout the Burkhart years, because disbursements in 1938 totaled $118,000. In that year $39,530 was spent on dental work, $40,259 on general treatment, $14,224 on repairing tooth irregularities, $11,536 on surgical work, and the remainder on extractions, x-rays, building expenses, library, clinics, lectures, and office expenses. Patient visits totaled 77,522, and prophylactic treatments in schools were given to 92,503 children. While Burkhart eschewed research and education (except for the hygienists and through the hygienists educating school children), he felt his main mission was preventive dentistry for children and the way to achieve this was through prophylactic treatments and filling cavities.

In subsequent years, the City of Rochester's contributions were increased to $25,000 per annum (1921) and then to $30,000 (1931–41), but at no time did these contributions cover the full costs of the program. Annual contributions by the early trustees continued well beyond the five years originally agreed upon with Eastman. All fifteen or sixteen trustees each donated $1,000 annually until Eastman's death in 1932. (Presumably with the additional $1 million bequest, annual contributions by trustees may have been discontinued.) Approximately $500,000 per annum was taken from the endowment for capital expenses up until the dental center moved in 1976. In spite of this, the endowment's market value increased from $9 million in 1955 to $27 million in 1975—slipping a bit from its peak of $35 million in 1973. During the same period, annual income from the endowment increased from $317,000 in 1955 to $600,000 in 1965 and to $1,050,000 in 1975.

In 1928, as we have seen, plans for the dental component of the School of Medicine and Dentistry were discontinued, and the University of Rochester developed the Dental Research Fellowship Program. At the same time, a consultation dental clinic was established in Strong Memorial Hospital's outpatient department. The Rockefeller grant—to support dental research and training in the fundamental biological background underlying dental health problems—that set up the fellowship program in 1929 expired after five years. Other sources of funding were found and this program became the foundation of the current Center for Oral Biology.

DEPRESSION, WAR, AND CRISIS

In 1955, Basil Bibby described the shortage of well-prepared dental investigators as the situation existed in 1930:

> There was little or no biological research in dentistry in this country and men trained in Europe were doing most of what was going on. Thus, the School of Medicine and Dentistry was unable to find for its faculty either dentists who could do worthwhile research in the biological sciences or scientists with a background in dental problems. . . . Because of the shortage of well-prepared dental investigators, funds, which might have been used for dental research, were spent for other purposes.

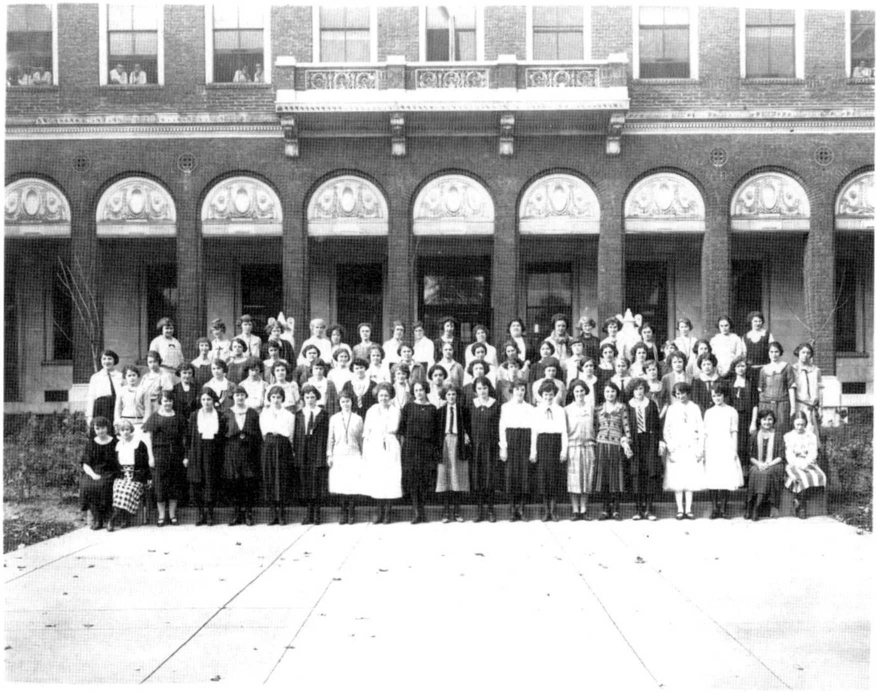

Probably a graduating class of the School of Dental Hygienists.
Note dentists in the windows.

Thus, "a vicious circle existed which prevented any forward movement in dental science. No scientific research was being done because there were no men trained to do scientific dental research; there were no men trained to do scientific dental research because no scientific research centers provided opportunity." Bibby continued:

> First-class research institutions could not afford to sacrifice going research programs until they were sure some research of scientific value would result. Fortunately, anxiety and isolation foster a sense of unity . . . and thus the feeling of not being wanted by dentistry contributed a group consciousness and sense of purpose. . . . To break the vicious circle, it was necessary to gamble that if dentists were given the opportunity some of them would develop the ability to do worthwhile research and dentists would ultimately organize their own research activities and training centers.

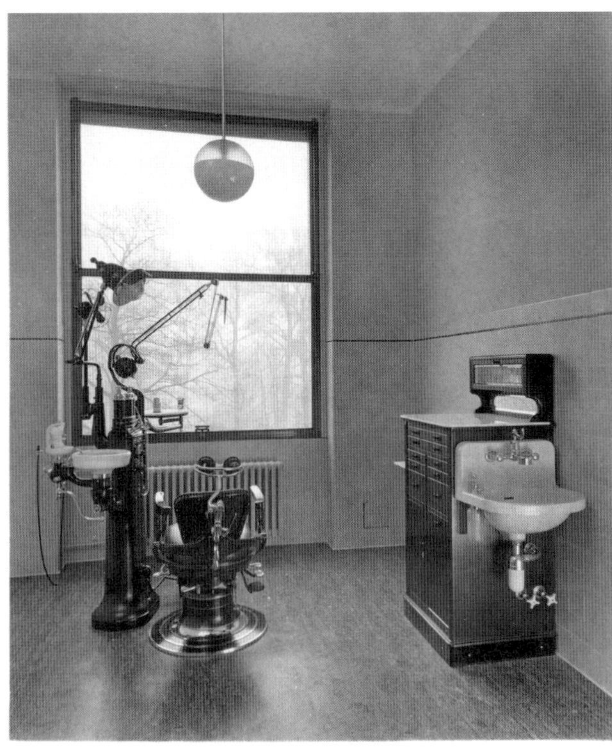

Dental operatory

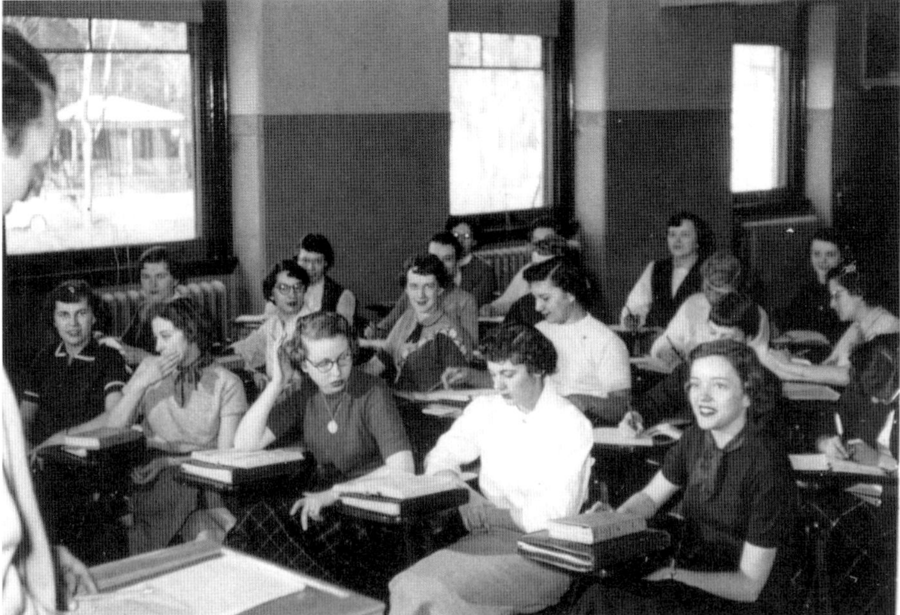

Hygienists in class

Dr. Whipple had the necessary faith in dentistry and was able to justify it by pointing out that a nucleus of research at Johns Hopkins University had stimulated research throughout America and brought about a science revolution in medicine. He believed that if some dentists were provided with a chance to develop as research workers the time would come to appreciate the importance of scientific research. It is only those of us who lived through the metamorphosis from lonely, almost suspect workers in an inconsequential and slightly disreputable field of investigation to full membership in respected scientific circles who can fully appreciate the progress which has been made to dental research. Among us are men who were the first dental members of some scientific societies and men who held the first full-time dental research appointments in American universities and who received the first professional and administrative appointments in dental schools on the basis of research rather than clinical skills.[7]

Since this was the state of dental research in a university research program, it is not particularly surprising that Burkhart did not want to divert funds from the Eastman endowment to something as suspect as research. According to Basil Bibby, the only time Burkhart's opposition to supporting the School of Medicine and Dentistry dental research program was overridden by the trustees (half of whom were also University of Rochester trustees) resulted in annual contributions in amounts ranging from $10,000 to $35,000. This began in the late 1930s after the original five-year Rockefeller grant had expired. The effort to make these contributions was spearheaded by Charles F. Hutchison, University of Rochester trustee, Eastman Dental Dispensary trustee, trustee member of the School of Medicine and Dentistry advisory committee, retired Kodak emulsion maker, George Eastman's next-door neighbor, and husband of Eastman's secretary of forty years, Alice K. Whitney Hutchison. Charles Hutchison was impressed by the research being done by the dental research fellows at the university and insisted that part of the Eastman endowment be used to support it.

Burkhart felt that his mission was to protect and further the interests of clinical and educational dentistry—including the school for hygienists and the training of interns. These interests would be damaged if the Rochester Dental Dispensary's endowment, the largest in dentistry, was allowed to pass into the control of the School of Medicine and Dentistry, which Burkhart felt had no real interest in dentistry beyond research.

Thus, and not surprisingly, money was at the root of the rocky quality of the relationship between the Eastman Dental Center and the School of Medicine and Dentistry. The school, despite Eastman's hopes and intention, never consistently used the funding allegedly set aside for things dental for that purpose. The dental center endowment and other of its funds and resources remained a temptation to the school. At the same time, the dental center has worried about being plundered by the school if the relationship got too close. In order to prevent this loss to the profession, according to Dr. Ralph Voorhis, a dentist and Burkhart's son-in-law, Burkhart decided that since he could find no one else besides himself who could do it, he would stay on his post of duty to the end.[8]

* * *

In 1940, Dr. Burkhart celebrated his fiftieth year as a dentist. At that time, the *Journal of the Dental Society of the State of New York* wrote, "He may well be considered at this time the outstanding leader of dentistry in the United States." By then, Burkhart was regularly referred to as "the famed director of the Rochester Dental Dispensary." (The name was changed to Eastman Dental Dispensary in 1941.) He was receiving awards, medals and testimonial dinners for his "distinguished contributions," "outstandingly wise and efficient administration," and "masterly piece of leadership down the years" at an astonishing rate. He was continually being honored by the American Dental Association, the U.S. Army Dental Corps, and the International Dental Congress for the "unique talents that he brought to a unique position," for "extending the prestige of American dentistry throughout the world," for "his outstanding accomplishments in the field of children's preventive dentistry," and "in recognition of his distinguished contributions to preventive dentistry and public health throughout the world."

By the late 1930s, Burkhart's principal duties, according to newspaper reports, "consist of seeing that [the European] clinics founded by Mr. Eastman are kept running according to the terms of their contracts. A close check on the operation of the European clinics is necessary . . . to insure their

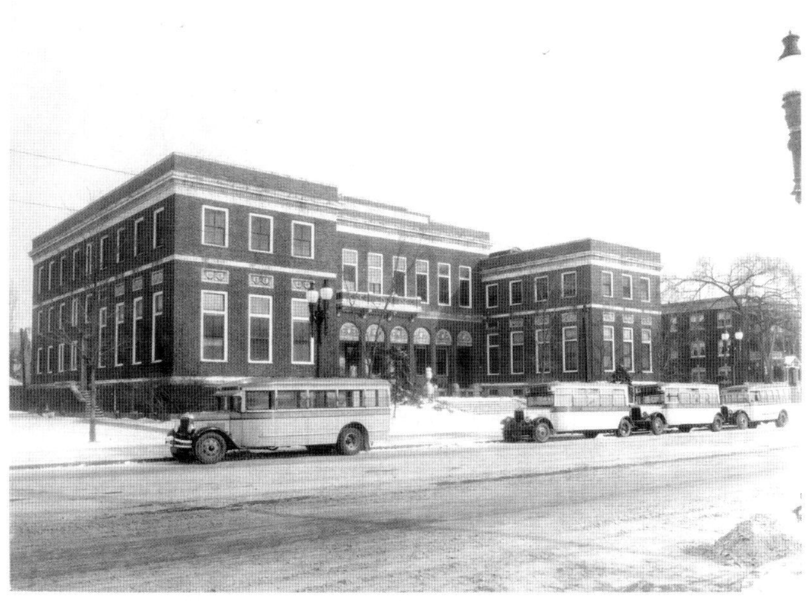

Buses deliver school children to the dispensary.

sound and proper regulation. This he usually accomplishes with the heads of respective governments in Italy, for instance, with his long-time friend, Benito Mussolini." For this purpose Burkhart traveled to Europe two or three times each year and clearly reveled in rubbing shoulders with royalty.

During the 1930s and 40s, he was presented to three kings of England—George V, Edward VIII, and George VI. He met with King Albert and Queen Elizabeth as well as King Leopold III and Queen Astrid of Belgium; King Victor Emanuel and Queen Helena of Italy; and was decorated by the King of Sweden. As late as 1939, he was referring to Benito Mussolini as his "long-term friend." He recalled the following dialogue from that visit when the Rome clinic director was a Blackshirt appointed by Mussolini:

Il Duce remarks upon the fine building in which the clinic was housed.

Burkhart: "But Your Excellency, bricks and stone and mortar make a fine building; they do not make an institution."

Il Duce: "I will see that they carry out your instructions." And he did.

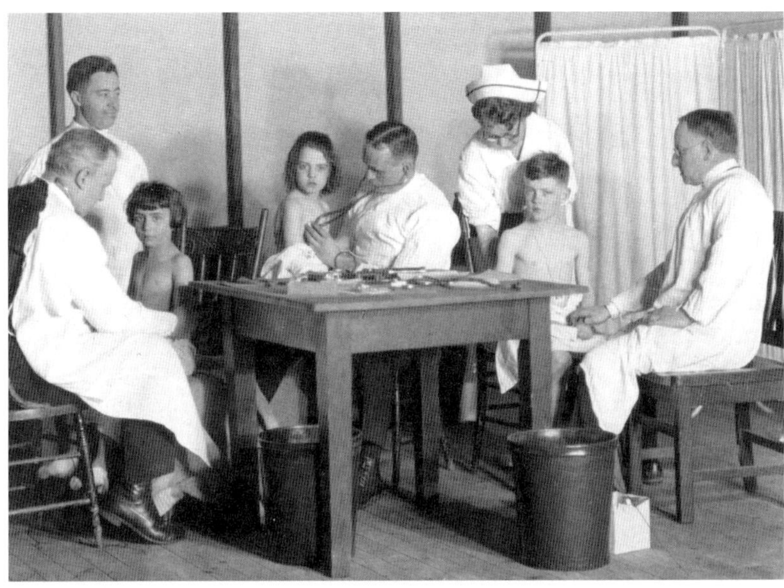

Checking in for a tonsillectomy (Author's collection)

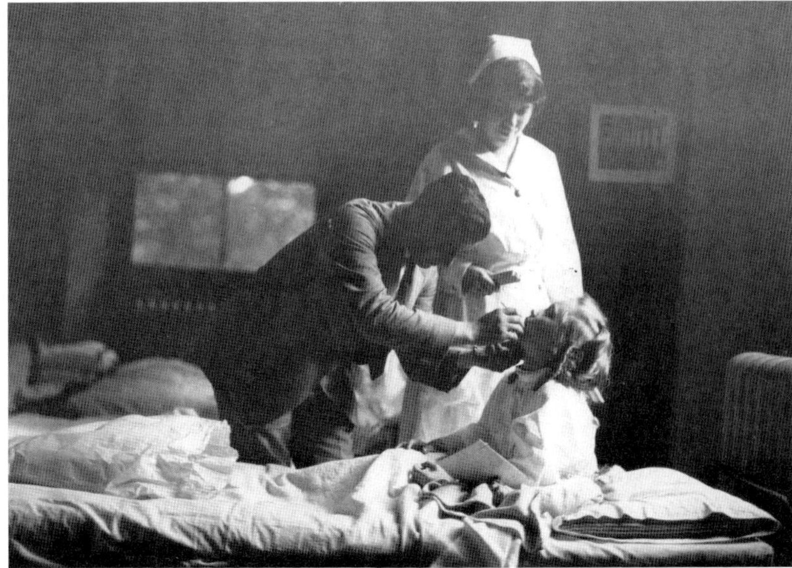

Checking a patient after a tonsillectomy (Author's collection)

THE CLINIC THRIVES—FOR A WHILE

The 1930s marked the high point for the Rochester Dental Dispensary in terms of clinical visits despite the fact that a shortage of interns and residents to staff the clinic was beginning to be its biggest problem. The Rochester Dental Dispensary and Forsyth Dental Infirmary in Boston had been the principal places for dental graduates to obtain postgraduate experience, but in the 1930s dental internships opened up in many hospitals. By 1950, there were 150 other hospitals offering internships and providing credit toward the new specialty boards. Most of the country's fifty dental schools offered postgraduate training. The U.S. Public Health Service offered fifty rotating internships with specialty board accreditation and higher salaries.

The nation went to war in 1941, and the military draft continued until the late 1950s. Recent dental graduates were needed in the armed services, and the clinical experience they received there surpassed what the dispensary could provide. Despite a two-thirds reduction in staff that forced the closing of two services—surgery and orthodontia—the Eastman Dental Dispensary reported record visits during 1943. At the annual meeting in January 1944, William Bausch, the original president of the board of trustees, was elected to yet another term.

Dr. Burkhart reported on the war years' activities. The Eastman Dental Dispensary was staffed by ten dentists, as compared to thirty-five before the Army and Navy made their demands. In March of 1943 the surgical department closed, but not before 145 operations had been performed, bringing the total since 1917 to 37,983. In July, the orthodontic department closed, leaving 500 patients without service. Teeth cleaning continued. Squads of hygienists still visited the schools twice a year, although many recent hygienist graduates did join the armed services. Emergency work was undertaken at the dispensary for the air cadets of the 51st College Training Detachment and the V12 unit of the University of Rochester.

Besides Bausch, the all-male board of trustees remained heavy with friends of the late George Eastman: F. Harper Sibley, grandson of the founder of Western Union; Charles F. Hutchison, Kodak emulsion maker and husband of Eastman's long-time secretary; Milton K. Robinson, Kodak attorney; Bernard Finucane, Kodak contractor; George H. Clark, son of an original Kodak director and a large Kodak stockholder himself; Sol Heumann and Charles

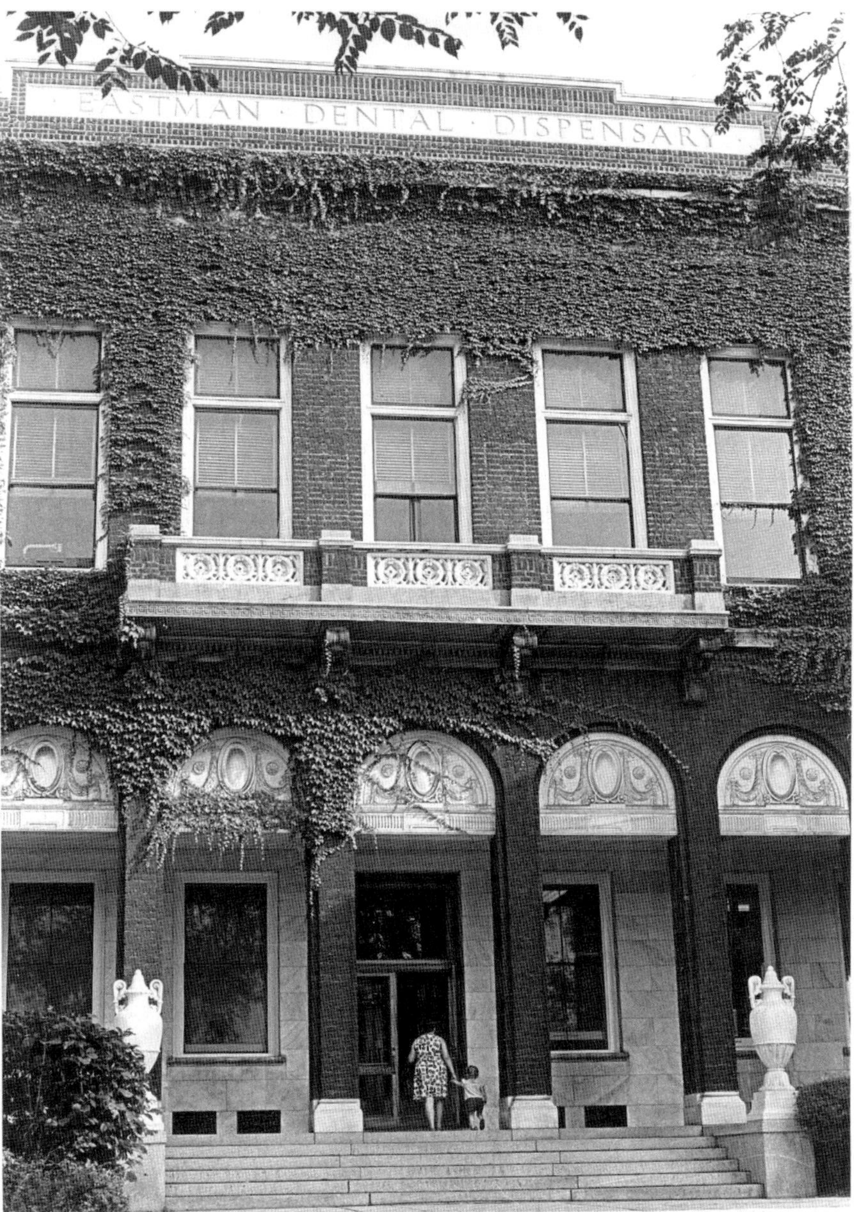

Ivy takes over.

Schlegel, Rochester businessmen; Alphonse Pieper, president of Ritter Manufacturing Company; Frank W. Lovejoy, president of Kodak; William G. Kaelber, architect or consulting architect of all Eastman dental clinics, the University of Rochester, Eastman Theatre and School of Music, and the Kodak office; Dr. Audley Stewart, Eastman's personal physician; Dr. Edward Ingersoll, surgeon in charge of tonsillectomies; and James Spinning, head of the city's school district.

When World War II was over and Britain was emerging with a socialist government that revamped its system of delivering medical and dental care, Dr. Harvey Burkhart took to the stump warning of socialism's evils. In April 1946, the *New York Herald Tribune* quoted him as asserting, "Preventive dentistry would be largely lost sight of in the socialized system of practice. The socialist setup might harm preventive work. . . . Since the English have inaugurated what they call 'panel dentists,' standards of professional practice have deteriorated."

In covering the same speech, the *New York Times* reported that the "dean of New York dentistry" was addressing 10,000 dentists at the seventy-eighth annual meeting of the Dental Society of New York State as a trustee of that group. He painted a dismal picture of returning to the state that existed before he and George Eastman reformed things. His reasoning was that socialized dentistry would make dentistry a "tooth-pulling profession." Under such regimentation, a dentist would not get paid for filling cavities, Burkhart articulated, and therefore would not bother with them. "Interest in preventive measures would be forgotten, along with the restorative processes, since a dentist would have a permanent job and be interested only in his stipend. . . . Even if there were arrangements made for dentists to care for inlay work, this country has not the manpower or facilities to do the job adequately."[9]

Burkhart urged the professionals to "exert their influence to the utmost to prevent legislation . . . enacting laws for socializing medicine, dentistry and other professions." But he ended his talk on an upbeat note, adding that he was not pessimistic about the future nor did he "believe that socialized medicine or dentistry would be established in the United States, but that private dental health insurance plans might be introduced to pay a large part of the cost of dental health."[10] Prepaid plans whereby a good part of the cost of reconstructive or restorative dentistry was underwritten by private insurance, Burkhart asserted, would be a good thing to come out of the "existing agitation."[11] Burkhart failed to understand the need and potential impact on dental

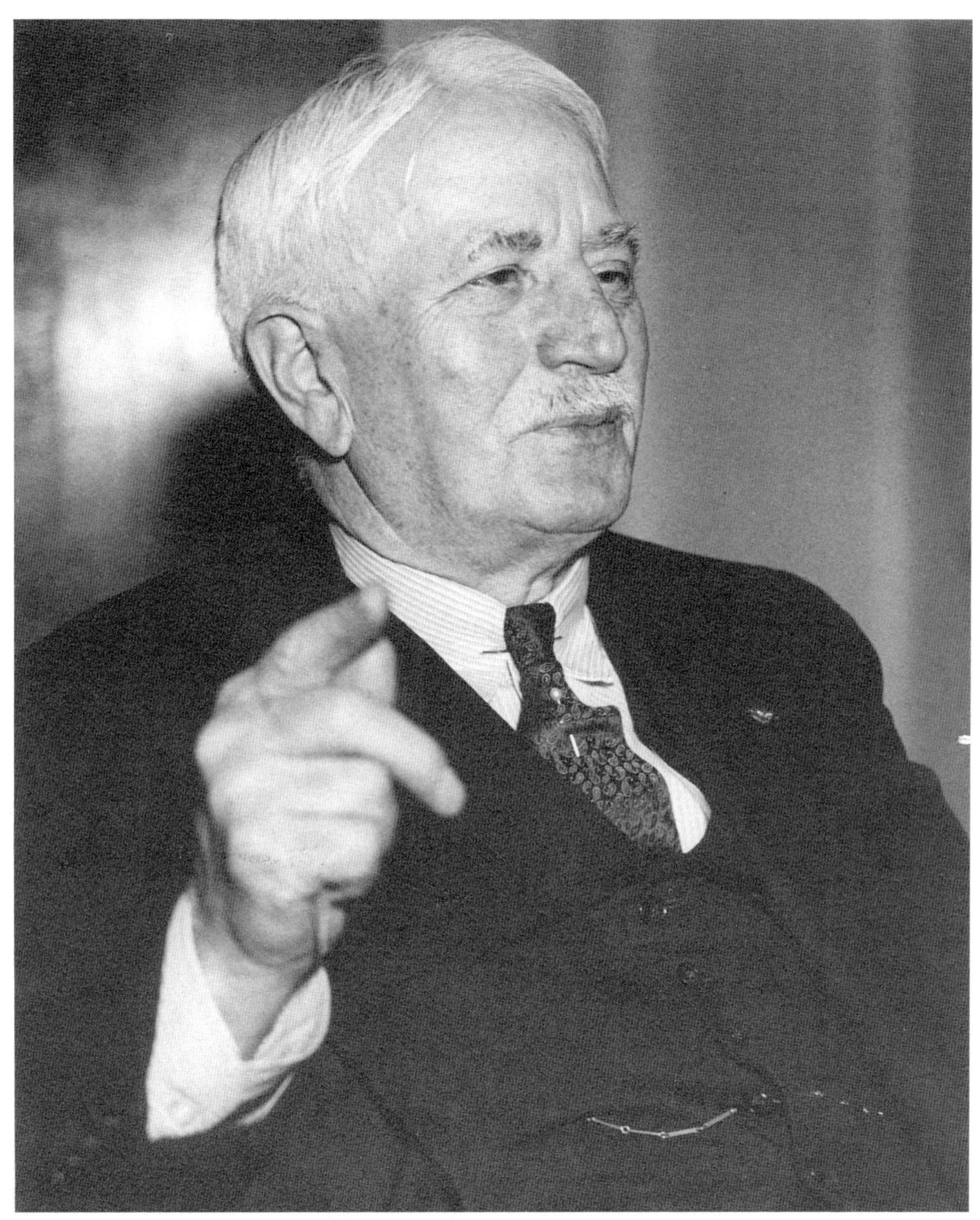

Dr. Burkhart in the 1940s

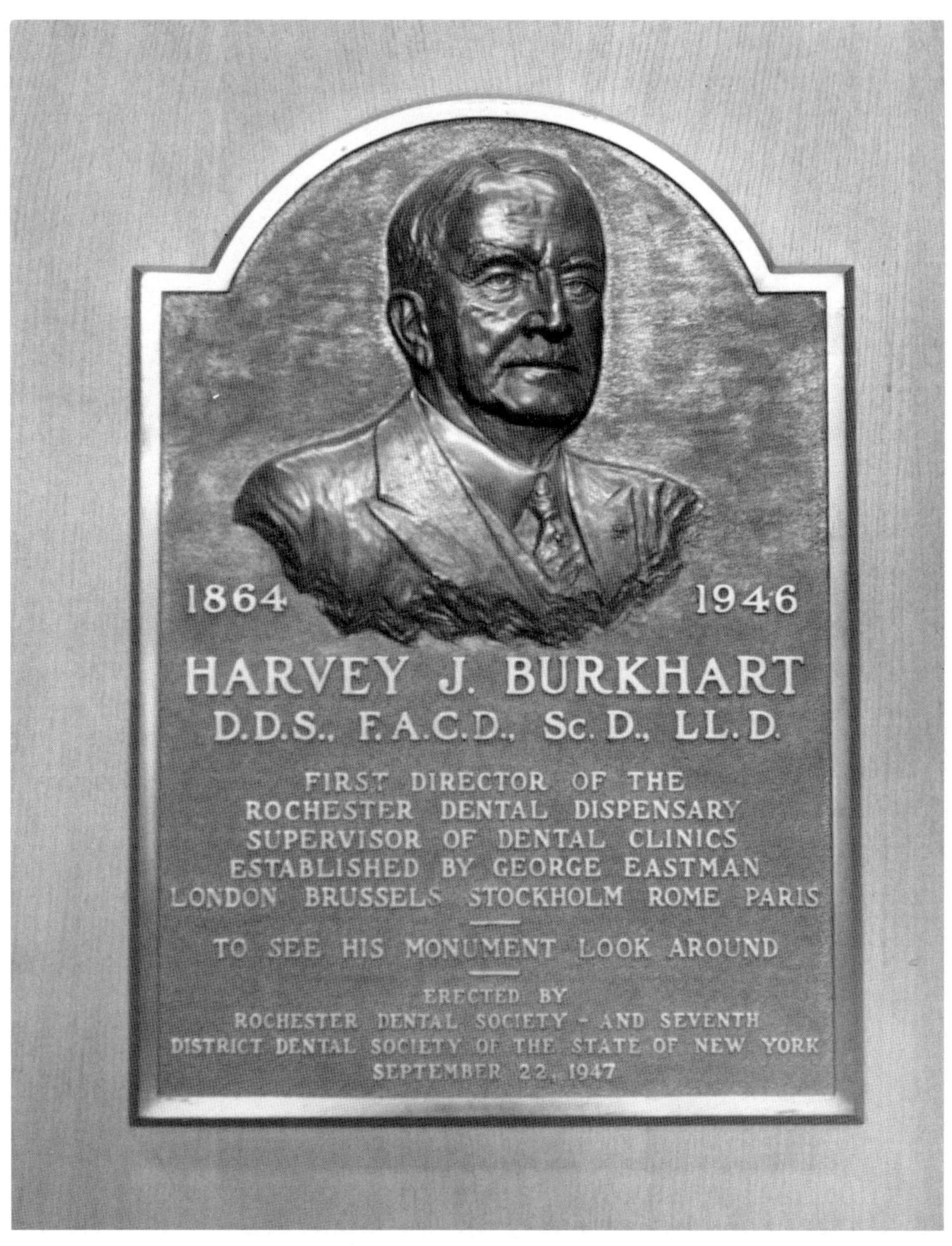

The plaque erected by the Rochester Dental Society and Seventh District Dental Society of the State of New York in 1947

disease and dental practice and in this he was not entirely alone. Until World War II, many people considered the loss of teeth and a full set of dentures the inevitable consequence of aging. With increasing affluence in the postwar period and the flowering of dental research, more teeth were restored and retained in the United States and other industrialized nations, though gum disease and tooth loss remained a serious problem among the poor.

Shortly after this April 1946 speech, it was announced in the Rochester newspapers of the day that Harvey Burkhart was planning a European trip to inspect the war damage and assist in the reorganization of the clinics: "Dr. Harvey J. Burkhart, 84, an international authority on dental surgery and a calm white-haired little man who met Hitler [at a Berlin Rotary Club meeting in 1934] and Mussolini in prewar years, is planning to return to Europe to take up his life's work where the Nazis interrupted it." The hobnail boots of Nazi soldiers had chewed up the floors of the Brussels and Paris clinics and the Allied bombing of the Rome railroad terminal damaged the Rome clinic. Worst hit of all was the London clinic. Burkhart applied for United Nations Relief and Rehabilitation Administration (UNNRA) grants to rebuild. "There is a tremendous field for dentistry among children in Europe," he said as he prepared to sail to Europe, "because European children have suffered from lack of proper nutrition and the absence of dentists in war."[12]

Dr. Burkhart never made that trip to Europe. In September 1946, a month after his eighty-fifth birthday, he was driving with his wife along Central Avenue in Rochester when he suffered a fatal heart attack.

EPILOGUE: THE COUP THAT FAILED

A year's delay followed Burkhart's death before a new Eastman Dental Dispensary director was appointed. During that period, University of Rochester representatives announced that they were taking over the Eastman Dental Dispensary. Dental trustees sought legal counsel. The Nixon Hargrave law firm determined that the School of Medicine and Dentistry had not activated its agreement to teach dentistry in more than twenty-five years, therefore the agreement was no longer binding and the university had no legal authority to appoint a director, take over the endowment, or use the dispensary for other than existing purposes. Writing some years later, Dr. Basil Bibby concluded that some Eastman Dental Dispensary trustees were "jealous of the independence of the [dispensary] and did not want it to become subservient to any other organization."[13] The age of the director (he was in his eighties at a time when the mandatory retirement age at the university was sixty-five) followed by a year's standoff resulted in a general decline of the plant—yet the new director would find it "adequately maintained." The war's decimation of the staff began at the end of Burkhart's tenure and was not reversed by a year's interregnum or the predatory inclinations of the School of Medicine and Dentistry.

Finally, a plan for preserving the interests of both the dispensary and the School of Medicine and Dentistry was developed. The University of Rochester would seek and nominate candidates for Eastman Dental Dispensary director. From among them, the Eastman Dental Dispensary board would choose a new director. Basil Bibby was chosen and invited to be the new director during the summer of 1947.

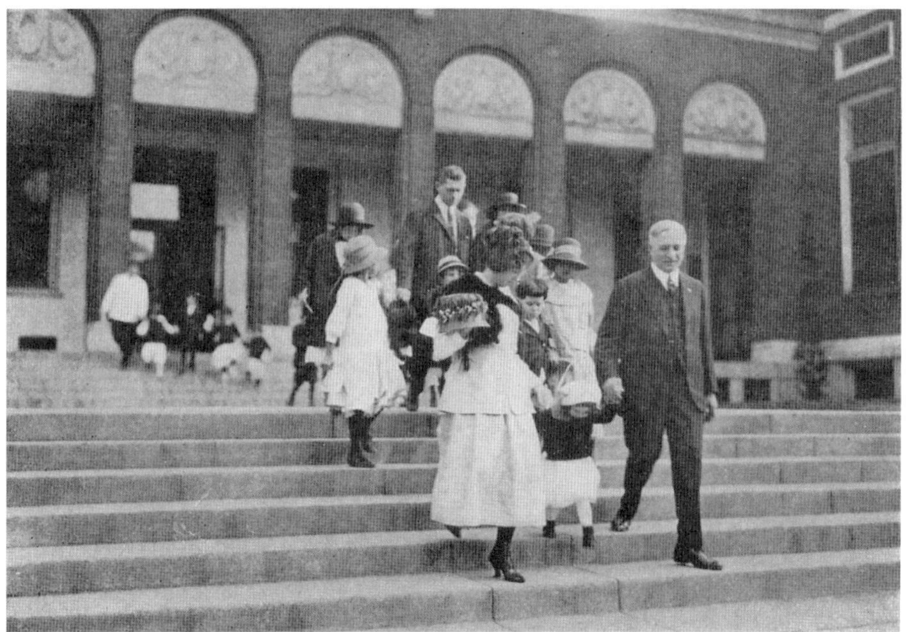

Dr. Burkhart, Director of the Dispensary, leading the group.

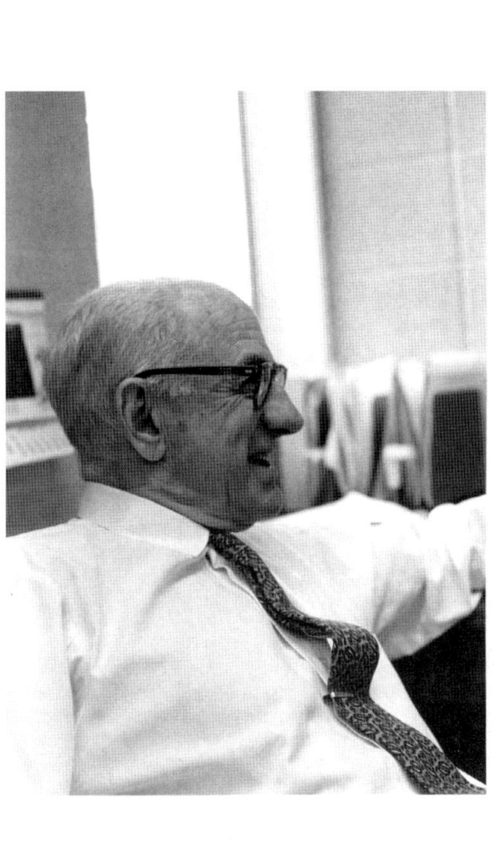
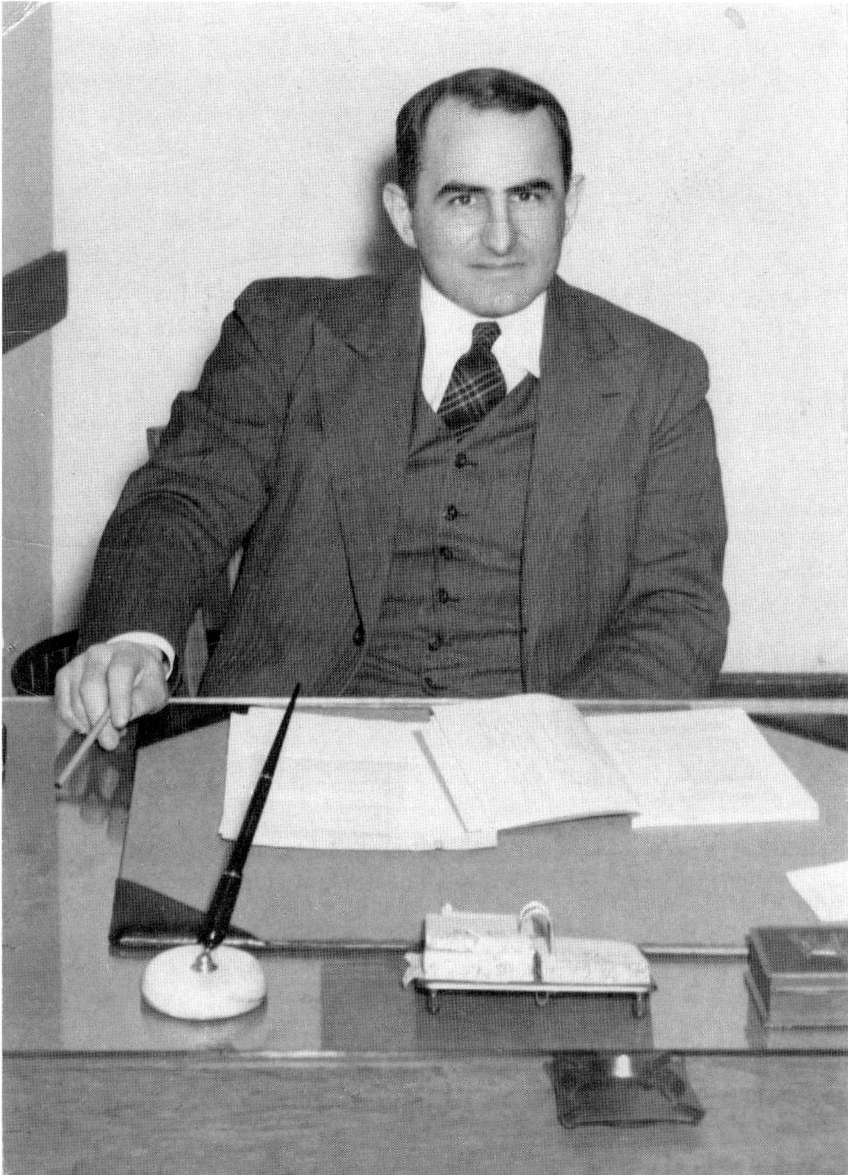
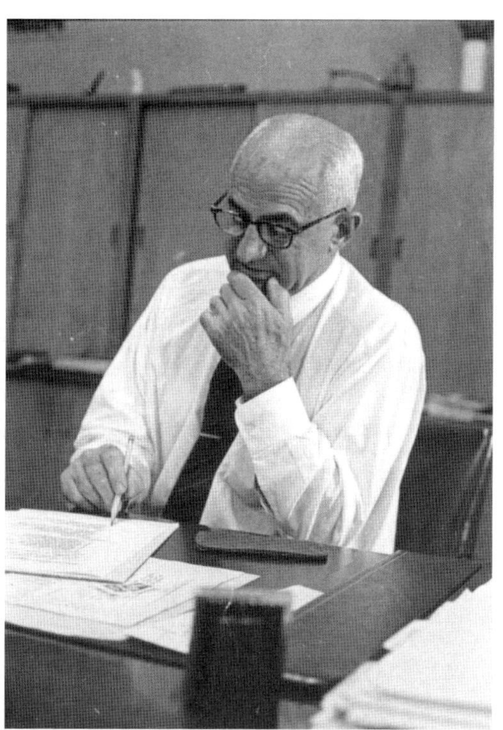

Dr. Basil Bibby

Chapter Five

THE BIBBY YEARS

CRADLE OF ACADEMIC DENTISTRY

It is worth emphasizing that activities which have been developed at the Dispensary are unique in American dentistry.
Nowhere else is there a dental institution which is combining, as do the teaching hospitals in medicine, responsibility for
community health, the training of graduate dentists and the carrying forward of basic clinically related research.

Basil Bibby, DMD, PhD, 1959

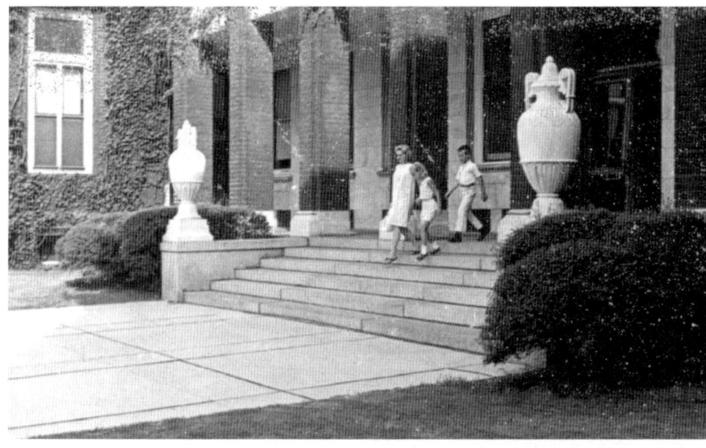

Patients and parent leaving the dispensary

WHEN VISITORS OR STAFF MEMBERS ENTERED HIS OFFICE, Dr. Basil Bibby characteristically had his feet on the desk and was chewing on the end of his glasses. Photographs often show him in a white lab coat—appropriate to one whose life centered on clinical research. Although he would enlarge the physical footprint of the Eastman Dental Dispensary (and change its name to the Eastman Dental Center in 1965) Bibby was fond of saying, "Bricks and mortar do not do research; it's people." Mentoring those people would be a hallmark of his tenure from 1947 to 1970.

The agreed-upon plan for choosing a new director preserved the interests of both the University of Rochester and the Eastman Dental Dispensary: The School of Medicine and Dentistry nominated candidates for director, and the Eastman Dental Dispensary board chose Basil Bibby from among the nominees.

Bibby arrived at (and returned to) the University of Rochester in 1947 from Tufts University dental school in Boston. At Tufts, Bibby had been professor of bacteriology and the school's youngest-ever (age thirty-five) dean. He also taught medical history, organized a major research program, and was active in building up the library. During World War II, he was a consultant to the Armed Forces Library and for projects involving the indexing of medical literature. Later, President Eisenhower named Bibby to the board of regents of a new National Library of Medicine (now the largest in the world). When Basil Bibby left Rochester in 1940, both George Whipple, dean of the School of Medicine and Dentistry, and Alan Valentine, president of the University of Rochester, had assured him "that he would be invited back to Rochester as soon as the university 'took over' the dispensary." But thanks to Dr. Burkhart, to the dispensary's endowment created by George Eastman, and to the determination of the Eastman Dental Dispensary's board that the dispensary not be swallowed up by the university, that takeover did not happen. However, the dispensary board saw that Bibby was the most qualified candidate, so in a sense he was the unanimous choice of both institutions.[1]

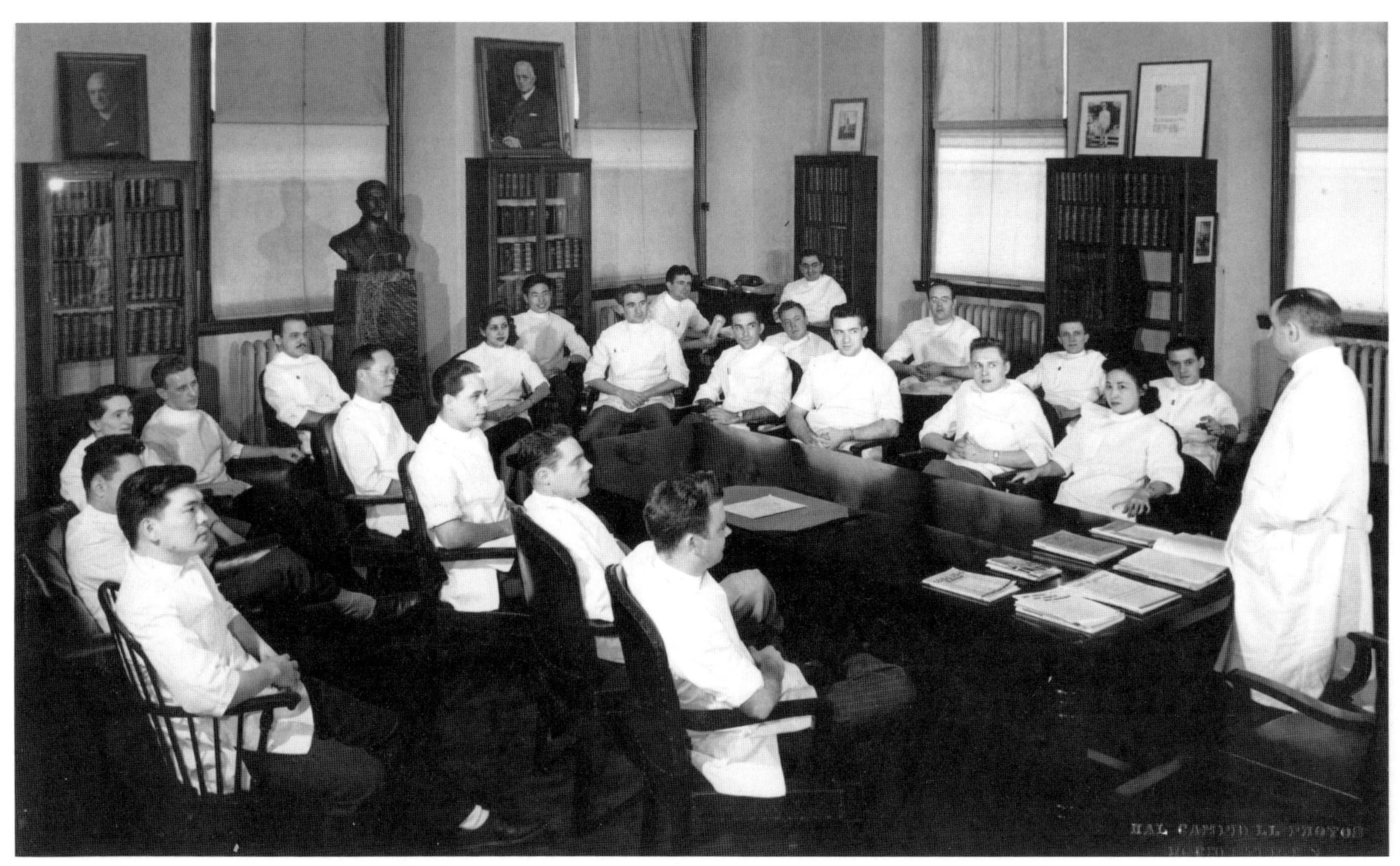

Intern staff with Dr. Bibby, 1948

The dispensary board also realized that Burkhart had stayed on too long and had neglected clinical research in order to maintain independence. The most explicit policy direction from the board was that Bibby "co-operate fully with School of Medicine and Dentistry and initiate research." Nevertheless, the providing of dental care for indigent children was to continue. And there was stronger interest by the trustees than Bibby anticipated in maintaining the training school for hygienists. Bibby's courtesy call on Whipple produced no recommendations from Whipple except an offer of any help the school could provide. Upon his return to Rochester as director of the dispensary, Bibby was also named professor of dentistry at the School of Medicine and Dentistry.

During his initial period, the new director received almost no support from local dentists or state agencies. Dentists were still smarting that they had not been consulted when the Rochester Dental Dispensary was set up, beyond a rudimentary check of preliminary architectural plans. According to Bibby, Burkhart ran the operation single-handedly, and other dentists were not allowed any opportunity to participate in the development of the dispensary. There is plenty of evidence that this was the case.

Many dentists were disappointed that a university-sponsored candidate rather than a local dental-society candidate was chosen as Burkhart's successor. Friends of Burkhart were disappointed that one of his associates, someone who would continue his policies, had not been appointed. Some dentists were suspicious of Bibby, whose brother in New Zealand had developed a successful public health dental nurses program that used young women, trained over two years, to staff school clinics and take care of the fillings and extractions needed by children. Even though Basil Bibby had said early on that this kind of program was not politically acceptable in the United States, dentists still feared that this might be the first step in weakening the American fee-for-service practice. New York State dentists even blocked Bibby from getting a state license to practice dentistry, but he remained a member of the American Dental Association through his Massachusetts membership. They insisted that he should sit for the state boards and did not offer him the courtesy of awarding him a New York State license.

In a 1966 address to the American Dental Association, Bibby pointed out fallacies in the three main preventive dentistry tenets—oral hygiene, proper diet, and regular visits to the dentist. Dentistry may have become "a victim of its own propaganda and is in danger of persuading itself that there is no possibility of anything better than what have become conventional beliefs." Visits to the dentists, per se, did not avert caries, he pointed out. Although early detection would obviate extraction, "it has never been shown that early treatment had any effect on caries in other teeth." Indeed, "during preparation of a proximal cavity, incidental abrasion or scratching can make the adjacent sound surface more susceptible to caries." He held that oral hygiene in the form of tooth brushing was not a major determinant of caries either, although it was effective against periodontal disease. As for diet, he put more emphasis on eating the more beneficial foods than on eating the least harmful foods, pointing to the fact that the poorly nourished populations of the world had the best teeth.[2]

Basil Bibby believed that the goal of any profession, including dentistry, was to put itself out of business. He held that caries could be prevented through the use of topical fluoride and by limiting the intake of carbohydrates, not by tooth brushing. Thus, while the filling and extraction of indigent children's teeth would continue at the dispensary, the goal of preventive dentistry was to make these procedures obsolete.

NEW VISIONS, NEW DIRECTIONS

William Bausch died at about the same time that Harvey Burkhart did, after having served as chairman of the board since the dispensary's inception in 1915. Bausch had been a primary influence in interesting George Eastman in preventive dentistry for indigent children. Businessman Harper Sibley, grandson of Hiram Sibley, founder and first president of Western Union, replaced Bausch as board chairman. He was a member—long before George Eastman's time—of Rochester's wealthiest family. Young Sibley and his wife, Georgiana Farr Sibley, were already well known in post-World War II benevolent circles worldwide through their support of the new United Nations and the international YMCA and YWCA. With new and energetic young board members, the Eastman Dental Dispensary was being revitalized.

Each year, Burkhart had prepared a beautifully printed and illustrated annual report, but the text was often the same An exception came during the 1930s when a few new paragraphs were added as each of the European clinics was built. Thwarted at home by circumstances and personalities in starting and leading a dental school, Burkhart spent the Depression years getting

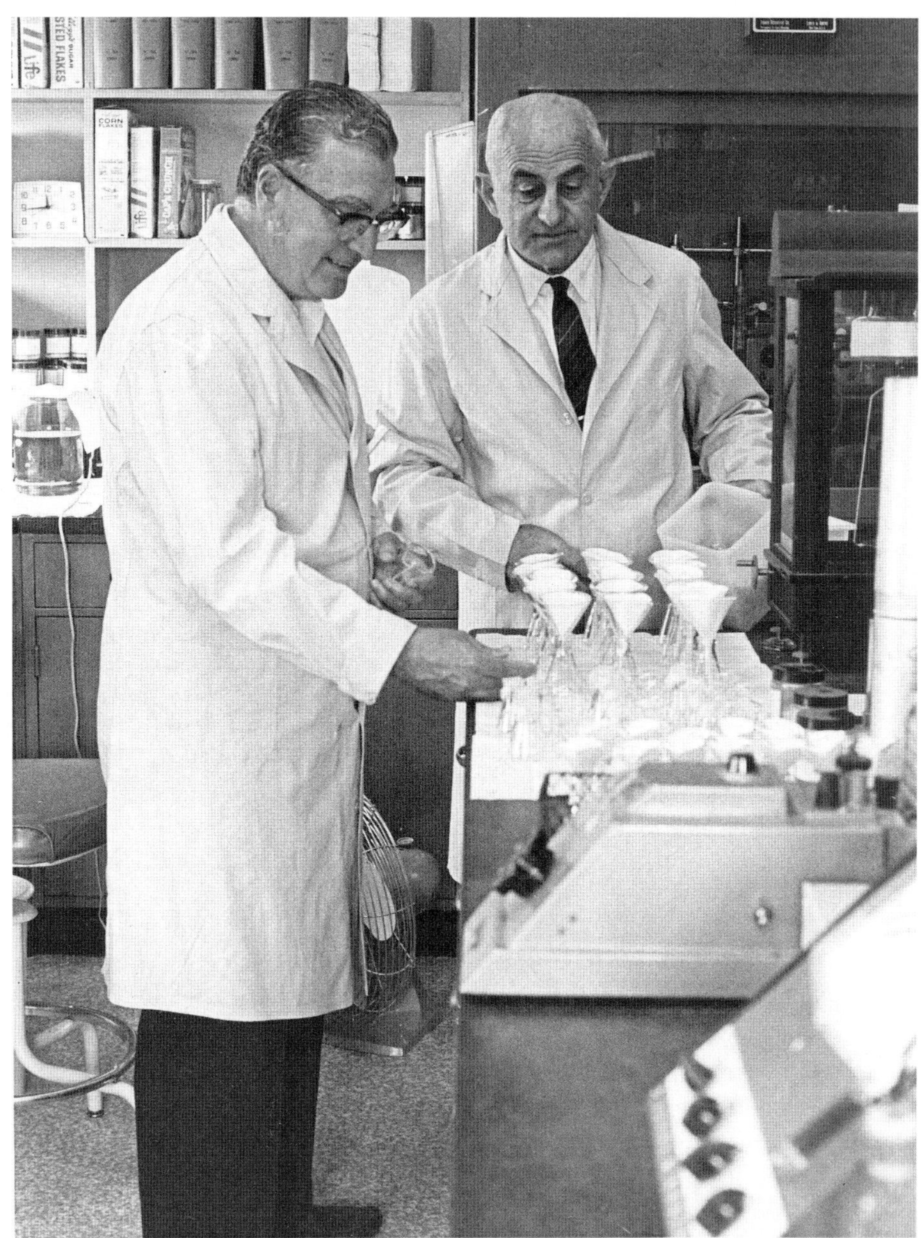

Research

the five European clinics built and operating—not a small achievement. The Rochester dispensary remained on hold, ossified, except that clinic visits increased each year and these statistics made the annual reports look as if all programs were growing. In the early 1930s it was not a problem to obtain young dentists to operate the clinic. World War II changed that, and when Bibby arrived, he was faced with a shortage of dentists.

Bibby asked for and received from the trustees time to assess the situation before he made a statement of basic policy and objectives. He took two years of "orientation and watchful waiting" before writing his first report—a ten-page typescript at the end of 1949 that would impress the trustees that he was on the right track. Then he began to recruit a teaching and research faculty.

DENTAL RESEARCH
DURING THE BIBBY YEARS[3]

Bibby envisioned a world-class center of dental research but he also realized he had to develop the center's clinical programs, create a first-rate postgraduate dental program, and modernize the dental hygienist program. His effort, he said at the time of his appointment, "enjoyed the highest level of cooperation with dental research and basic science departments at the medical school." Bibby proposed an active research program by full-time salaried researchers and a program for training them. He outlined eight possible sources of financial support: income from endowment securities; annual grants from the City of Rochester; grants from the U.S, Public Health Service and National Institute of Dental Research; tuition; research grants from private sources; private endowments; annual state education grants; and grants from industrial plants.

In 1950, the administrative structure for dental research and postgraduate programs of the dispensary and the School of Medicine and Dentistry assumed the form that continued until the merger of the two institutions in 1995. The Department of Dentistry and Dental Research was formed at SMD. Eastman Dental Dispensary developed a parallel department of dental research. The dispensary was not able to grant degrees or directly sponsor postdoctoral clinical programs. This had to be done under the auspices of the University of Rochester in conformity with New York State law. This was

accomplished, and the dispensary was added to the American Dental Association list of graduate training centers.

Bibby's first order of business was to recruit a teaching and research faculty. He had established a wide network of contacts as a result of his initial activity at the University of Rochester, involvement in the International Association of Dental Research, and as dean at Tufts, but a career in research did not have the cache that it enjoys at present, at least for those interested in an academic career. Dentists weren't beating down the doors to come to the Eastman Dental Dispensary to train for a career in dental research, but Bibby had confidence in his vision and became exceedingly successful.

In July 1949 Dr. Finn Brudevold became the first director of dental research to work at the dispensary under Bibby, taking over the chemical research position (investigating bacteriology of the mouth) vacated by Dr. David Marshall-Day. The Brudevold appointment ushered in a broad range of innovative research initiatives. These included studies of ammoniated dentifrices; the development of a micro anticavity electrode for intraoral pH measurements; studies on the mechanism of action of fluoride; chemical studies of the levels of copper, lead, tin, and strontium in human enamel; acid reducing effect of anti-enzymes in plaque; abrasion of toothbrush bristles on tooth structure; polarized light studies of fluoride in enamel; microradiographic studies of pits and fissures; and trace element studies in ancient incisor teeth.

Brudevold developed an important technique that was subsequently used by many other investigators involving extracted teeth both for bench experiments and experiments in the mouth. On each tooth a standard area was outlined, and the rest of the surface was covered in wax or varnish. The clear area was then subjected to varying concentrations of different acids, foodstuffs, or oral conditions. This Brudevold research led to the strong recommendation by dentists to prescribe brushing immediately after meals and to reduce between-meal munching. Even one little sugar-containing snack may leave as much acid-forming residue as a seven-course dinner, he discovered. Brudevold left the dispensary in 1958 to become professor of dentistry at Forsyth, which had recently merged with Harvard's School of Dental Medicine. Brudevold was a competent, broad ranging, and imaginative researcher and was very successful in securing grants from the National Institute of Dental Research. His departure from Eastman Dental Dispensary was a loss. Scuttlebutt indicated that he would rather have stayed at the dispensary, but

Dr. Bibby (who had a reputation for being frugal both with his and institutional money) declined to meet Forsyth's financial offer. Consequently, in 1959, Dr. Michael Buonocore, who had followed Bibby to Rochester from Tufts, took over as research coordinator. Dr. Hugh Averill, a highly respected local dentist who received a master's degree in public health at Harvard, was hired to head the dental health programs in the public schools and promote preventive programs in the community. For example, Rochester was one of the earliest communities to fluoridate its water supplies.

Although Bibby continued to be actively engaged in research on the relationship of foodstuffs, fluoride, and dental caries, he still had a strong interest in promoting the study of oral microorganisms. He recruited bacteriologist Marion Gilmour, PhD. Gilmour did innovative work on filamentous organisms and set up a sophisticated, state-of-the-art bacteriologic laboratory. Although she aspired to do more, her major contribution was as mentor to two postdoctoral students who went on to establish internationally recognized careers, William Bowen and Dorothy Geddes. Gilmour was also helpful to Stanley Handelman in setting up his laboratory and in establishing his research career in microbiology. Although he hired full-time research faculty throughout his directorship, when he recruited faculty to lead clinical programs he selected individuals with research credentials on the assumption they could delegate teaching responsibilities on to qualified part-time teachers.

Dr. Helmut Zander was recruited by Bibby from Minnesota in 1956. Bibby knew him from Tufts, where Zander had done pediatric research on pulp therapy with calcium hydroxide. While at Minnesota Zander transformed himself into a periodontist. His strength was his ability to recruit outstanding students, many of who became deans of dental schools (for example: Stan Hazen, Jim Kennedy, and Richard Ranney). By designating salaries that were budgeted for clinical administration and supervision but were in fact primarily for research, Bibby maximized research productivity and promoted the primacy of research as a dominant institutional mission. This approach exists to day.

Some considered Helmut Zander the father of periodontology. But while his research was well funded by National Institute of Dental Research and he was highly regarded, he was only one of a constellation of periodontology researchers that also included Glickman, Goldman, and Ramfjord. Dr. Zander enjoyed provoking controversy and debate. At scientific meetings, usually

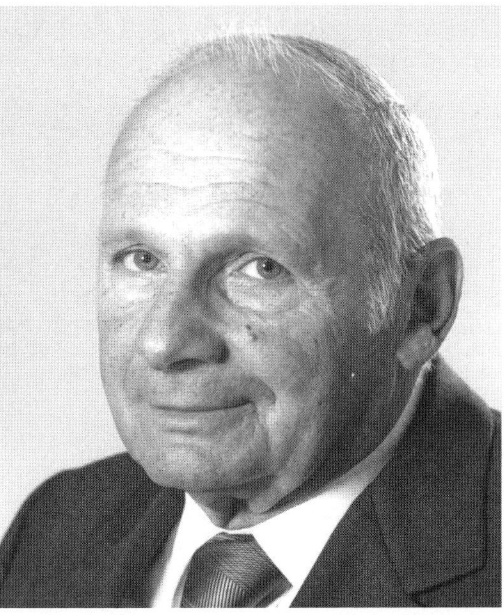

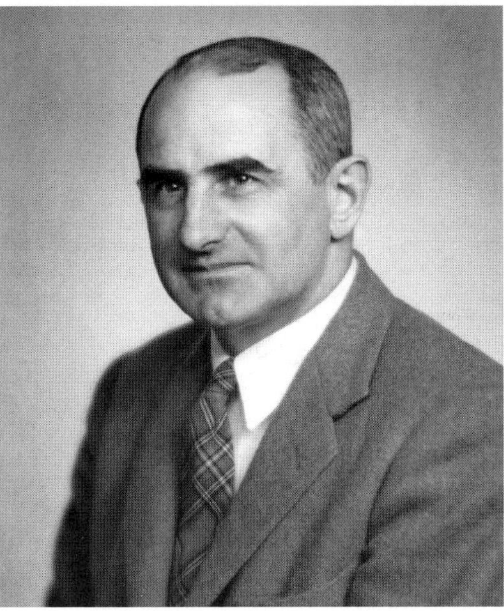

Drs. Helmut Zander (top) and Basil Bibby (bottom)

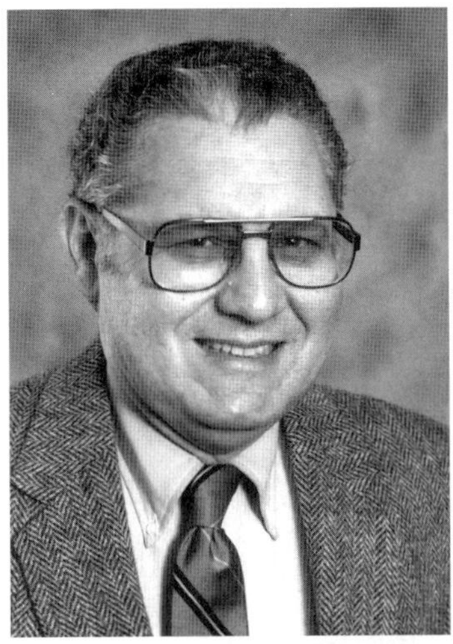
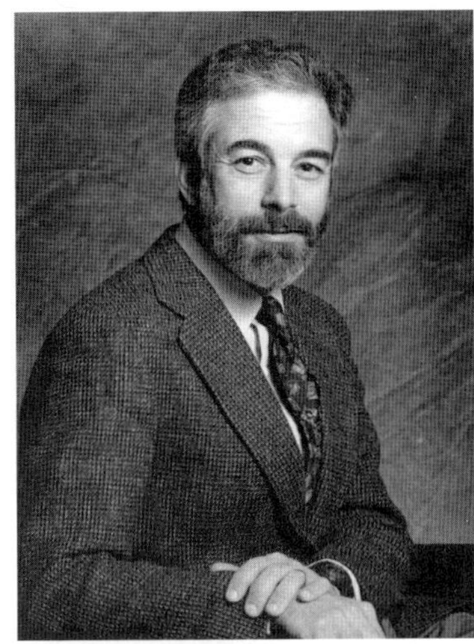
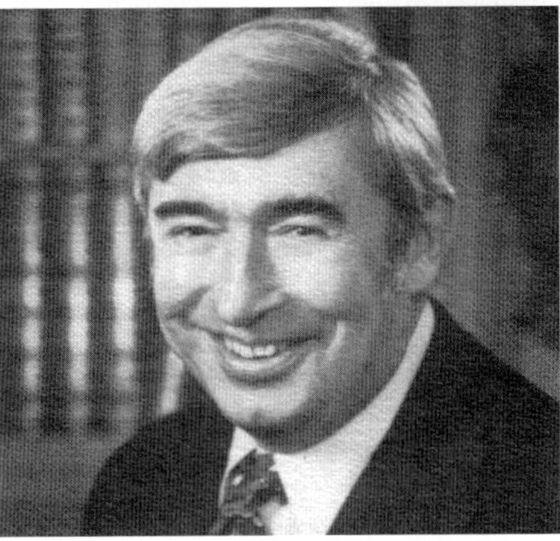

*Clockwise from top, left: Drs. Stanley Handelman,
Domenick Zero, and J. Daniel Subtelny*

with Glickman (Tufts) and Goldman (Boston University), the audience frequently overflowed into the hallways in anticipation of the heated and often times personal debate.

Many academically oriented dentists who studied under Zander, Buonocore, Handelman, Bibby, and other Eastman or university faculty went on to become leaders in dental research, dental education, and general dentistry. Former students and residents include Jay Gershen, Cyril Meyerowitz, Domenick Zero, Paul Desjardins, Eric Solomon, Glenn Clark, and others who achieved high academic rank. These former students are notable for their general dentistry credentials rather than a specialty.

Bibby recruited J. Daniel Subtelny from the National Institute of Dental Research. His wife, Joanne Subtelny, a speech pathologist, became another productive member of the research faculty. Roland Hawes followed Bibby from Tufts after a stint in the Air Force; he led the one-year pediatric intern program and had a strong interest in dental research. Hawes is best remembered for establishing the highly regarded accredited pediatric dentistry program.

While Bibby was hiring a team of outstanding researchers, many students who enrolled in the clinical programs at Eastman had little or no interest in research when they first arrived at 800 East Main Street. For them, the work at the dispensary was a break between the intensity of dental school and the real world of private clinical practice. For some foreign dental students it was an opportunity to visit the United States. Some individuals clearly came for a clinical or research education, but others did not. What was remarkable among the latter group, Dr. Handelman notes, was that the challenge that research provided and the personal encouragement that Dr. Bibby and his faculty offered inspired numbers of these bright young dentists who were ambivalent about their choice of dentistry to pursue careers in dental research and academics. During Bibby's years foreign students tended to come from the Commonwealth countries, Europe, and Latin America. Some stayed on in the United States after their time at the dispensary, especially those who met and married Rochesterians; others returned to their homelands. The tradition of recruiting international students continues to this day.

Other well-considered research efforts that were supported by the National Institute of Dental Research grants were studies conducted by Hawes and Handelman on the long-term effect of antibiotics on dental caries and oral bacteria. Two unique populations receiving long-term antibiotic therapy for prevention of recurrent rheumatic fever attacks and upper respiratory disease, respectively, were identified. Human studies confirmed the caries inhibition findings of antibiotic studies in laboratory animals and clearly supported the hypothesis that dental caries was an infectious disease caused by bacteria. These investigations determined that long-term antibiotic therapy in humans reduced caries increment by two-thirds. Salivary samples from this population demonstrated higher levels of antibiotic resistance in salivary bacteria but comparable number of salivary organisms between antibiotic users and sibling non-users.

Bibby's interest in fluoride started when he was a dental fellow under Whipple and continued during his deanship at Tufts. Among the first projects he initiated when he returned was a clinical study by Marshall-Day, through a National Institutes of Health grant, leading to more efficient use of fluorine. Marshall-Day subsequently became dean of the dental school at Tufts. Rochester was one of the earliest cities to incorporate fluoride in its water supplies, and Averill, the head of Community Dentistry at Eastman Dental Dispensary, and Bibby reported on the beneficial results for the city's children. Their views on the mechanism of action of fluoride were controversial in the early 1950s. The prevailing view at that time was that fluoride from the drinking water and foods was incorporated in tooth structure systemically during the body's growth and formed a fluorapatite that was more acid resistant than normal enamel. Bibby disagreed and felt that the topical application of fluoride was the mechanism of action. Although he and other investigators at the university and Eastman Dental Dispensary published numerous papers demonstrating the topical effect of fluoride, some public community health officials were concerned that these investigations supporting the topical effect of fluoride in toothpastes, mouth rinses, and professional applications would undermine public support of fluoridation of public water supplies. The controversy was largely laid to rest by the elegant studies of a number of investigators working at Eastman during the McHugh years, including John Featherstone. These studies established the fact that in addition to its antimicrobial effects, the most significant mechanism of fluoride's action was the enhancement of remineralization of tooth structure that had been demineralized by acid attack.

Bibby's work on foodstuffs continued to gain him international recognition. He demonstrated that "cereals" (Bibby's word for grains) from different areas of the world suggested that minerals incorporated in the cereals from the soil may have an inhibitory effect on dental caries. He worked with Brudevold, Beck, Goldberg, Losee, Curzon, and others to develop techniques to measure pH, acid production, and decalcification using different oral organisms and various foodstuff mixtures. He continued to work well after his official retirement as director to develop an artificial mouth to simulate oral conditions as a more efficient way of studying the carious process compared to using laboratory animal and human studies.

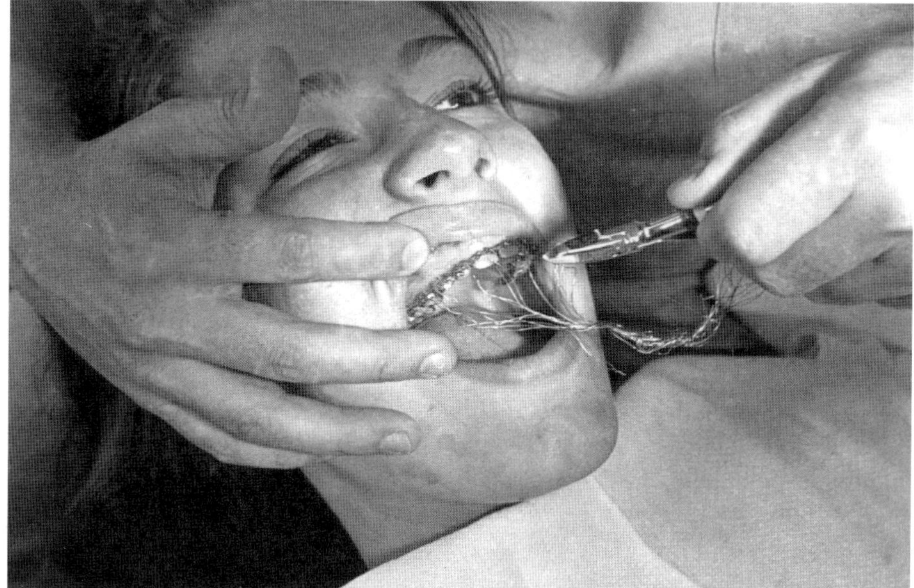

A patient receives orthodontic treatment.

One of Bibby's graduate students was Barry Gillings from Australia. Gillings developed a cutting machine that sectioned thin slices of tooth structure. Buonocore and others used the machine in dye penetration studies to determine whether there was leakage around sealants and restorations. Gillings also implanted a tiny radio transmitter in the mouth to determine if an individual had a normal or abnormal bite or how a child grinds his or her teeth at night. The transmitter fit into an appliance resembling a removable or fixed bridge and was designed to be worn in the mouth in the area of a patient's missing teeth. Earlier methods of measuring bite patterns were hampered because they interfered with normal functioning of the patient's jaws.

MICHAEL BUONOCORE

Perhaps the most noteworthy achievement in research while Bibby was director was research in adhesive dentistry. In 1967, Michael Buonocore discovered that etching the enamel surface of the tooth with a weak acid would enhance the adhesion of plastic fillings to the teeth, revolutionizing the field

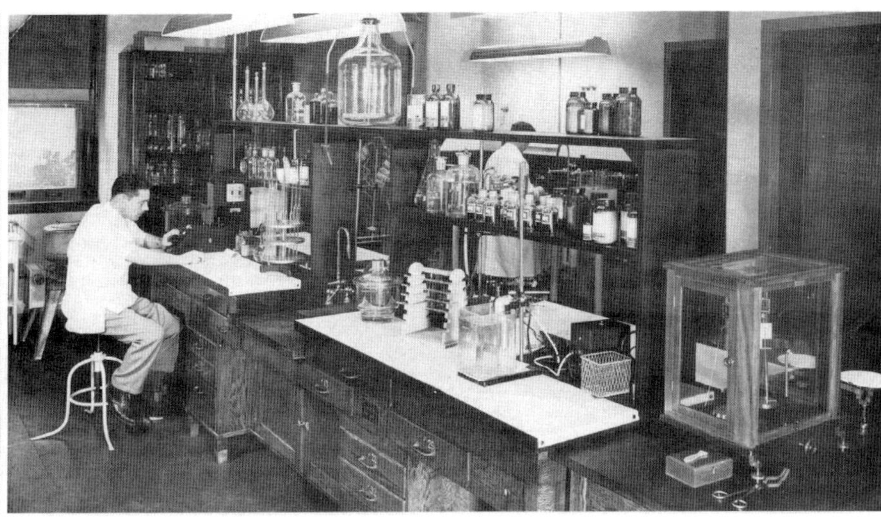

Dr. Michael Buonocore in laboratory

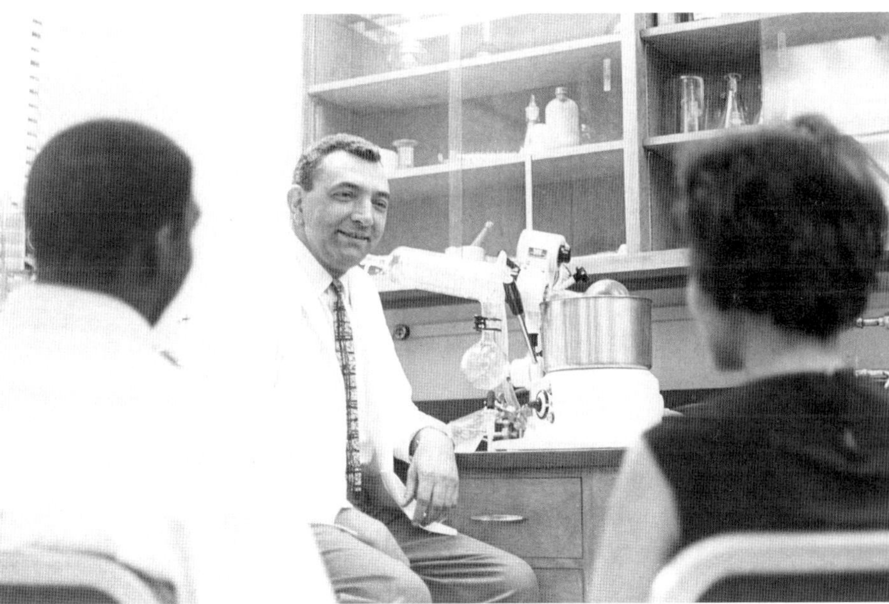

Dr. Buonocore with students

of restorative and esthetic dentistry. Actually, Buonocore's first report on acid etching was published in 1955 while he was still at Tufts. His studies also advanced the prevention of dental caries through the development of dental sealants. As a result, Buonocore is considered the father of the adhesive dentistry.

Most cavities occur on the biting surfaces of teeth. Small pits and fissures, or grooves, trap decay-causing bacteria that toothbrush bristles can't reach. "These teeth decay very early in life, generally shortly after the teeth come in," Buonocore said in 1971, and his seventeen-year search for a sealant ended in the announcement of what has been called "the most important advance in preventing cavities since fluoridated water."

The Buonocore sealant, available to dentists since April 1971, seals pits and fissures with a hard plastic coating. Sealants prevent dental decay by physically separating the decay-causing bacteria from their nutritional source of sugar and other refined carbohydrates and they physically protect against acid attack. This mechanism is different from the remineralizing action of fluoride, which is more effective in reducing dental decay between teeth.

A former student of Buonocore, Dr. Louis Ripa, chairman of the Department of Children's Dentistry at SUNY at Stony Brook, said in 1990, "Dr. Buonocore used to sit down and say things like, 'Think about it: why don't we have a procedure to treat a fractured anterior tooth by using a material with which we, like an artist with a brush, could build that tooth up to its natural form, rather than using a pin or large crown? And why can't we use a light to harden the material so that you would have all the working time you needed to place the material exactly where you wanted it?'" Buonocore flowed with ideas, but also had a steely determination to test them with the most carefully designed and executed experiments. "He had two things," said Dr. Ripa. "He had a visionary's dream and he had the scientific acumen to make that dream a reality."

The usefulness of the acid-etch adhesive technique influenced a cadre of students and colleagues and encouraged the development of new restorative and aesthetic dental materials and procedures, composite retained bridges, the splinting of teeth, and ceramic veneers. Daniel Subtelny, the chair of the orthodontic department and a close friend of Michael Buonocore, said that the acid-etch technique had a major impact on orthodontic treatment. Hitherto metallic bands with attachments for the arch wires had to be fitted around the tooth and cemented into place to move teeth. Direct banding of attachments to enamel simplified the process, was more aesthetically acceptable, and reduced the washout of cement and resultant decalcification around the bands. Some of the individuals at the Eastman Dental Center who worked with Buonocore included Eriberto Ceuto, John Gwinnette, Stanley Handelman, John Hinding, Oivind Jensen, Dennis Leverett, Hugo Retief, Louis Ripa, and Zia Shey.

Buonocore considered patenting his bonding procedure. "Poor Mike, everybody took his material," one colleague sympathized. Ironically, patents could have made not only Buonocore but also dentistry at the university and at Eastman financially independent, as other medical inventions have done in other places. There are two divergent opinions as to why the patent process was never pursued. Martin Curzon and Daniel Subtelny stated that Bibby considered the patent process too commercial and said in effect, "No, this is a university. We don't do patents." Martin Curzon speculates as to why this happened: "The New Zealanders have a very strong socialist background. They are a bit more socialist than the British but far more than the Americans. So Basil would have a strong sense of responsibility to society and therefore something as revolutionary as the fissure sealants should be available to all, and not restricted, which a patent would do. His generation would think that way."[4]

However, Stanley Handelman recollects that Bibby said his decision was based on considered legal opinion. With the publication of the acid-etching technique, this knowledge entered the public domain and undermined the patent process. Secondly, the curing of a resin with a light source was a known process. A clever patent attorney may have found a unique part of the process to patent, but there was the risk of investing large sums of money in legal fees with no payoff. In today's world, the university may have taken the risk of putting up the money since the payoff could have been very substantial.

Sealants never became as popular as Buonocore anticipated for two reasons. First there was the issue of inadvertently or purposefully sealing dental decay. A major six-year study funded by the National Institute of Dental Research and led by Stanley Handelman entitled "Effect of Fissure Sealant on Progress of Dental Caries" addressed this issue. The study determined that the bacteria in sealed carious lesions dramatically declined and that dental caries did not progress and in fact sometimes regressed as long as the sealant was intact. Second, and perhaps more important, was the issue of payment in private clinical practice. Sealants were introduced after dental

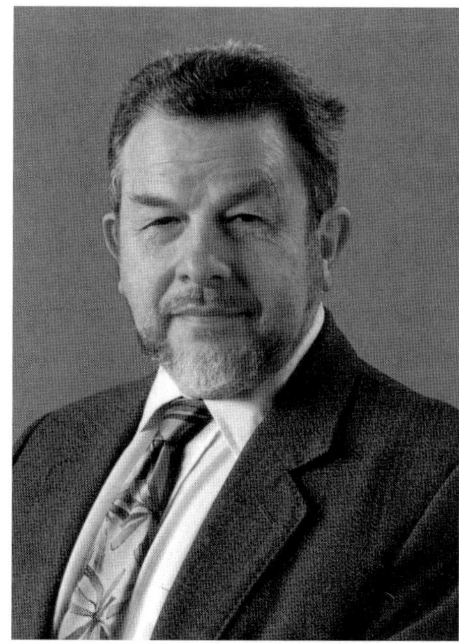

Dr. Martin Curzon

insurance was established, and insurance companies hesitated to fund this new procedure which they thought dentists would use indiscriminately. Dentists found it more acceptable to do a composite restoration sealant combination that was fully covered by insurance than to have a sealant that was not covered by insurance. In contrast to private clinical practice, advocates of public health programs generally advocated using auxiliary personnel to perform the sealing of all posterior permanent teeth in underserved and poor populations for both prevention and treatment.

Annual reports from 1949 on list research projects that grew each year. Financial support for research and for a major addition to the research labs would most often come from outside agencies such as the National Institute of Dental Research. Under Bibby, research continued to grow. By 1966, for example, forty-three original research articles and reviews were being published annually—the most in Eastman Dental Center history up to that point—and a budget of about $700,000 was spent, which was a substantial amount for that time. The scope of research activity was also demonstrated by the publication of 261 papers by postdoctoral students while they were enrolled in the program. The number of published papers continued to be twenty to thirty-five per year up to the present time. Although the senior investigators may have changed, the baton has been passed on successfully from year to year.

What was unique about research activity during Bibby's directorship? Dental research was centered on the potential and interest of the individual rather than on a strategic plan. Although he identified and fostered diverse research themes, such as foodstuffs, fluoride, bacteriology, trace elements, and periodontology, Bibby's major strength was generative and facilitative. He had the knack of recruiting talented people, such as Andlaw, Brown, Caldwell, Curzon, Cutress, Koulorides, and many others, and provided them with laboratory space and modest financial support. The number of papers published under Basil Bibby's leadership and by those individuals trained in Rochester accounted for a significant percentage of all dental research conducted during that period. Some regard this period under Dr. Bibby as "golden years."[5]

A REAPPRAISAL OF PRINCIPLES

"The most fundamental question which had to be raised was whether the principles on which the dispensary was organized more than thirty years ago were still valid and whether they were still fully effective in furthering the purposes of the institution."[6] Bibby wrote in 1949. If not, he felt that he might need to recommend far-reaching reorganization and even abandonment of an independent existence. In his 1949 annual report, Bibby proposed that the large, independent, centralized clinic that concentrated on clinical community dentistry for children and that had initially led the way in dentistry in the 1915 world might be outmoded. Those services, Bibby maintained, were now being provided more efficiently in smaller dispersed clinics in places such as Bibby's native New Zealand. This model for dispersed clinical service was the direct opposite of what George Eastman proposed to William Bausch, who had been engaged in starting dispersed clinics in various Rochester schools between 1901 and 1914.

"To fully justify itself, [the central clinic] must do more than provide just routine dental service," Bibby wrote. "If we accept a broader objective than the supplying of routine dental care, then the central clinic is easy to justify."[7] It can provide orthodontic service and other special treatment clinics, experimental service programs, or preventive service not offered elsewhere and not possible in a decentralized clinic program. "However," Bibby continued, "it is when we move out of the area of direct clinical service into that of long range service for children in general that the central clinic can make its greatest contribution. It is only in a central clinic that the significant educational or research programs can be organized that will ultimately benefit the community and the dental profession . . . [and] can serve the dental profession in the way in which good hospitals now serve the medical profession." Finally, Bibby concluded in his landmark 1949 annual report, "the independence of the dispensary, which could have been a liability, is proving to be a real asset. Freedom from the overly complex organization and divergent functions of a large medical center makes it less easy to lose sight of the patients and the basic purpose of the institution. Smallness increases unity and permits a flexibility . . . that simplifies the making of changes at the most profitable time."[8]

According to Harper Sibley, all of the trustees agreed with Bibby's de-emphasis of the service aspects and the highlighting of the educational and research aspects. In January 1950, Sibley complimented Bibby and noted, "The trustees were very disappointed by the limited scope of the work before you came, in light of our splendid facilities and equipment. However, we were helpless as Mr. Burkhart was clearly too old to take on any new aspects to our program. We all approve of the broadened research activities. . . . Your suggestion . . . of broadening the education of the interns and holding out for a higher quality of usefulness will certainly have results."[9]

CLINICAL DENTISTRY

Lack of interns and residents to staff the clinic was the biggest problem of the late 1940s and early 1950s. Looked at a different way, there were too many underserved children needing treatment.

The nation had slipped quickly from 1930s Depression to 1940s World War II to the Cold War and then to the Korean War in the late 1940s. A military draft was still operating and recent dental graduates were needed in the armed services. Bibby hoped to counter this with part-time staff, short-term

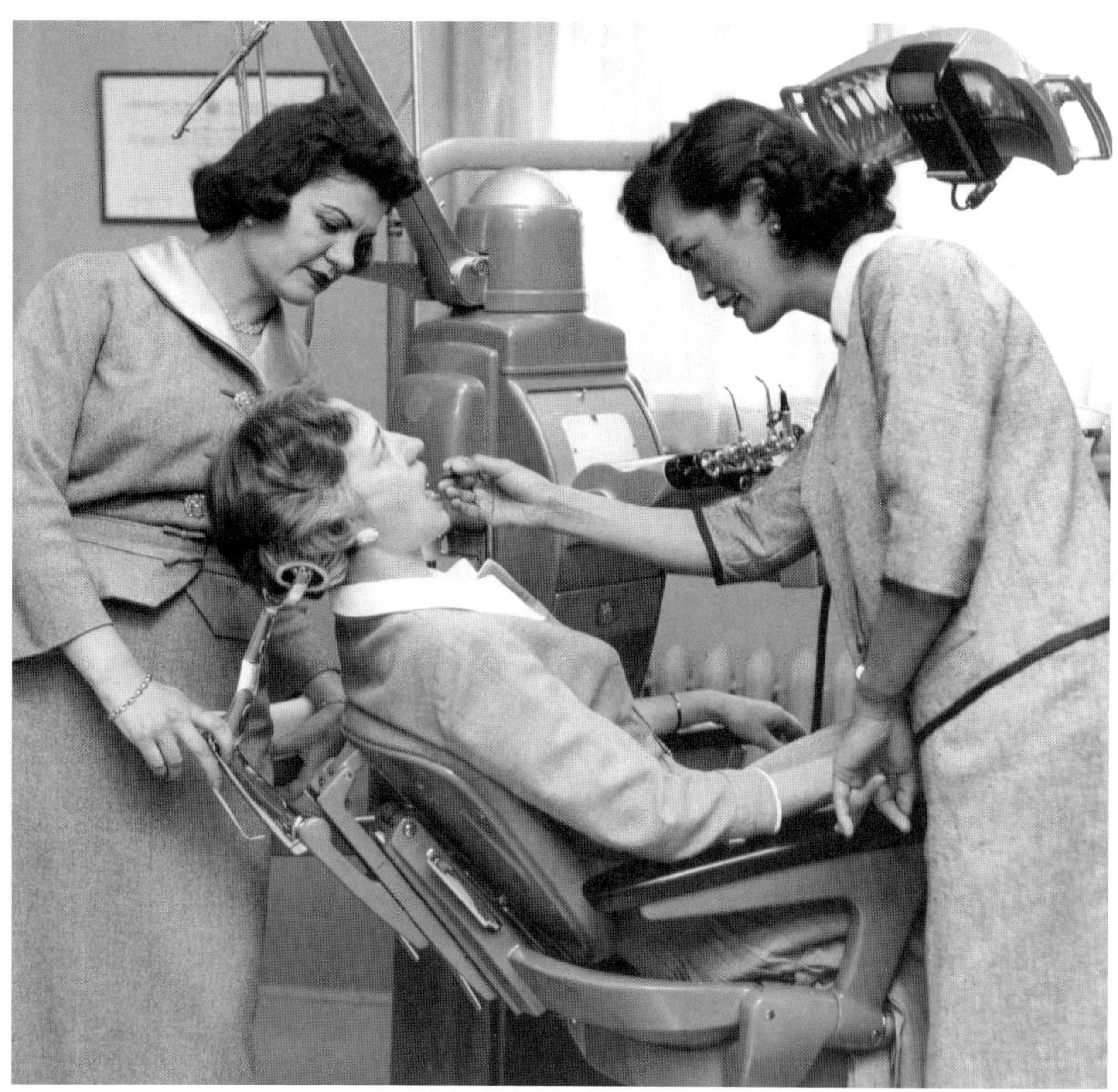

Clinical dentistry, 1958

appointments before or after military service, and by "stimulating a sense of responsibility in private practitioners for caring for children." Bibby maintained that local dentists were "unwilling or unable to spend sufficient time to control the behavior of children" under a fee-for-service arrangement. He suggested that the Eastman Dental Dispensary could contribute by "training 'good dental patients' in the pre-school group." Then, "the dentists should be more willing to increase their acceptance of child patients for maintenance purposes."[10]

The amount of pediatric dental service declined somewhat after the Burkhart years—and had been declining since the high point in 1934, partially because interns and residents went off to war. The quality of service, however, was improved by the introduction of a new innovation, bitewing x-rays of all patients, and a new policy of assigning each patient to a specific dentist. These advances increased the finding of dental disease and eventually lowered the number of visits required per patient to six—from ten the previous year and from fifteen ten years previous. The relationship between the number of teeth filled and the number extracted also improved. Yet Bibby felt, "Service of this sort cannot be given to more than a fraction of the children of Rochester." He cited the number of dentists that would be needed to treat the increasing incidence of pediatric caries. He initially found conditions at the dispensary "somewhat depressing. The physical plant was adequately maintained but drab, out of date, and devoid of any bright touches. Only a portion of it was in use. The large central cage of canaries designed, as in all Eastman dental clinics, to provide a cheerful atmosphere in the waiting room, was no longer equal to the task."[11]

DIFFICULTIES IN CLINICAL CARE

Tonsillectomy, perhaps the most common surgical operation in Western civilization for 2500 years, probably fell out of medical fashion because it was overused, particularly in the United States and Canada. The new techniques of anesthesia and surgery had triggered the mass acceptance of tonsillectomy. Previously indicated only for severe inflammation of the throat, tonsillectomy in the early twentieth century became the routine treatment for almost all throat infections and was undertaken prophylactically, even when there was no obvious infection. This operation achieved bandwagon[12]

status after the Johns Hopkins medical school revamped the procedure in 1907, making it safer, more comfortable, and less likely to be followed by a recurrence of infection. Studies by surgeons (such as Dr. Albert David Kaiser[13]) reported striking improvement in symptoms that led to the operation, while other studies in which tonsillectomized children were compared with unoperated controls were far less impressive. However, as Bibby wrote in an early report, "Penicillin and changes in medical thinking had driven the tonsillectomy program into limbo."

There were other difficulties. When Dr. Pammenter applied for specialty board qualification in pedontics, he was not approved because his treatment methods consisted of rampant caries being treated by gross removal and the topical application of silver nitrate, a primitive nonscientific method. Dr. Schulman supervised the general pedontic clinic on a half-time basis while a part-time dentist supervised the hygienists and student hygienists. Dr. Schlenker, head of orthodontics, divided her time between the dispensary and the dental practice. As the clinic developed under Bibby, there would be less emphasis on the number of patients treated and more emphasis on research and educational activities.

The dental operating staff at that time numbered twenty-one. Of these, nineteen were from Cuba and the other two had substandard qualifications. The Cubans' difficulties with English made them somewhat less effective with children and their continued availability was made uncertain, Bibby wrote, by reason of the ugly noises Fidel Castro was making. More than half of the foreign-trained dentists at Eastman Dental Dispensary graduated from schools other than those registered as qualifying for dental practice in New York State. By 1957 Bibby had solved the problem and had a balanced staff of U.S. and internationally trained dentists.

Most patients were transported from city schools by school buses. Reliance on bus schedules forced less than desirable operating conditions. Dentists and hygienists criticized the schedules to no avail; eventually, the bus service was cancelled.

Moreover, Bibby felt the level of clinical dental services in the Rochester area institutions had not developed in parallel with advances in research. He pushed for upgrading the dental services not only at the Eastman Dental Dispensary but also those offered at Strong Memorial Hospital and Genesee Hospital and for improving the quality of dentistry available to the community.

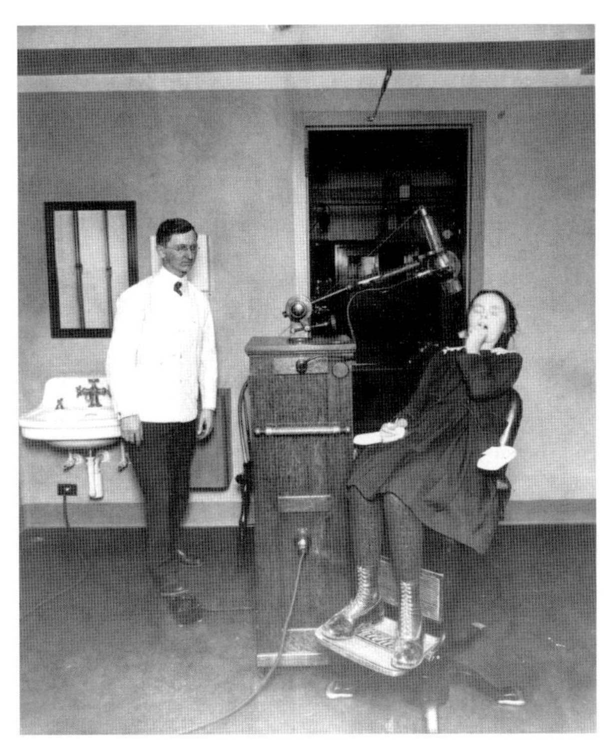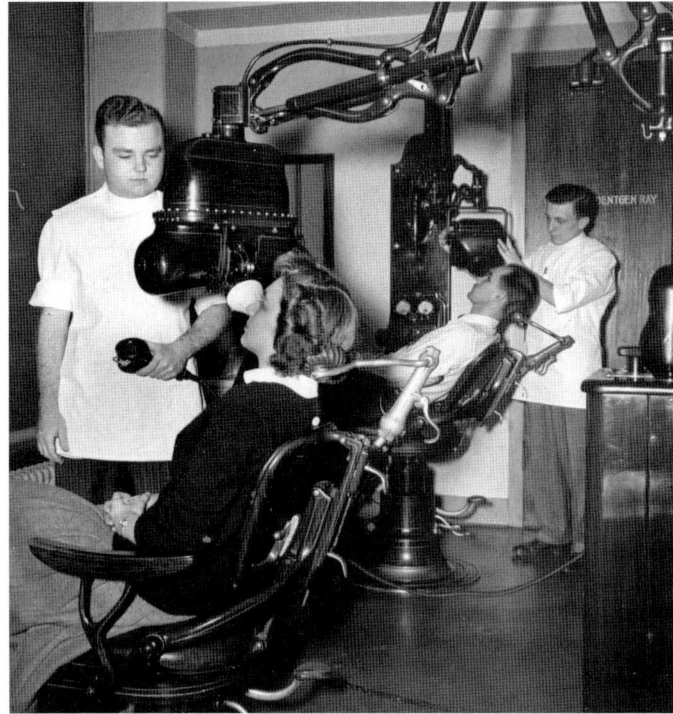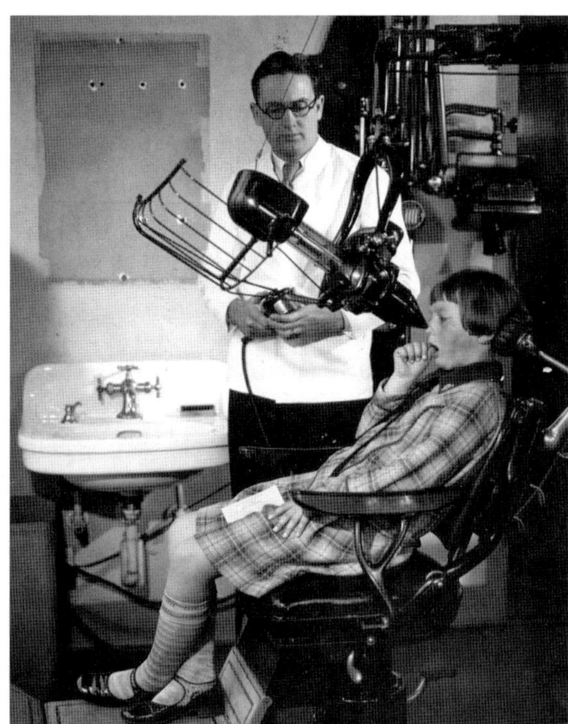

X-rays in 1917 and 1950

Despite the difficulties related to clinical care, the historic mission of the Eastman Dental Center continued even while Bibby's new emphasis on research was emerging. In the 1960s, Genesee Hospital, which was more conveniently located for city residents than was Strong Memorial Hospital, asked the center for help in developing its dental services. After Genesee Hospital appointed a member of the center faculty, Dr. Bejan Iranpour, as chief of its dental service, Genesee replaced Strong as the hospital called upon when special diagnostic or treatment services were needed. It continued to serve in this capacity until the School of Medicine and Dentistry dental service was reorganized and the Eastman Dental Center moved to the medical center.

In 1968, the Rochester Neighborhood Health Center was opened under university auspices, with three dentists on staff who held appointments either at Eastman Dental Center or the university. The next year, formal affiliation between the Genesee Hospital's dental department and the School of Medicine and Dentistry took place. The American Dental Association approved a three-year oral surgery program, jointly developed with the School of Medicine and Dentistry and Genesee Hospital. The City of Rochester already had a vested interest in the maintenance of dental health through fluoridation of its drinking water and an annual grant of $50,000 to the Eastman Dental Dispensary. Dr. Hugh Averill, a local dentist, headed up a program to expend the oral hygiene program in the schools that was funded at over $120,000.

Along with fluoride, the introduction of Medicaid in the 1960s created major changes in the clinical program. Bibby wrote in anticipation: "The coming of Medicaid with its undertaking to provide dental care for the entire socioeconomic group that the dental center is serving, in a sense deprives the center of what has been its central function." But this did not turn out to be true. Medicaid in New York State paid for routine dental services for economically disadvantaged adults and children. In effect, it served to offset the subsidy that the Eastman Dental Center underwrote for dental services to poor children but significantly expanded the role of the center as the provider of dental services to the same children. The full potential of Medicaid payment was not realized until the 1970s, when Dr. William McHugh became the director.

EDUCATION

The dispensary faced increasing challenges in its educational program during Bibby's tenure. At one time the Eastman Dental Dispensary and Forsyth Dental Infirmary were the principal places for dental graduates to obtain postgraduate experience and education. By 1950, however, there were 150 hospitals offering internships and providing credit toward the new specialty boards. By then, most of the nation's fifty dental schools offered postgraduate training. The U.S. Public Health Service also offered fifty rotating internships with specialty board accreditation and higher stipends.

The Eastman Dental Dispensary internship program was a ten-month program for graduates of American and foreign dental schools. Patients that they treated in the main clinic were children and adolescents, many of who were referred by dental hygienists in the Rochester school system. Under Bibby's leadership, to meet the increasing competition for dental interns, the intern education program was expanded by the addition of a morning lecture series on dental medicine and the prevention of dental decay. If all this came together, Bibby told his trustees, "it will probably represent something unique in American dental education."

In his 1948 annual report, covering the first full year after he became director, Bibby described the education program he had devised for the intern staff. It consisted of films, lectures, and conferences on dental topics as well as presentations in the more general field of medicine. He wanted to increase awareness of the early signs of systemic disease that so frequently appear in the mouth. Bibby also reorganized the education program for the clinical staff—lectures, visual education, and seminars—fulfilling the legal requirements of the State Education Department. Bibby thought the greatest need in dental education was teachers who had both clinical skills and research experience.

To make Eastman Dental Dispensary more attractive to young dentists looking toward graduate degrees, Bibby organized a series of special lectures and seminars that were presented by staff or visiting authorities. The University of Rochester graduate school agreed to accept the lectures and seminars along with research done at the Eastman Dental Dispensary as credits toward a master of science. These opportunities proved attractive to foreign dentists and led to increased applications from Scandinavia, Great Britain, New Zealand, Australia, Asia, Latin America, and the Indian Dental Society. The visiting dentists could work in dental clinics caring for children with the option of spending time in research laboratories and university classes. They could earn credits that could be applied towards a master of science or specialty board qualification. After five years of the Bibby plan, the problem of attracting dentists and interns to the Eastman Dental Dispensary had been solved.

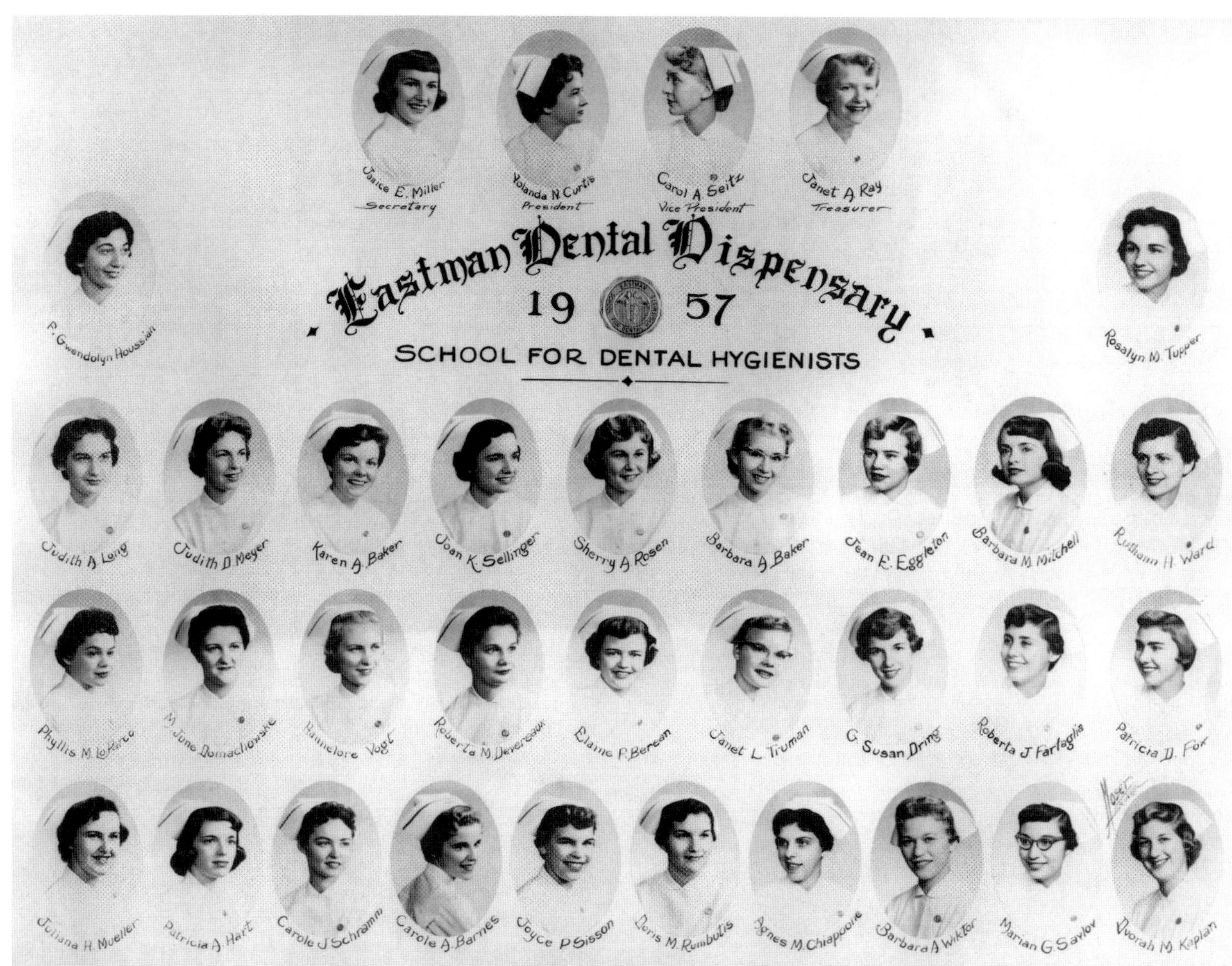

One of the last classes before the move to Monroe Community College

SCHOOL FOR DENTAL HYGIENISTS

At the beginning of Bibby's tenure, the School for Dental Hygienists was a two-year course, but the costs of instruction were not matched by increased tuition and patient care income. Smaller graduating classes did not meet the demand of regional dentists or school systems. In 1964, the administration of the school was transferred to Monroe Community College. The new program provided for students to do classroom work at the college and clinical work at both Eastman and Monroe Community College.

The new association created a new position of dean in Monroe Community College's department of dental hygiene—one of the twelve career programs at the college. Dr. Kjellaug "Chell" L. Gilda, who had completed her predental education in her native Norway in 1942, was appointed to this with the rank of full professor. Bibby said that the new arrangement with Monroe Community College would permit students to transfer credits to four-year colleges more easily and enable them to receive state financial aid. For years, Bibby and Dr. Ruth Vann, principal of the Eastman Dental Dispensary's School for Dental Hygienists had been looking for the opportunity that presented itself through the establishment of the community college and its department of dental hygiene. After two years, students would get an associate's degree in applied science and would be able to take the state licensing test. After successfully passing the test, they could practice, apply for a provisional teaching certificate, or transfer to a four-year institution.

Bibby predicted: "In future years, the prevention of periodontal disease will become accepted as the major contribution which dental hygienists can make to public health." Dr. Gilda concurred and felt that to achieve total preventive dentistry, the main emphasis should be on patient education. The new curriculum was to emphasize the correlation of didactic and clinical training and the hygienist's role in preventive dentistry.

FLUORIDATION WARS UPDATE

By the 1950s, the fluoridation wars were raging nationwide. The battle reached Rochester, and within a few years, most of the communities of central and western New York State. The fluoridation controversy centered on the mandatory addition of fluoride, which is toxic when ingested at high levels or at one time, to the drinking water of whole communities. Skeptics who did not want to apply fluoride topically could opt out of doing so; it was much more difficult to avoid if it was in the drinking water. The fierce opposition came from an unusual combination of forces including Christian Scientists, skeptical scientists and clinicians, chiropractors, health food advocates, and right-wing groups that viewed fluoridation as a communist conspiracy to usurp individual rights and impose socialized medicine. The continuing political controversy led to only 62 percent of communities in the U.S. having fluoridated water in 1992. Proponents of water fluoridation continue to support it as the effective method of choice for controlling mankind's most prevalent disease—dental caries. The safety and effectiveness of water fluoridation have been reevaluated frequently, and no credible evidence associated fluoridation with any of the conditions that opponents have claimed it produces.

A NEW RESEARCH WING

A National Institutes of Health grant of $254,666 combined with fundraising and interest from the Eastman endowment to build a new research wing. The wing, which also included some treatment facilities, was built on the west side of the original Main Street building and announced in July 1962. It was the first construction since the building opened in 1917. The $730,000 structure, fronting on Main Street and running along Alexander Street, was opened in May 1964. The 15,000-square-foot wing, connected by corridor to the original building, was dedicated in ceremonies led by J. Wallace Ely, president of the board of trustees. When the new wing opened, the staff numbered 140. During the school year, it had classes for about forty hygienists in training and twenty-three dental interns or fellows.

Designed by Waasdorp, Northrup, and Kaelber, successor to the architectural firm that designed the original building, the four-story wing allowed for a fifth floor to be added at a later date. One newspaper claimed that the new wing "bristles with the stuff of modern dentistry" while providing for an expanded program of dental research. The reporter found that "research today is a thing of electronics and modern science," citing a "one-way window where scientists can watch a person's reactions to what's being done to his mouth," sensors to record blood pressure, expensive panoramic x-ray machines, tiny radio transmitters to send out signals concerning a person's

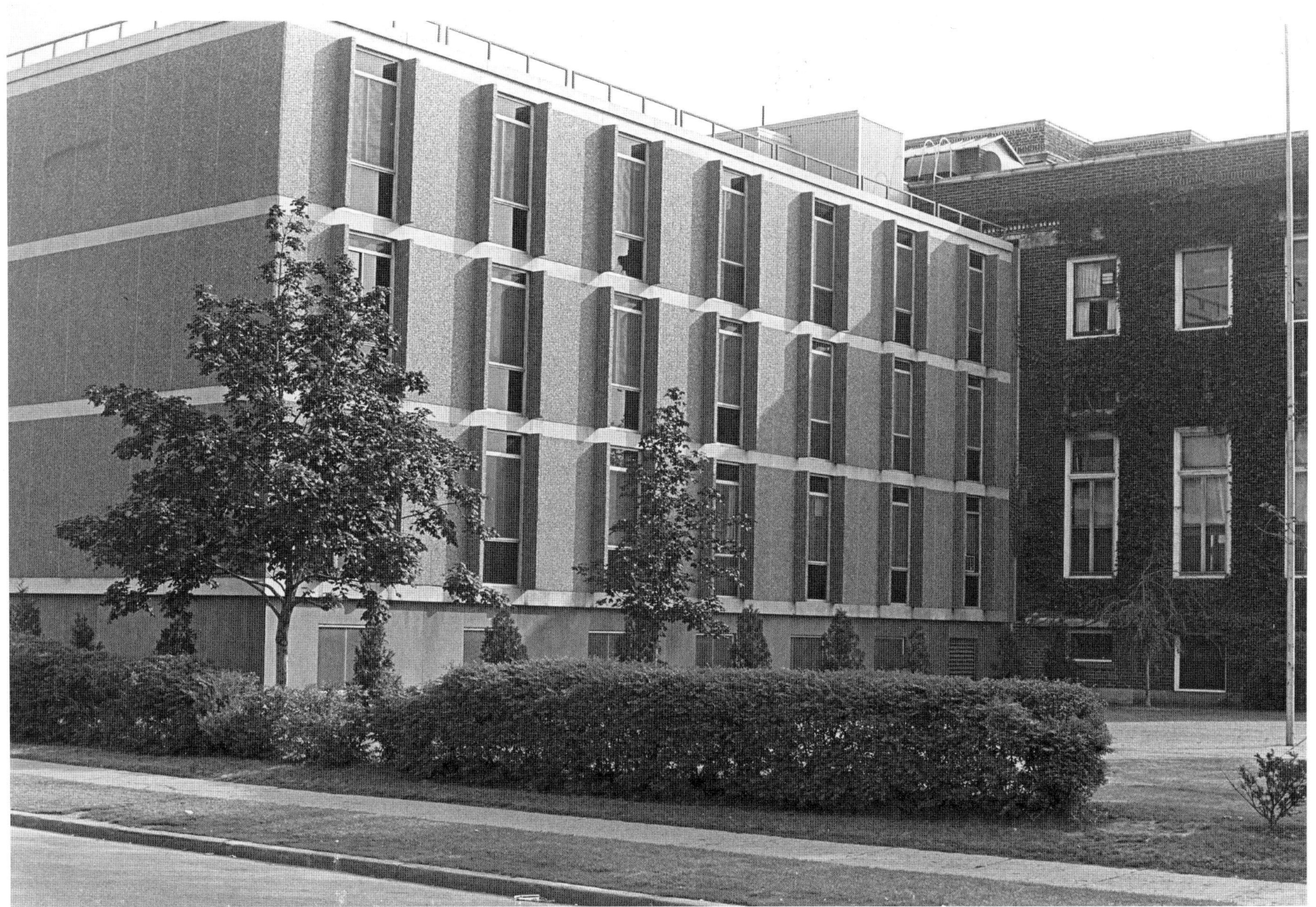

The new research wing opened in 1964.

bite, a basement lab with an x-ray motion picture camera, a lab where tooth transplantation is studied, and tiny, sensitive devices to record air pressure as part of a project on cleft palates.

Basic research on the little-understood act of swallowing was conducted in a room constructed so that sensitive equipment inside would not record outside vibrations. In another room, electronic equipment measured electrical current given off by muscle movement. A nearby computer, surely one of the first, could make a complex analysis of the information. The research conducted in this state-of-the art wing would reach the rest of the world through research reports. At the time the wing opened in 1964, the dispensary ranked at the top among institutions giving reports to the International Association of Dental Research. "A large number of government grants helps support some of the work," a 1964 newspaper account noted.

A NEW NAME: EASTMAN DENTAL CENTER

On its fiftieth anniversary, the dispensary became the Eastman Dental Center. The name change came in 1965 after the new wing opened and was meant to reflect the diversity of academic, research, and patient care activities. More than just a name change, it represented an important historical moment—the maturation and concretization of the Bibby vision. "The function of words, like that of institutions, changes with time," Bibby wrote, as he traced the history of the word *dispensary*. In colonial times dispensaries provided practically all medical services. But by the mid-twentieth century, the earlier dignity of the title of dispensary had fallen from grace. "Dispensary sounds like the back room of a drug store," Bibby wrote when the name was changed.

Bibby further noted that George Eastman expected the trustees of any company or organization that he founded to make any changes they deemed advisable. The charter that Eastman approved for the dispensary in 1915 gave its purposes as "to own, maintain, and operate a dispensary for the prevention, treatment, and cure of diseases of the eye, ear, nose, mouth, throat, and any part of the head by medical, surgical, or prophylactic methods." The trustees voted unanimously in 1965 that the purpose of the dispensary was to provide dental care, offer training for dentists and auxiliary personnel, and conduct research. This action confirmed what had evolved over the years and established an identifiable starting point for future developments. In 1965, the Eastman Dental Center carried out

between $600,000 and $700,000 worth of dental research annually. It attracted about fifty dentists yearly from throughout the country and many foreign nations for advanced training in specialized dental fields.

THE BIBBY LEGACY: RESEARCH, TEACHING, AND COMMUNITY SERVICE

Basil Bibby, upon becoming director, identified dental research, dental education, and clinical/community dentistry as the tripartite objective of the Eastman Dental Dispensary.

Dr. Stanley Handelman, professor emeritus of the Eastman Dental Center, is perhaps typical of those who considered Bibby a mentor. Handelman was chairman of the Department of General Dentistry for twenty-four years (1970–94) and before that, a research associate and clinical instructor from 1958 to 1970. Handelman created a faculty, wrote a manual, and conducted workshops on the development of general practice residency dentistry programs. During these years, there was significant expansion of graduate programs in dental specialties.

At age twenty-seven, Handelman and his wife, Estelle, came to Rochester in search of a private practice in a medium-sized city with all of the cultural and educational perks of larger cities—such as Estelle's hometown of Boston. Stanley had completed a general practice residency with the U.S. Public Health Service. Handelman recalls vividly his initial meeting with Basil Bibby at the Eastman Dental Dispensary in the 1950s.

"I seemed to answer things in a favorable way," Handelman recalls. "He then took me around and introduced me to people that I could possibly work with on a volunteer basis." Handelman decided he could learn a great deal from being associated with the Eastman Dental Dispensary and could offer something too. "I had no idea as to my direction. But the people that I met were very, very helpful."[14]

Bibby directed Handelman and many others toward research. As with all successful mentors, he had the knack of making them feel an increasing sense of ownership of the research ideas and activities that were emerging. Handelman describes his research as examining the "population in Rochester who were receiving antibiotics for chronic respiratory disease . . . [to see whether] antibiotics had any effect on the dental decay rates and on the oral bacteria" of that population.

The Eastman Dental Dispensary had an international flavor in the 1950s, Handelman recalls. "There were people here from all over the world. I found it to be a very exciting atmosphere, primarily because of Basil's personality."

Martin Curzon recalls that there were "lots of people—Brian Clarkson, John Brown, Ramon Castillo, and many others [then at the Eastman Dental Dispensary]—we all went to the Eastman to do clinical training and then ended up doing master's degrees. Basil had the great skill of watching people and picking those who would be receptive to his ideas." He continued:

> I used to sit at the end of the table in great wonderment, watching all these interactions and learning how to manage people positively and how not to do things. But I'd also had the basis, you see, of being a pupil of Basil. And Basil was the consummate leader. His style, I thought, was the best style and in fact I have always tried to adopt it myself.[15]

Curzon thinks of the Bibby years as "forty years of international leadership, being a powerhouse of research, but also the development of people. There was a period when . . . there were hardly any good dental schools around the world that didn't have an Eastman person heading a department, if not being the dean. . . . Everyone keeps referring back to Basil. . . . Now, some of that was the impetus of George Eastman. The money he donated was conditional upon things happening. Burkhart did drive it on, and he did keep its independence. . . . You could say because he stayed on too long, that made it just right for Basil Bibby."

This is in contrast to the Forsyth Institute, which started out as strictly a community service provider, later added research, and ended up as solely a research institution. Bibby saw the contribution of both the Forsyth and the early Rochester Dental Dispensary as "popularizing children's dentistry amongst parents and through the dental profession. For many years, they alone taught children's dentistry." That changed as almost all dental schools began to offer courses in children's dentistry and as the need for it became more widely appreciated. The very success of centralized dental clinics made them less important than they used to be.

In his 1959 annual report, Bibby would write:

> It is worth emphasizing that activities, which have been developed at the Dispensary, are unique in American dentistry. Nowhere else is there a dental institution

which is combining, as do the teaching hospitals in medicine, responsibility for community health, the training of graduate dentists and the carrying forward of basic clinically related research.

And so, the tripartite mission of patient care, education, and research; the name change; and his overall inspirational vision are all part of the Bibby legacy

"What did he like best about the job?" an interviewer asked Beatrice Bibby in 2004 about her husband. Mrs. Bibby replied:

> I think just seeing things grow, seeing people grow and become interested in doing research. . . . A lot of people . . . told me that he turned their lives around. They had no interest in research, didn't know they were interested in research when they first came. And then, they became interested in research and went into academics. A lot of people of that original group became teachers and deans and presidents in dental schools. . . . Some of them even became presidents of universities.

Dr. Bibby retired in 1970 from administrative duties to devote his time to research as senior scientist emeritus, a post he held almost to the time of his death in 1998. On the occasion of the dental center's fiftieth anniversary in 1967, an assessment of the status of clinical/community dentistry found that "virtually no legal restrictions are placed on the age or economic status of patients treated by the Eastman Dental Center." In practice, however, the center still "emphasizes care for underprivileged children through high school age."[16] Fifty years out, dental research, dental education, and clinical/community dentistry were all represented: "The major program includes complete dental care for needy children and adults; programs of dental education and prophylaxis in both public and parochial schools; assistance in the training of dental hygienists; the provision of postgraduate education for dental school graduates, and carrying on of clinical and laboratory research."[17]

Dr. Stanley Handelman may have captured the essence of Bibby years when he wrote:

> The Bibby years redefined the legacy of George Eastman and established the Eastman Dental Center as a leading dental postgraduate educational and research institution. But more than his unquestionable intellectual impact on the growth of the Eastman Dental Center's stature and his impact on the profession, Bibby's facilitative personality has placed young dental professionals at the very center of the learning process.

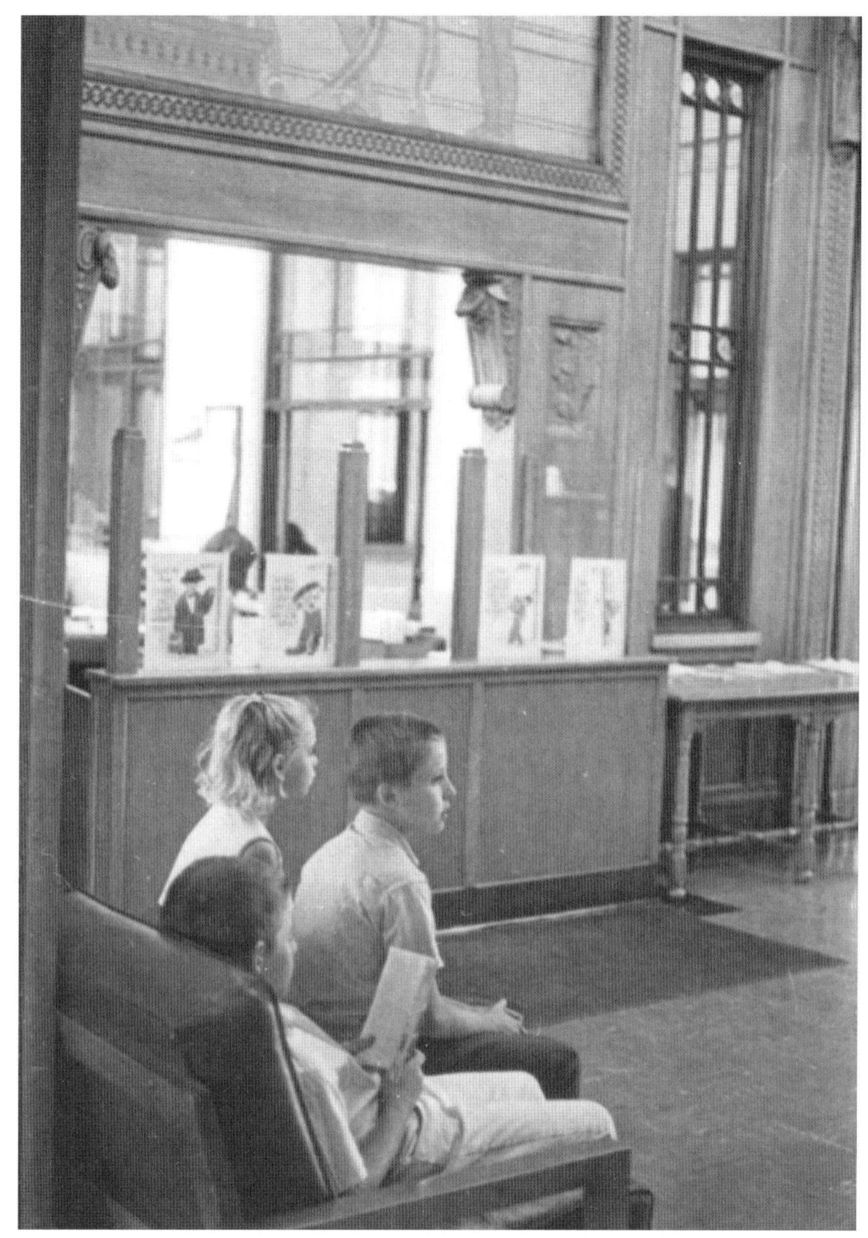

The waiting room in the 1950s

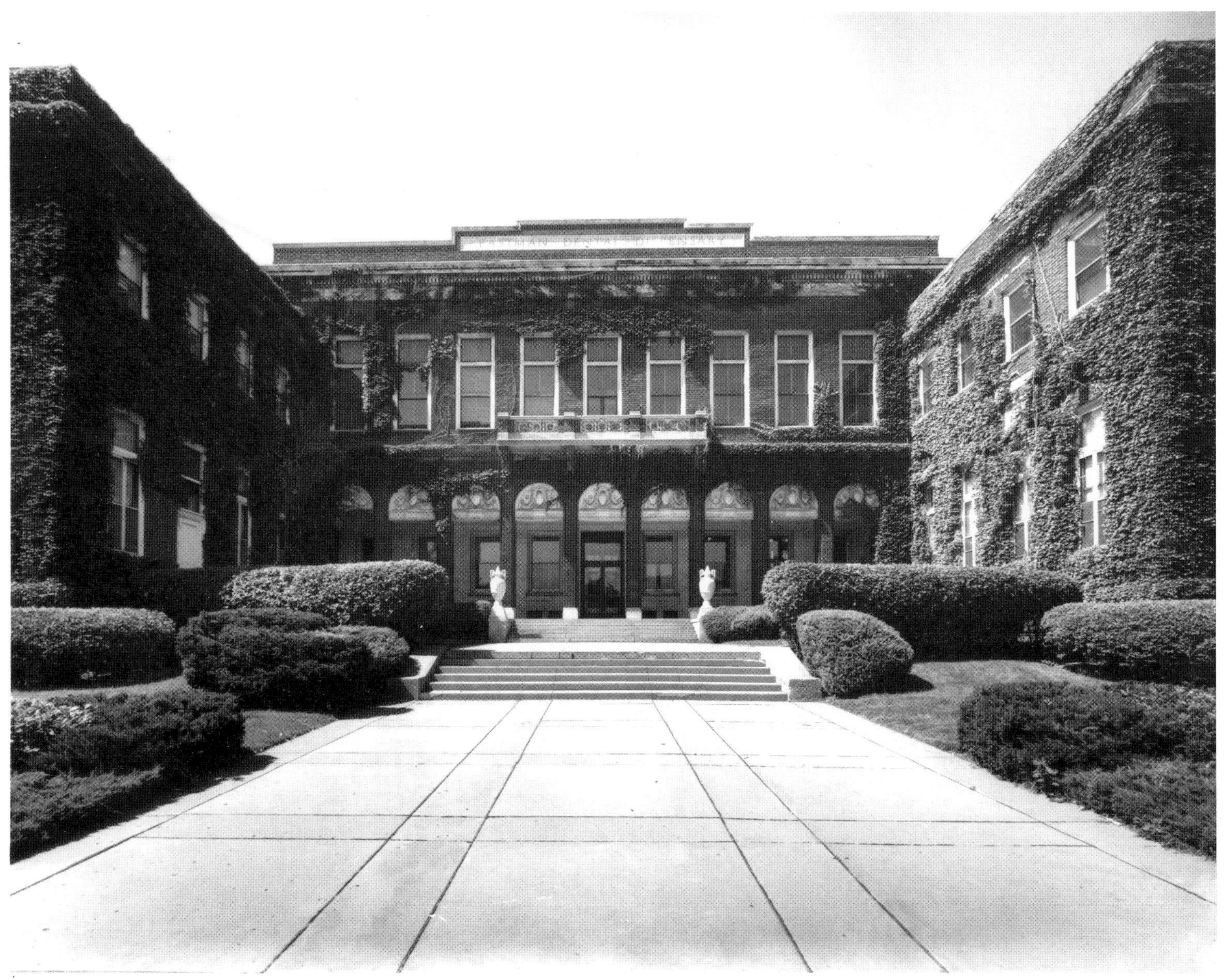

Eastman Dental Center

Chapter Six

EDC AND SMD

CLASH OF CULTURES AND PERSONALITIES

*Mr. Eastman expressed great interest in the possibility of developing a medical
school which would allow his plans for a dental school to be realized.*

Harvey Burkhart, DDS, LLD

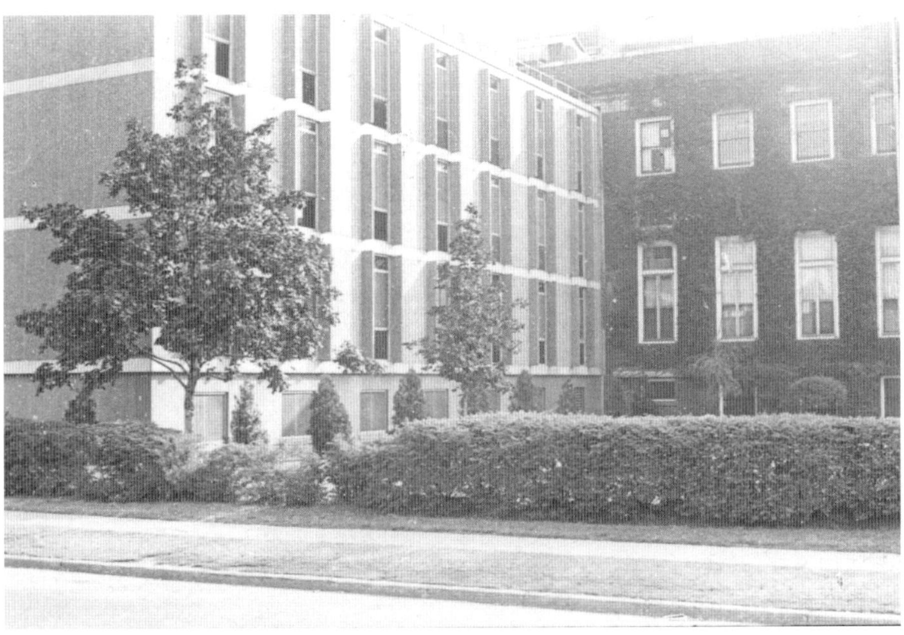

The new research wing at 800 Main Street, Rochester

Dr. JOHN HEIN RECEIVED HIS PhD FROM THE UNIVERSITY OF ROCHESTER in 1952, the same year that the university decided that a formal structure for the dental program was required. Hein was appointed as the first director of the new Department of Dentistry and Dental Research. A new administrative structure divided dentistry into three components: dental research would be carried out at the School of Medicine and Dentistry, clinical dentistry at Strong Memorial Hospital, and various graduate and postgraduate programs at the Eastman Dental Center.

Bibby found Hein to be a progressive associate whom he wanted to keep in Rochester, and when Hein's salary was found lacking, Bibby wanted to ask the Eastman trustees to supplement Hein's university salary with a special stipend using Eastman Dental Center funds. But Hein preferred to bring in grants to support his programs. Only then would he try to persuade the university to increase its support for dental research. Hein was successful in seeking grants from industry, but this had its downside. Products had to be tested, and this drew dentists away from basic research in the medical science departments into which they had been accepted. Department chairmen became unhappy with the increasing demands that testing commercial products made on laboratory space and support services. Bibby saw that by using so many medical students and university personnel for product-testing projects that posed no questions of scientific interest, test subjects were unfavorably impressed with the purpose and merit of the dental research program in the School of Medicine and Dentistry and dental research in general. Still, personalities meshed well and tension was generally absent.

In 1953, Hein wrote an unusually frank history of dentistry at the Eastman Dental Dispensary and School of Medicine and Dentistry and circulated it to the university trustees without Bibby's approval and against his advice.[1] In this document, Hein analyzed "the role dentistry played in establishing the Medical Center, the initiation and the collapse of the undergraduate dental school, and the development of the graduate dental program." According to Hein, his was the first completely honest assessment of the relationship between the Eastman Dental Dispensary and the School of Medicine and Dentistry. He undertook the appraisal at that time, he said, because "the graduate dental program is in a critical period and the decisions of the next few months will profoundly affect its future."[2]

Hein's presentation included suggestions of how several million dollars could be used for the benefit of dentistry at the University of Rochester. He asked the trustees to keep in mind the following points:

Mr. Eastman was primarily motivated by an interest in the dental phase of the School of Medicine and Dentistry when he donated $6.5 million to the institution during his lifetime.

Dental interests have never been fully represented in the uses made of the donations from Mr. Eastman.

The graduate dental program while officially a substitute for the undergraduate dental program has been in reality considered only as a temporary measure.

The university and its medical school have never taken any concrete steps to assure the graduate dental program of a secure and adequate financial future.

In spite of existing under adverse circumstances, the graduate dental program has been eminently successful and has and is filling a unique need in dental education.

The graduate dental program has the moral and just right to expect that its needs be met now, even if this means transferring the burden to those who have benefited from dentistry's interests in the past.

Not surprisingly, this severe assessment of how dentistry had been "cheated" from the beginning did not endear Hein to university trustees nor to his superiors. A new medical dean, Dr. Donald Anderson[3] had just come on board, and Hein's blunt approach contributed to souring Anderson on Hein and perhaps on Bibby—who was not directly involved. In addition, Dean Emeritus Whipple, who had conceived and started the fellows program, was offended by Hein's harsh words. In his report, Hein reiterated the history of the School of Medicine and Dentistry, noting that Abraham Flexner[4] had said at the school's inception: "The new school will undertake to place training in dentistry on the same academic and scientific level as training in medicine and surgery." Hein further noted that when Dr. Burkhart informed the donor of his letter to Dr. Simon Flexner, "Mr. Eastman expressed great interest in the possibility of developing a medical school which *would allow his plans for a dental school to be realized* [emphasis added]." Hein quoted Eastman as saying: "The dispensary is the best clinic in the world for dental surgery . . . [and] will make possible a combination of dental with medical education which is ideal and will set a new standard for training in dentistry as Johns Hopkins did for training in medicine a generation ago." Another Eastman quote that Hein reiterated was: "The carrying out of such an alliance will call for a very high degree of cooperation between the trustees of the dispensary and the trustees of the university." That high degree of cooperation would prove elusive.

Hein put his finger on the chief reason that efforts to found an undergraduate school of dentistry failed: The required preparation for entrance to medical school was three years of college, but for dentistry, only high school graduation. Yet it was only on the basis of absolute parity that the doors of the School of Medicine and Dentistry were to be opened to interested dental applicants. Catalogs from the years 1925 through 1929 stated: "Absolutely the same standards will be applied in rating the qualifications of applicants for the course in dentistry and the course in medicine," which to many looked like a not-too-subtle way of discouraging dental applicants. "One would have to be very naive to expect a rush of [dental] candidates," Hein concluded, and then added: "It certainly must have been anticipated by those interested in the program, that considerable time would elapse before the program could begin to function. If this had not been anticipated, then it must be assumed that those responsible either were not sincerely interested in the ultimate success of the endeavor, or were completely unfamiliar with the problems of dentistry at that time."

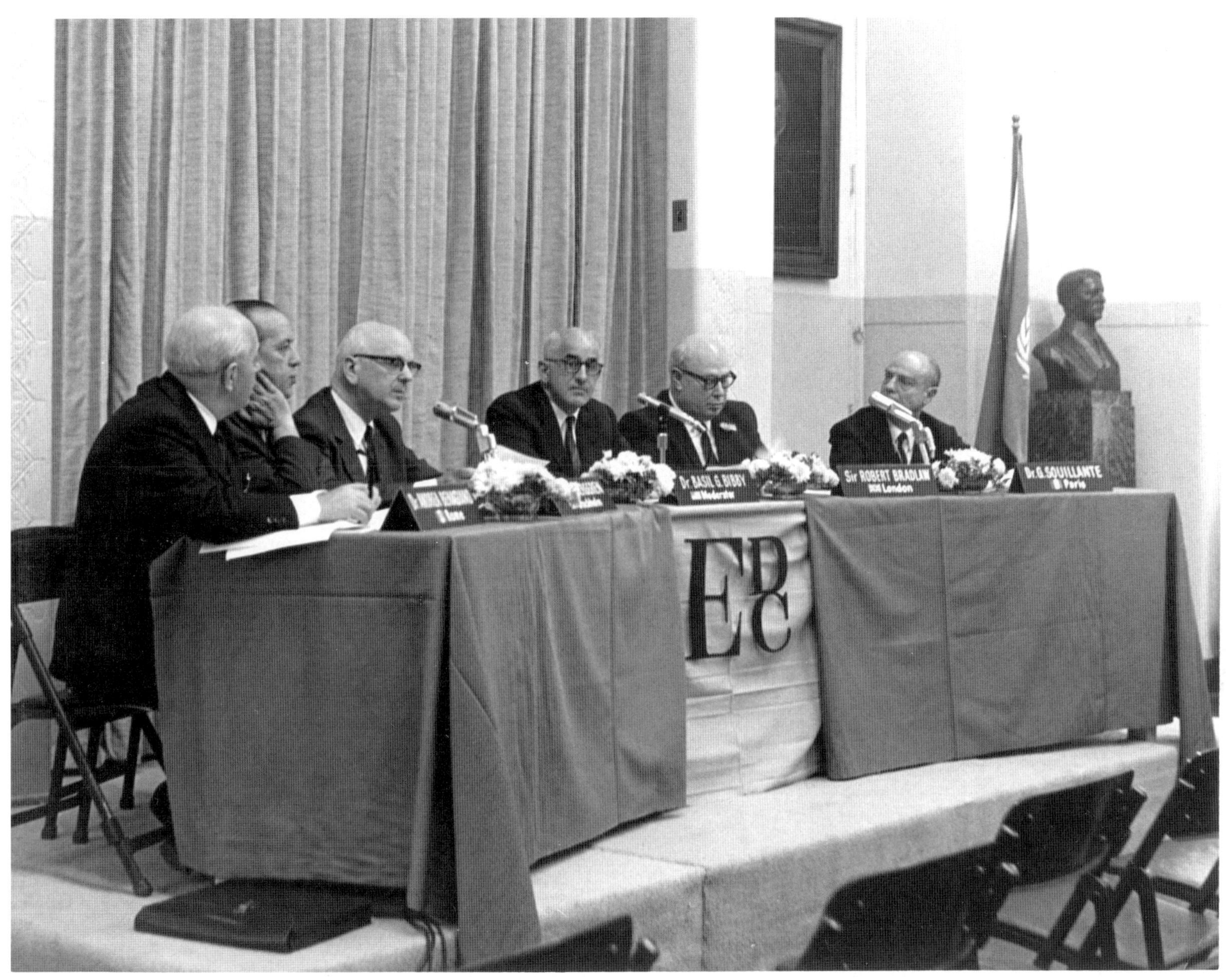

Dr. Bibby and panel of directors of European clinics in 1967 on the occasion of the fiftieth anniversary of the opening of the Rochester Dental Dispensary

Hein saw a diminished and minor emphasis on dentistry at the university from the beginning. The early catalogs averaged thirteen sections on such topics as the advantages of Rochester, housing and recreation, public health, libraries, and the school of nursing. Only one of the thirteen catalog sections was about dentistry. Hein thought the lack of support for dentistry that had been part of the physician-dominated medical school was exemplified from the very beginning in President Rhees's 1929 announcement: "It now seems to me wise that we discontinue the offer of undergraduate instruction in dentistry for which there seems to be no demand."

Hein saw this as closing the doors of the dental school, replacing it with an "outside-supported program"—the Dental Research Fellowship Program that was supported by the Rockefeller Foundation. He argued that dentistry's interests were never equally represented. Although Dr. Burkhart held the title Dean of Clinical Dentistry from 1925 to 29, neither he nor any dentist was on the advisory board of the School of Medicine and Dentistry (only medical departments were represented) or on the powerful University Council. Also, Hein claimed, there were irregularities in some of the PhD programs that had been worked out for the dental fellows. Some were transferred from one science department where their research or academic progress was questionable, to another department, where less was expected of them.

Hein attempted to involve the new university president, Cornelis W. de Kiewiet, in an effort to gain additional support for the dental research program in the face of what he believed was the new medical dean's diminishing interest in dental research. Despite Eastman's stated intention of "doing something else for dentistry," none of the $29 million that he willed to the university was being set aside to meet the needs of the dental research program in the School of Medicine and Dentistry or the dental service in Strong Memorial Hospital. Hein's attempt to force the university to take action favorable to dentistry had no positive effect, Bibby concluded. Instead, its failure persuaded Hein to resign. From that point onward, relations between the School of Medicine and Dentistry and the Eastman Dental Center went south. Dr. Stanley Handelman identifies some of the sources of discord and tension as physicians versus dentists in a medical center setting, basic science researchers versus clinical researchers, and both of the latter versus clinicians.

A thirteen-page history titled "Eastman Dental Center and School Of Medicine and Dentistry" written in March 1976 by Basil Bibby, then in his retirement, begins with the three areas of interest that gave rise to the University of Rochester School of Medicine and Dentistry: patient care, education, and research. He noted, "Shortly after the dispensary opened, Mr. Eastman expressed interest in training dentists in Rochester and was encouraged in that possibility by Dr. Burkhart. Whether the motivation was purely educational or mixed with practical considerations of providing dentists for the dispensary is not known. Mr. Eastman is reported to have said that he wanted a dental school but if the only way he could get it was with a medical school then he would support that too."

Bibby also quotes pediatrician Dr. Albert D. Kaiser, city health officer, friend, and traveling companion of Eastman, who cites Eastman's interest in founding a permanent children's hospital in conjunction with a dispensary for tonsillectomies. Kaiser advised Eastman that "such a hospital service should be planned in the broader context of a general hospital or medical center." Bibby further writes that the Rockefeller money was "matched by five million dollars from Mr. Eastman, one million dollars of which was represented by the money Mr. Eastman had vested in the dental dispensary. The dispensary's endowment and independence was a recurrent temptation for the School of Medicine and Dentistry." The founders also anticipated they were breaking new ground in attempting to educate physicians and dentists together in a medical center setting: "Both Mr. Eastman and Dr. Burkhart anticipated that the dental school would have higher educational standards than those then current in the United States," Bibby wrote.

COOPERATIVE EDC / SMD PROGRAMS

During the Bibby years, several cooperative research projects were carried forward with the university dental fellows or by faculty at the medical school. In 1957, the university received a $175,000 grant from the U.S. Public Health Service, the largest grant to that date received by the School of Medicine and Dentistry. The grant provided for the addition of three more dental research fellows and the purchase of research equipment. In addition, on the heels of that grant, the Colgate Palmolive Company gave two equal grants to the school and dispensary of $4,500 each. The university grant was to fund a $4,000 fellowship plus $500 to cover research costs; the grant to the dispensary was to assist its program of training dental graduates for careers in

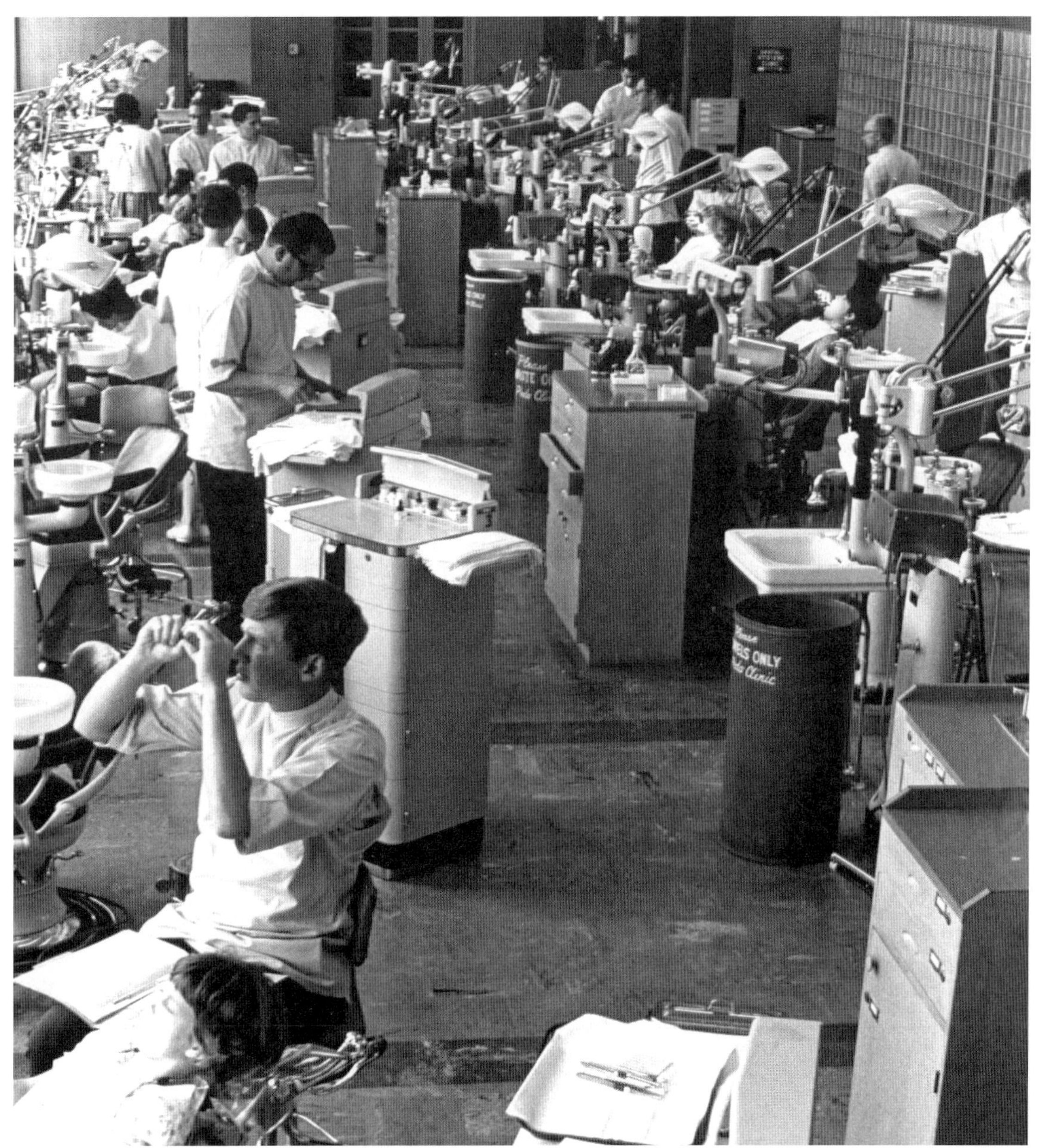

The Eastman Dental Center in operation

teaching and research. Dentists from abroad on the junior trainee staff at the dispensary were required to participate in course work, seminars, or research for which a master of science degree in dental science from the university could be earned. They were registered at the dispensary as clinical dental fellows in a combined School of Medicine and Dentistry/Eastman Dental Dispensary program with approval of registration resting with the university rather than the state Board of Dental Examiners. Dean Donald Anderson, who succeeded Whipple as dean of the School of Medicine and Dentistry and who was director of the Medical Center when Whipple retired in 1953, obtained approval for this cooperative program from the State Education Department. After the program was initiated, some of the dentists treating patients at the dispensary were registered as clinical dental fellows in this combined program. Over the years, this unique dental fellowship program attracted dentists from many parts of the world.

In 1955, Dean Anderson spoke of an extra benefit of the program: "The research contribution is noteworthy even though the main emphasis of the program is preparation for teaching and research careers rather than in pursuit of research itself."[5]

> They have shown that dentists can do high-grade research; they have established that dentistry does have a scientific content which is worth the attention of good non-dental scientists; and they have demonstrated that research experience is valuable training for teachers in a changing profession. Twenty years ago, these ideas were completely strange to dentistry, but now largely as a result of the dental experiment in Rochester, they are widely accepted, and many universities and governmental agencies are now offering dentists training and research fellowships in the medical sciences.[6]

Other examples of positive collaboration between Eastman Dental Center and the School of Medicine and Dentistry include the formalization of the university's master's degree program in dentistry and five graduate courses focusing on dental caries, periodontal disease, saliva, mucus membrane lesions, and head and neck anatomy. These carried credit on par with other graduate school courses and were required for master's candidates at the dental center.

Bibby, however, maintained that his group did the best research: "These golden days at the Eastman Dental Dispensary were not paralleled by dental research developments at the University of Rochester." Nevertheless, there

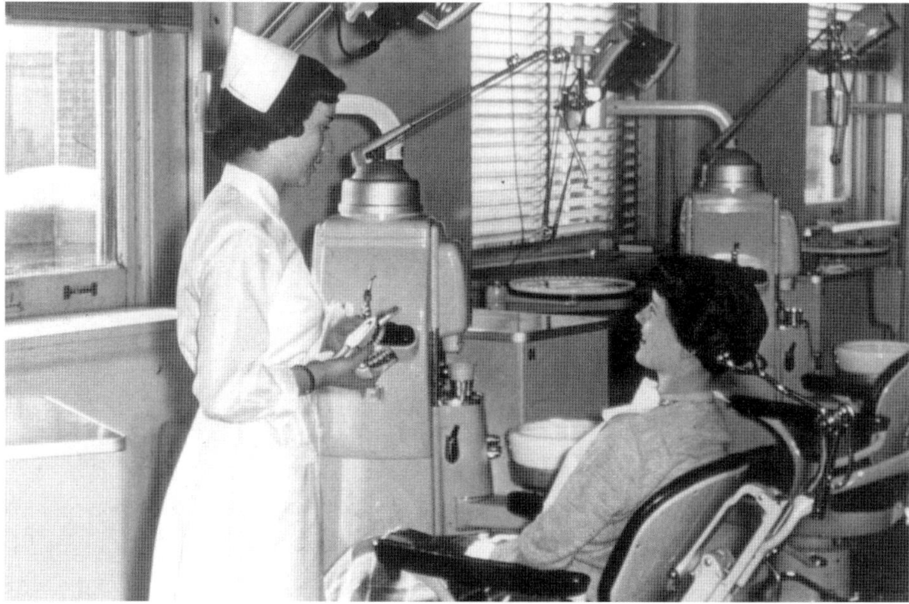

Advice from a hygienist: "Floss, floss, floss"

are examples of significant research at the School of Medicine and Dentistry, such as Harold Hodge's work on fluoride. Two university scientists and a former assistant dean of the school were part of a six-person task force studying ways of combating tooth decay.

In 1955, Bibby commissioned an independent "appreciation" of the Eastman Dental Dispensary by G. N. Davies, who reported: "Dental education and public health dentistry received their initial stimulus from independent institutions—such as the Eastman Dental Dispensary and Forsyth Dental Infirmary. [These] have now become so organized that the independents have become of progressively decreasing significance." This was a radical change of focus, and Bibby realized that a reappraisal of the role of the independent institution was needed. He envisioned an Eastman graduate school of dentistry operating under the auspices of the University of Rochester. "It is unfortunate for dentistry," he wrote in his annual report in 1957, "that so far the university has shown little interest in exploring such possibilities."

But Bibby soldiered on. He wrote, "To be registered as a graduate school . . . it is necessary for it to work out an agreement with the University of Rochester so that the Eastman Dental Dispensary becomes recognized as a graduate division of dentistry. . . . For this purpose it is necessary for the Eastman Dental Dispensary to accept a limited number of adult patients." And so, a limited number of adult patients referred by practitioners were enrolled. But other impediments remained: the physical separation of the campuses, the clash of personalities, and the questions of who would head the department and who would control the sizable Eastman endowment.

ERLING JOHANSEN SUCCEEDS HEIN

The close relationship between Bibby and Jack Hein produced an active exchange of research, information, facilities, and staff. Hein's successor, Dr. Erling Johansen, made this appraisal:

> John Hein was a fearless fighter and he prepared and circulated his, at the time, famous document outlining the needs of the department relating it to the history of dentistry at the University of Rochester. . . . It created a major stir at all levels in the university, resulting in renewed scrutiny of dentistry's relevance and place in the School of Medicine and Dentistry. There did not seem to be resolution forthcoming in the spring of 1955, and John Hein resigned to take a position at the Colgate Company.

With Hein's departure, Johansen was appointed chairman of the Department of Dentistry and Dental Research on the same day that he finished his PhD defense. Some thought that he was too young and inexperienced. Suddenly, all of the problems were right in his lap. Johansen determined to continue his good personal relations with the retiring Dr. Whipple as well as with Dr. Bibby and with Harold Hodge of School of Medicine and Dentistry's pharmacology department, and to establish good relations with the new dean, Dr. Anderson. To this end, Johansen developed the idea of a major celebration of the twenty-fifth anniversary of the dental research program, including a reunion of past fellows participating in a symposium on dental research on October 8, 1955. The event was deemed a rousing success and contributed to calming the situation temporarily.

As a youth, Dr. Erling Johansen had been in the Norwegian resistance movement from 1940 to 1943, from age seventeen to twenty. He had studied German for three years and so was one of the few in his country town, heavily occupied by Germans, who could translate back and forth. He drove a taxi and reported on strategic troop movements and documents for the resistance. Radios were verboten and listening to broadcasts from London, where the legitimate Norwegian government was in exile, was punishable by death. It was a dangerous time, Johansen remembered:

> I carried with me . . . enhanced power of observation, analysis of the environment in which I was functioning, deductions on what was said versus actuality, separation of friend from foe, and absolute emotional self-control and ability to keep silent when that seemed to be called for in the situation and the virtual persistence and optimism in spite of insurmountable obstacles and danger. At Rochester, I soon became a friend of the chairman of the department of dentistry and dental research, Dr. John Hein, who also served as my best man [in his 1952 marriage].

Johansen came to the School of Medicine and Dentistry in 1950 as a graduate student fellow and PhD candidate in the pathology department. He had spent one year as a dental officer in the Norwegian contingent of the allied occupation force in Germany and four years as a dental student at Tufts. He found that the new research department where he was enrolled did not have any space, laboratory, or office of its own. Its budget was totally inadequate and it was not represented in the governing body of the School of Medicine and Dentistry. At the Eastman Dental Dispensary, Dr. Bibby was moving fast to establish and expand research programs and graduate training programs in cooperation with the new Department of Dentistry and Dental Research. Early in his tenure, Johansen told Bibby that, as a result of his war experiences, he had learned to trust no one. Bibby assumed this would include the director of the Eastman Dental Dispensary. The two had diametrically opposed memories of the twenty-year period from 1950 to 1970.

Johansen recalls warm relations and friendships with his chief advisor, Dr. William Hopkins, professor of pathology, with George Hoyt Whipple, chairman of pathology and the dean while Johansen was a graduate student, and with Dean Anderson. Anderson appointed Johansen to an endowed professorship in 1966—only the third endowed professorship in the whole medical center—to dissuade Johansen from taking a leadership position at the

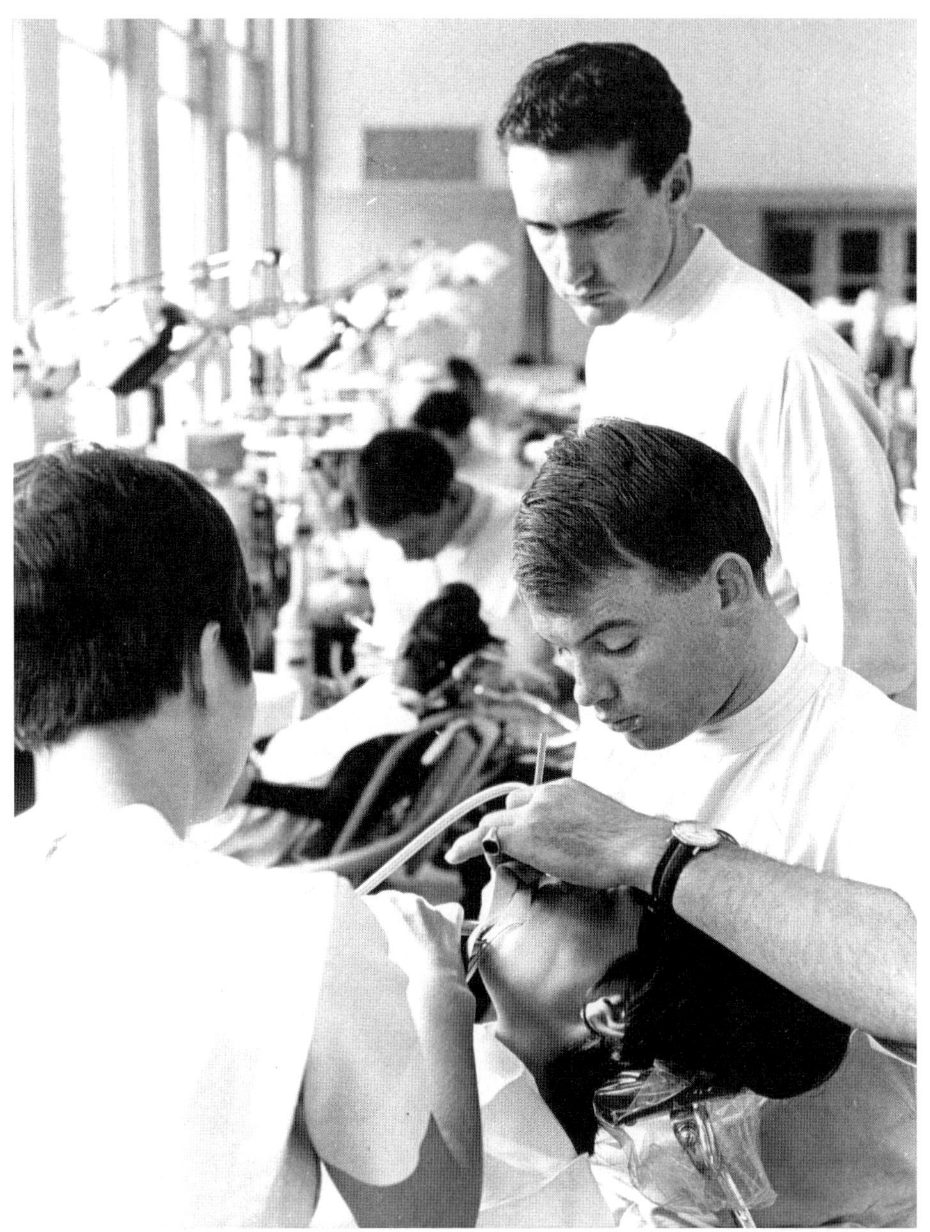

Supervising the work of interns

Harvard School of Dental Medicine. Johansen remembers the relationship with Bibby as one of mutually supportive, friendly cooperation. "Both Dr. Bibby and I had the same basic interest and concern, namely to advance dentistry, that is dental education, research and patient care, to the fullest extent made possible by our resources." Johansen said tensions between the School of Medicine and Dentistry and the Eastman Dental Center began in 1970 after Bibby's retirement. Bibby, on the other hand, wrote that stress was present from the time that Hein left in the early 1950s.

One thing seems clear: The relationship between the school and the dispensary was never clearly defined or properly structured nor a chain of command established until the twenty-first century. When inevitable personality clashes and turf wars arose, competition rather than cooperation became the norm.

COOPERATION AND TENSIONS

With the goodwill that had developed, Johansen believed he had largely achieved the goals outlined by Hein—space for laboratories and offices, a budget to support the department, and representation on the advisory board or the governing body of the school—although this was not fully realized until William McHugh's tenure as director of the Eastman Dental Center. Johansen asserts that "with major funding by obtaining grants from the National Institute of Health, industry, and corporations, the department flourished until Dr. Bibby's retirement."

Bibby had a different take. From the time of Dr. Hein's dramatic departure from Rochester in 1955, things changed. An era of fledgling cooperation ended. He and Johansen did not always see eye-to-eye, and uncertain support for the Eastman Dental Dispensary from the new medical dean, Donald Anderson, added to funding problems. There was difficulty in obtaining approval for appointments; the lack of a source of animals and animal quarters suitable for dispensary research dried up research projects. Dr. Daniel Subtelny's cinefluorography study in x-ray orthodontic dissection in anatomy was blocked, and university faculty did not consult dental center staff. The physical separation of the dispensary from the medical school and Strong Memorial Hospital reflected "the separation of medicine and dentistry which in the United States is wider than anywhere else in the world," Bibby wrote. He believed that Flexner and Eastman had organized the School of Medicine

and Dentistry as a single school for the "purpose of narrowing this unhealthy educational gap." When the experiment failed, the fellows program was established, which largely closed the gap in scientific research but not in training opportunities for clinical teachers. Bibby saw a "musical comedy quality" about the fact that after many years when Burkhart "avoided committing to any cooperative program . . . the roles have been reversed, and the Dispensary has become the ardent suitor, while the University plays the part of the coy maiden fearing despoilment."[7]

That the subject of cooperation between the two entities was foremost in everyone's mind is evident from the many archival documents exploring the subject. A 1952 conference held by Bibby, Hein, and Elmer. J. Pammenter, of the Strong Memorial Hospital dental clinic, concluded that the dental clinic in the surgery department had not produced clinicians with a broad background and training in dentistry. Programs in other institutions had equaled or surpassed the formerly renowned dental fellows program. Rochester had limited financial resources—excepting the dispensary endowment. Pooling resources into an integrated program of dental education, research, and service leading to the development of a graduate school of dentistry could attract outside support and funding.

Within two or three years of Hein's report and the appointment of Johansen, issues and tensions had moved front and center. In 1957, Dean Anderson, Harper Sibley, civic leader and dispensary trustee, and university president de Kiewiet asked Bibby to prepare a proposal for expanded cooperation between the dispensary and university. For the purposes of achieving educational leadership and community benefit, his proposal stated, "the recruitment and training of *clinical dental teachers* should be added to the graduate dental program." That same year, Bibby invited himself to the executive committee meeting of the American Association of Dental Schools to present plans for a joint Society for a Graduate Study Center in dentistry, which he thought the university had agreed to, only to find that Johansen, representing Anderson, was present at the meeting and denied that the university would participate in the plan.

A comment on relations written by Bibby in 1959 begins, "The staff of the Dispensary is confused as to what type of relationship the University wishes to have . . . Formal and informal approaches have failed to produce definition." Bibby concludes by suggesting that the dispensary be constituted as a "separate dental department parallel to but independent of the university's

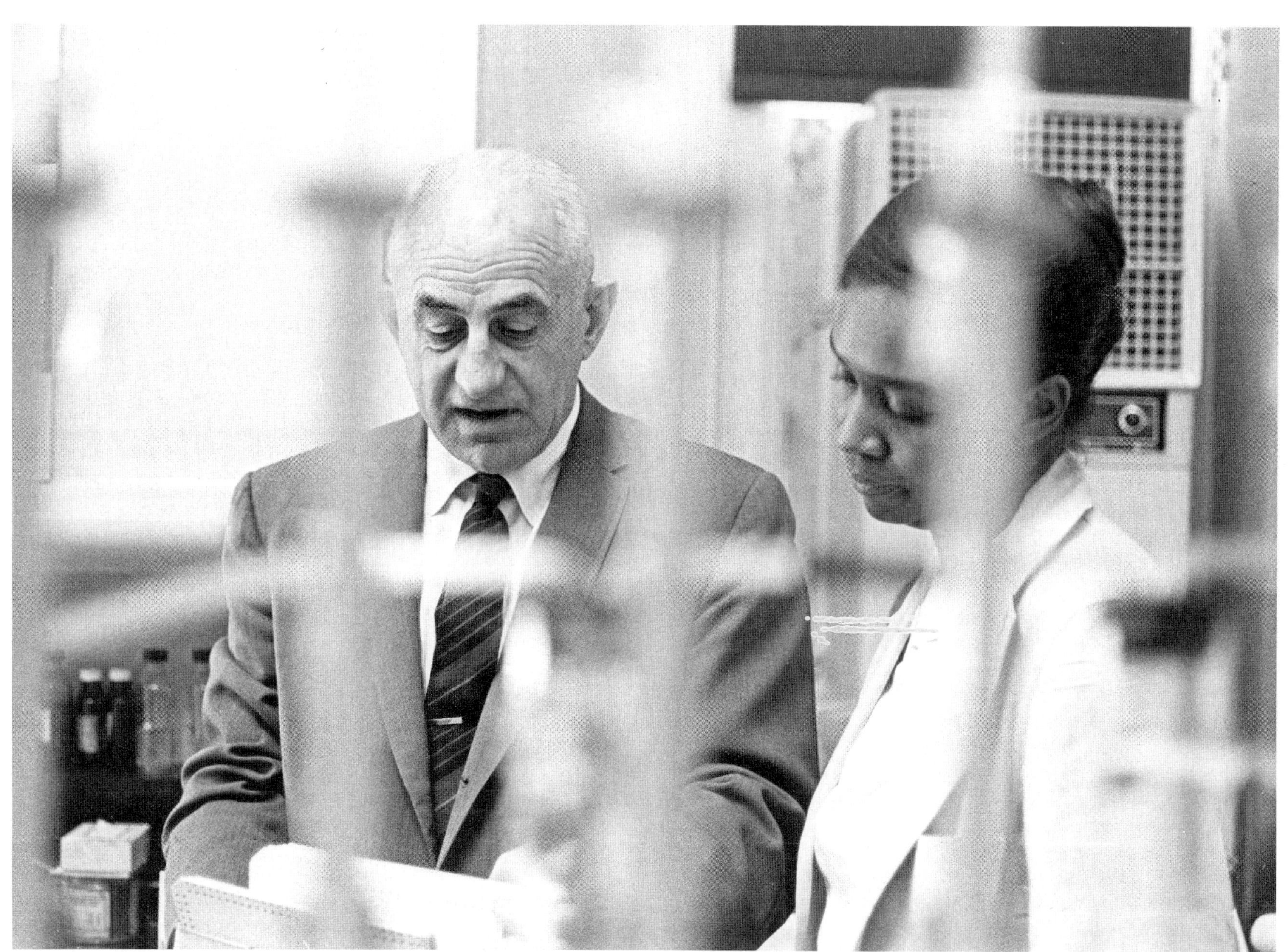

Dr. Bibby in the research laboratory with a technician

Department of Dental Research." An alternative suggestion advanced by Bibby was that the pattern of affiliation entered into by Harvard and the Forsyth Infirmary, in which Forsyth gave up clinical dentistry to become the dental research arm of Harvard, be considered. This memorandum was also circulated to dental trustees Bernard Finucane, M. Herbert Eisenhart, and Charles Hutchison—all close friends of George Eastman.

In 1961 Bibby wrote a memorandum to file entitled "Cooperation." These three pages listed areas of "disappearing cooperation" and concluded: "The loss to dentistry of an almost unequaled opportunity to develop a unique clinical research and training activity gives the situation the air of tragedy rather than comedy." That same year, visiting dental consultants urged "closer collaboration" and the formation of a joint committee to study and make recommendations. Bibby noted on his copy of the report: "By Product of some prompting by BGB & from above." Dean Anderson wrote a cover letter endorsing the idea of closer collaboration, while at the same time he and Johansen authored a confidential memorandum to William S. Vaughn, president of the Eastman Kodak Company, and Marion B. Folsom, the Kodak official who became Secretary of Health, Education, and Welfare under President Eisenhower. Anderson and Johansen's "Outline of Background of University's Program in Dentistry and Its relationship to the Eastman Dental Dispensary" stated, "Today the University of Rochester is considered the outstanding center for the training of dental teachers and investigators." It further admitted, "The cooperation between the two dental programs has not been as effective as might have been hoped. . . . The university's educational contribution to the joint graduate program represents an activity of considerable magnitude. . . . The organization of a clinical teachers program may depend on Eastman Dental Dispensary cooperation, as the University of Rochester is not in a position to commit funds for this purpose."

For his part during the early 1960s, Bibby suggested joint activities in clinical areas (joint appointments, referral of patients, training, instruction, and clinical research), in laboratory research areas, and in the instructional program. Once the new dental center research wing was completed to accommodate the greatly expanded research activities and the institutional name changed, Bibby returned to reviewing on paper the dental activities in the two institutions. A 1967 memorandum to file, "Cooperative activity with U of R," he frankly admitted, placed "emphasis on their present weaknesses rather than their past achievements." In it, Bibby compared the mission of

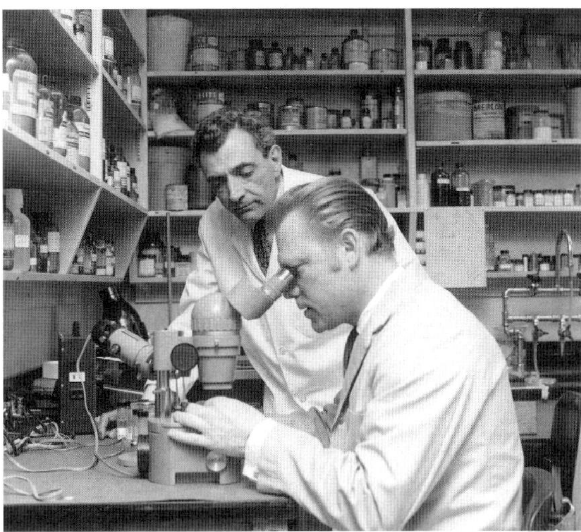

Dr. Buonocore (standing) with research technician Dick Glena

the dental center to that of a teaching hospital in medicine. The philosophy behind patient care had changed from the Burkhart years and the center now emphasized providing "quality service to interested patients rather than supplying larger numbers of poorly motivated persons with less adequate treatment." As with many documents in the archives, there is no indication of whether this memo was meant for a specific person or publication or whether it was simply Bibby's own musings in preparation for a board meeting or annual report.

Bibby came to believe that many dental center activities suffered disadvantages because they were not under university sponsorship. "The national patterns of support for research and training and educational accreditation have been tailored to fit universities," he concluded. "Independent institutions start at a disadvantage. While there is questioning of university centripetalism, it must be accepted as fact in present-day society." The Eastman Dental Center had advanced to the point where it could not move forward without dependence on the University of Rochester.

Consultants recommended university cooperation with the dental center in training teachers for clinical dentistry. Problems of oral biology needed to be presented in a more challenging manner. The clinical dental program at Strong Memorial Hospital was undistinguished and contributed little to

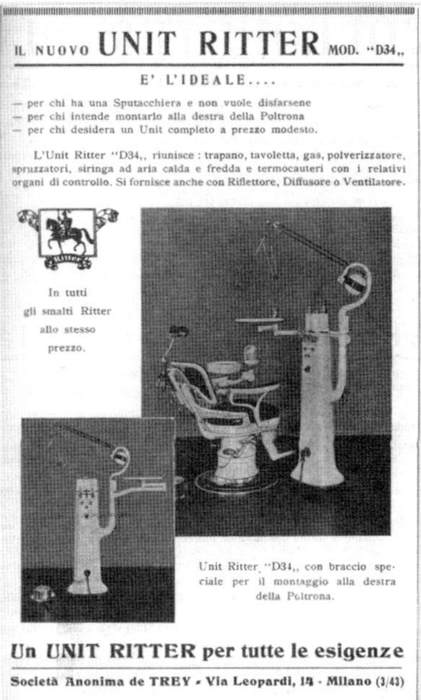

Ritter ad, Milan, Italy

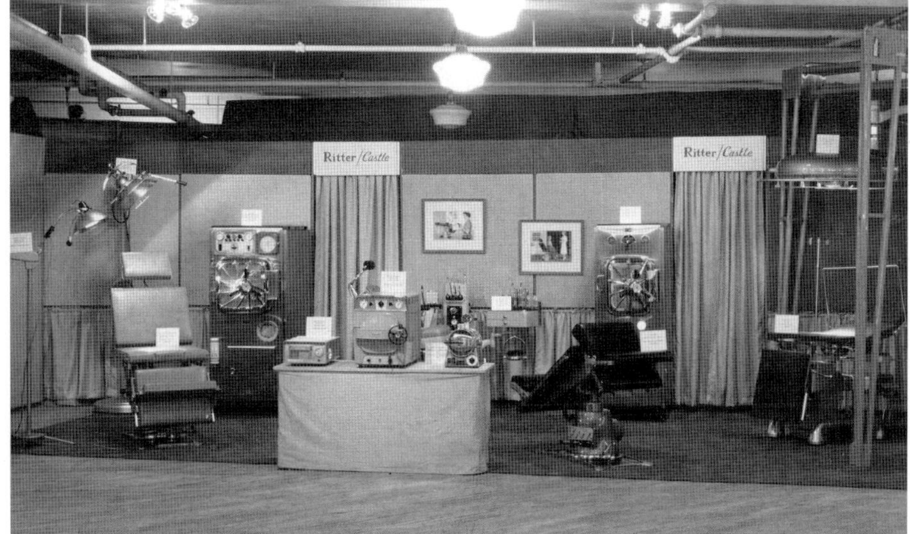

Ritter/Castle exhibit

dentistry in the community, they reported. It was the only clinical department that did not have a full-time head. Most Rochester-trained physicians held dentistry in lower esteem than it deserved, the consultants concluded. Bibby proposed that the weaknesses in the dental programs of both institutions could be overcome by coordinating and expanding under defined management to develop a graduate school of dentistry under a board of control composed of equal numbers of university and dental center trustees. This board would appoint a dean for joint dental activities. The dean would hold senior rank at both the School of Medicine and Dentistry and the Eastman Dental Center.

Johansen's concept of academic management was based on his European background, Bibby concluded. The dental research group was in need of a period of tighter administration than Dr. Hein had provided, according to Bibby, and "to Dr. Johansen's credit," he provided that. Without this "'in line' direction it is probable that School of Medicine and Dentistry support of the dental research group would have evaporated and the program discontinued."[8] Instead, by not being committed to supplying special opportunities for senior staff or trainees at the Eastman Dental Dispensary and by rigid control of the dental program at the School of Medicine and Dentistry, Johansen may have helped build the dental research group more firmly than previously into the school's table of organization.[9] However, Johansen's tight administration also frustrated Bibby, as when Johansen cancelled existing cooperative arrangements established under Hein, substituting School of Medicine and Dentistry courses that he himself organized for the cooperative courses.

According to Bibby, Johansen indicated that he did not want dental center people working out arrangements for special instruction or laboratory activities with the heads of the medical science departments (for example, head and neck dissection arranged by the Department of Anatomy). And no Eastman dentist would be allowed to work in any department of the School of Medicine and Dentistry without Johansen's permission. Bibby decided that either Johansen did not want research and teaching activities at the dental center, or that Johansen knew of the clause indicating George Eastman's wish that if the dispensary were unable to continue, all assets would be transferred to the university. Nevertheless, the basic science departments of the School of Medicine and Dentistry that were not under Johansen's control did work with the Eastman Dental Dispensary on important research on the reactions between fluoride and teeth in the prevention of caries. Full cooperation of the

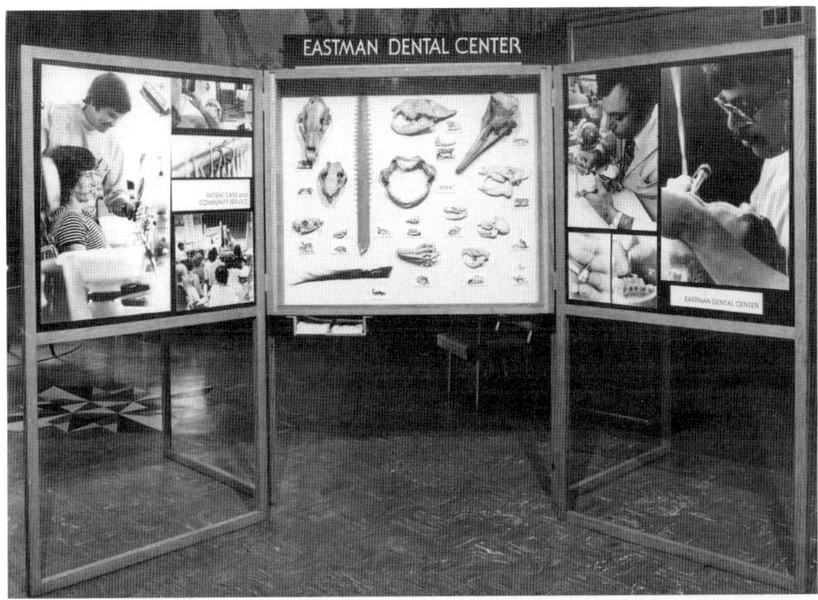

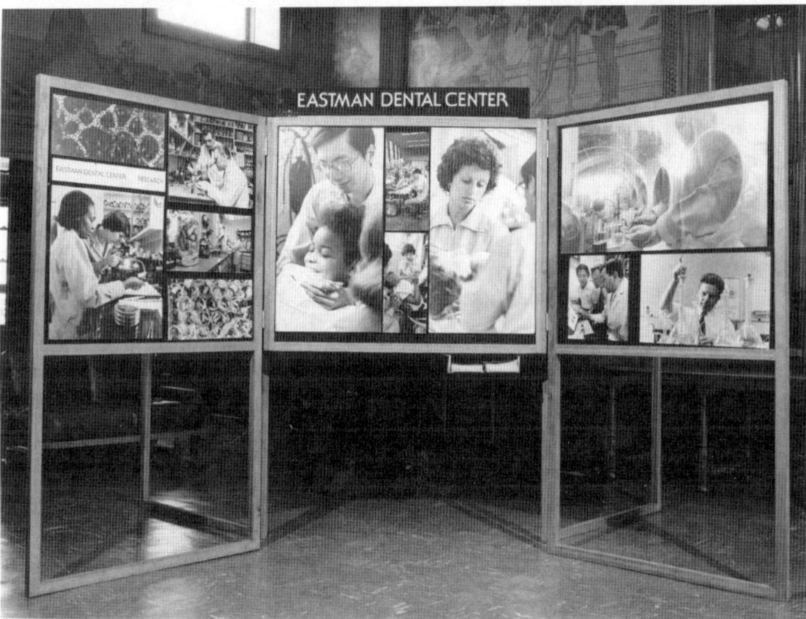

Eastman Dental Center exhibits

nondental staff of the School of Medicine and Dentistry was maintained in obtaining research grants. Charles Hutchison had been the dispensary trustee primarily responsible during the Burkhart years for having the Eastman Dental Dispensary annually contribute to the support of the research training program at the School of Medicine and Dentistry. But Hutchison now asked whether, in view of the National Institutes of Health support of the university training program, the board should continue to make this contribution. The dental trustees instructed Bibby to find out how the Eastman contribution was being used. Dean Anderson agreed that the contribution was no longer used for fellowship support but not that the unused portion should be used for support of research fellowships at dental center. Needless to say, this did not please Bibby.

Since the Eastman Dental Center was in a period of expanding growth and activity in research and clinical teaching, Bibby tried to reach an understanding with Johansen so that school developments would supplement rather than compete with Eastman developments. Even within this framework, Johansen had no interest in discussing coordination of long-range developments.

From the vantage of 2004, Beatrice Bibby commented on the spirit of cooperation during these years: "One of the things Basil had hoped would be achieved would be good rapport with the university, which I think was just fine for a while. Jack Hein was director of the dental research group when Basil became director of the dental center. But then personalities intervened and that kind of close relationship didn't work out. . . . You change the dean and the whole dynamic changes," Mrs. Bibby continued. "Or you change the man who is the head of the dental group and the whole dynamic changes. I think they just saw things from different angles. So, it was hard for them to cooperate."[10]

"Personalities," Beatrice Bibby says. She indicates that Whipple was Basil Bibby's mentor and that Whipple was instrumental in Bibby becoming director of the Eastman Dental Dispensary. That close relationship did not exist between Bibby and Whipple's successor, Donald Anderson, after 1952. Cooperative effort also broke down on the selecting of senior faculty that would be most useful to both institutions. In keeping with the understanding that had existed with Dr. Hein, appointments of dentists qualified to head up an oral surgery and periodontal clinic at the Eastman Dental Dispensary/Center were discussed with Johansen. However, after the appointed men, Dr. Don Robinson and Dr. Helmut Zander, had moved to Rochester, Johansen

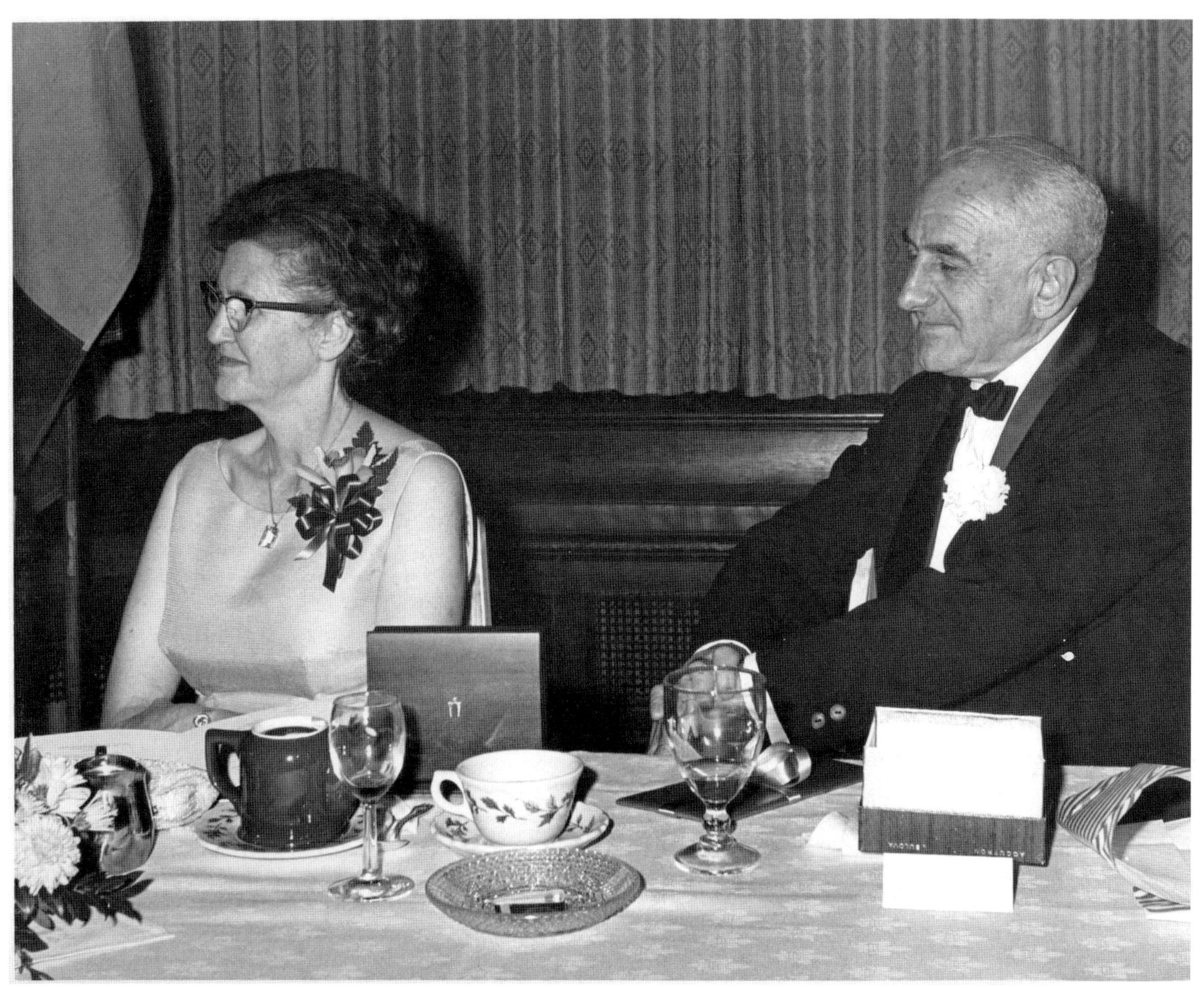

Mrs. Bibby and Dr. Bibby

maintained that the appointments had been made without his knowledge. Robinson received such a cool welcome that he went elsewhere. Zander brought several research grants to Rochester, but did not get a professional appointment to the medical center until Johansen had left. After informal discussions yielded nothing, Johansen agreed to consider written proposals for closer cooperation. Several were prepared. One Bibby proposal outlined long-range developments in dentistry at the two institutions that would lead to a graduate school of dentistry. Another proposal suggested that plans for developments in one or another field of dentistry supplement rather than compete. For example, a needed major activity in periodontia could be developed at Strong hospital while the major responsibility for prosthetic dentistry could be assigned to the dental dispensary. Johansen acknowledged neither of these proposals; only after Bibby circumvented him and sent them to Dean Anderson were indefinite and negative responses received.

Secrecy reigned. Dental fellows and dentists at Strong Memorial Hospital's dental clinic were told to keep clear of the Eastman Dental Dispensary and faculty or their appointments would be at risk. Clinical services provided by Eastman to Strong's dental clinic broke down after Dr. Elmer J. Pammenter retired from Strong Memorial and Johansen did not favor his replacement. The arrangements under which Eastman patients whose diagnoses or treatments needed a medical opinion and who were referred to Strong Memorial Hospital began to slow while exchange of services in the opposite direction was unaffected. Active research continued with nondental faculty at the School of Medicine and Dentistry who were not under Johansen's leadership.

Johansen refused to recommend a research application from the School of Medicine and Dentistry's x-ray department and the Eastman Dental Center's orthodontics department to the National Institute for Dental Research requesting support for making a cineradiography study of swallowing and speech in patients with cleft palate. (By rewriting the application so that the special x-ray apparatus was installed in the dental center instead of the school, the grant was obtained.) Later grants to the dental center for research and teacher training were a vote of confidence that the National Institutes of Health considered the dental center as capable of conducting its own research and teacher training.

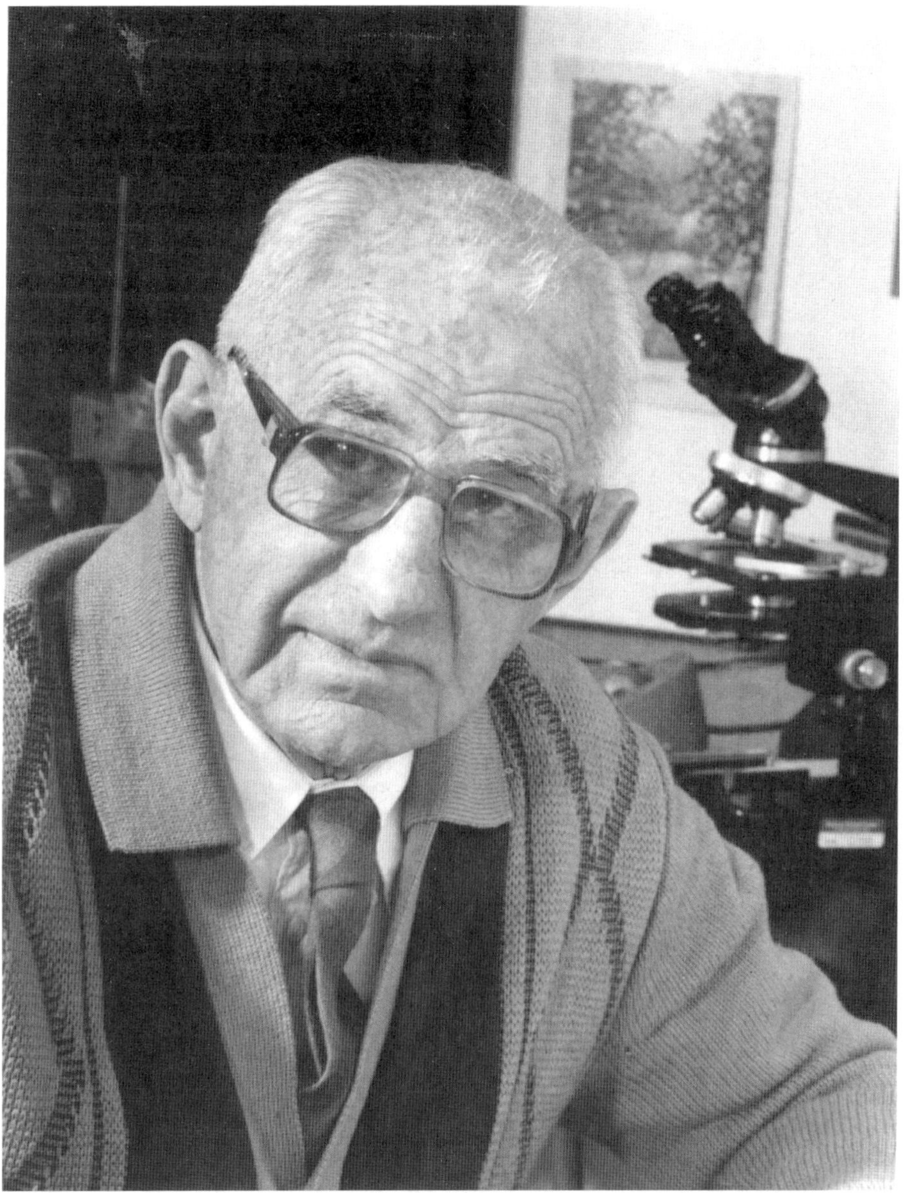

Dr. Basil Bibby

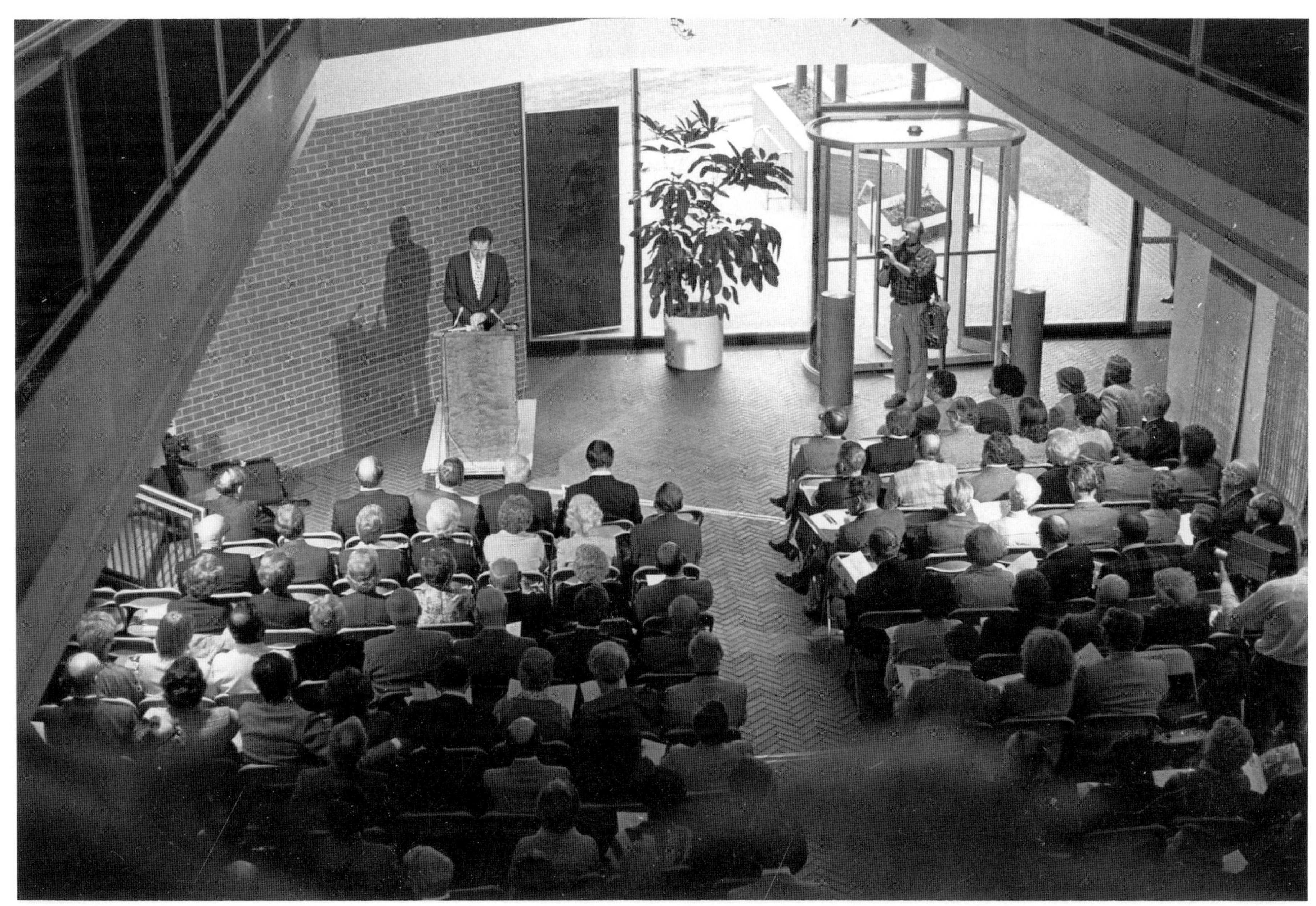

Dedication of Elmwood Avenue building in 1976

MOVING TOGETHER

DESTINY AT THE MEDICAL CENTER CAMPUS

It was felt at the time of the move, completed in 1977, that the organizational framework for closer collaboration had been established. The benefits were threefold—for the dental center, the medical center, and the community.

William D. McHugh, DDS

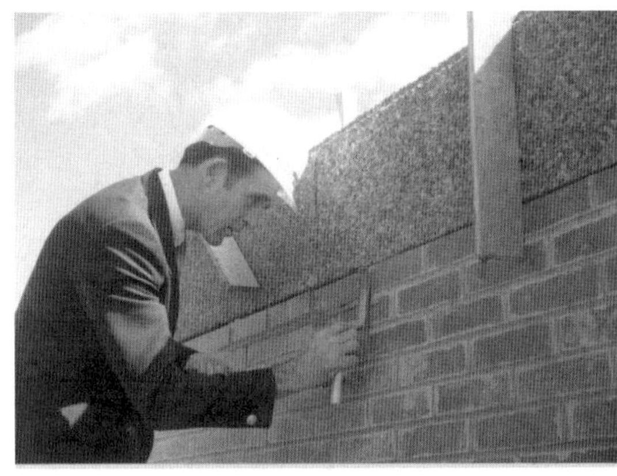

Dr. William D. McHugh applies the mortar.

ASSOCIATE DEAN FOR DENTAL AFFAIRS

IN 1969, BASIL BIBBY PREPARED TO RETIRE AFTER TWENTY-THREE YEARS as director of the Eastman Dental Center so that he could to devote his time to research. The Eastman Dental Center board and faculty along with Bibby supported the opinion that his replacement should hold the position of associate dean for dental affairs at the School of Medicine and Dentistry as well as being head of Eastman Dental Center. A joint committee composed of university personnel and the trustees of the dental center, prompted by the

Eastman Dental Center faculty and administration, made the recommendation. The recommendation stipulated that the position be held by the director of the Eastman Dental Center in order to maintain effective academic ties between the two institutions. The stated goal was to move the two institutions closer together, perhaps sealing an eventual merger. Then, as earlier, there was no unanimity on the desirability of a merger. Most Eastman Dental Center trustees were leery of losing independence and endowment, whereas students assumed that the entities had already merged. A built-in weakness was present from the start in that the heads of dental departments at the School of Medicine and Dentistry would have to report to an associate dean when previously they had reported to the medical dean of the School of Medicine and Dentistry. Furthermore, the associate dean was not given authority over the department budgets.

Dr. William D. McHugh, DDS., chair of the Department of Dental Health at the University of Dundee in Scotland, was appointed to both positions in 1970. McHugh had a long-standing interest in dental education, especially at the postdoctoral level. He had been educated the University of St. Andrews at Dundee and undertook advanced training in research and periodontology at dental schools in Malmö, Sweden, and in London and Birmingham, U.K. In 1963, he spent a sabbatical year in Rochester. Considering that three of the six directors of the Eastman Dental Center (in fifty-one of the past ninety-one years) have not been Americans, something could be presumed about the international repute of the Eastman Dental Center. Along the same lines, one of the unique marks of the Advanced Education in General Dentistry program developed during the

McHugh years was the number of highly qualified foreign residents. Beginning during the Bibby years, there had been a constant flow of foreign scientists on sabbatical, which, with the postdoctoral students from every continent, has created a unique international and intellectual ambience.

According to Stanley Handelman, who was at the Eastman Dental Center through both the Bibby and McHugh administrations, it was not an easy task for McHugh to follow in the footsteps of someone who was as universally respected as Basil Bibby. Bibby's board of trustees was cooperative and rarely questioned his decisions. The endowment was almost entirely invested in Kodak stock and enjoyed a remarkably high return in the postwar years, and there were no significant budget pressures on the clinical programs to increase their productivity.

In contrast, McHugh's board of trustees frequently challenged him. Part of this was related to the tenor of the times. Boards were increasingly expected to take a more active role in overseeing the financial management of institutions. Furthermore, Kodak stock was no longer a solid investment. To the credit of McHugh and the board, the endowment, which was over $30 million at that time and had been passively and conservatively managed by a local bank, was divided in three parts and now managed by three investment firms to facilitate the board monitoring their comparative returns.

EASTMAN DENTAL CENTER / SCHOOL OF MEDICINE AND DENTISTRY RELATIONS

"Eastman Center to Join U of R" was the newspaper headline that announced a merger of sorts in 1971. The text continued:

> The Eastman Dental Center has become formally affiliated with the University of Rochester, the institutions announced. Under terms of the affiliation, which has been approved by boards of trustees of both institutions, both institutions will work to develop programs of advanced dental education, research and service. Faculty appointments relating to cooperative activities will be made jointly by the university and the dental center.[1]

Thus, by December 1971, the Eastman Dental Center was officially *affiliated* with the School of Medicine and Dentistry "in order to provide a formal basis for joint activity in developing programs of advanced dental education, research and service."[2] In the years that followed, it became obvious that affiliation and cooperation were easier to declare than to practice. In 1993, twenty-two years later, the joint Eastman Dental Center /University of Rochester Affiliation Committee was still discussing "the role of the Eastman Dental Center director and staff in the School of Medicine and Dentistry, including the appointments, privileges, responsibilities and obligations." The 1993 committee further reported, "If agreement can be reached on these subjects the committee will have overcome a major obstacle to successful affiliation."[3]

Under McHugh's leadership in his role as School of Medicine and Dentistry associate dean for dental affairs and with the encouragement of Dr. Lowell Orbison, dean of the School of Medicine and Dentistry, a Department of Clinical Dentistry was formed. Dr. Fred Emmings was named chair. As McHugh wrote in 1975: "It was but a short step from the joint appointment of a senior administrator to the formalization in 1971 of the affiliation between the university and the Eastman Dental Center . . . for the joint development of programs of advanced dental education and research."[4] The creation of the new clinical department at Strong was a symptom of Dr. Johansen's diminishing credibility. The Department of Dental Research was having difficulty attracting graduate students and securing grants from the National Institute of Dental Research.

For the next three years, the strongest—indeed, the only—dental power in town was the Eastman Dental Center. Nevertheless, the opportunity was not taken to consolidate Eastman Dental Center's leadership role. The creation of the position of associate dean for dental affairs at the School of Medicine and Dentistry for McHugh was meant to draw the Eastman Dental Center and School of Medicine and Dentistry closer to a legal merger. Instead, or in addition, it interjected an impediment. Previously, the chair of the Department of Dentistry and Dental Research had reported to the dean of the School of Medicine and Dentistry. The new plan that he report to the new associate dean for dental affairs created difficulties. In this case, Erling Johansen felt that he was the senior person who had done a tremendous job for the university for twenty years in terms of teaching, research, getting grants, and organizing the very successful Dental Fellows reunion of 1955 in honor of the retired George Hoyt Whipple. "It was demeaning," he has said of the new plans that were emerging. "My wartime-acquired attributes were rekindled in response to the new leadership. Another atmosphere prevailed, quite different from what it was during the preceding twenty years. I found it to be insensitive and at times mean."[5] From Johansen's vantage, working with Dr. McHugh was much more difficult than working with Dr. Bibby had been. As associate dean for dental affairs, McHugh was intended to bring the two dental programs closer together, but from the beginning, he was in conflict with Johansen.

Perhaps history was repeating itself. As we have seen, Burkhart had difficulty knuckling under to the younger Whipple after being a unitary CEO for five years. Johansen may not have found Bibby a threat because they were equals (or maybe he even had a leg up on the older Bibby). But after twenty years of equality, McHugh's arrival as associate dean and therefore Johansen's boss was perceived as a threat. Bibby may have been more diplomatic too.

At the same time that Johansen gained a new boss, his department was split in two—with the new Department of Clinical Dentistry falling under Fred Emmings's leadership. From Johansen's perspective, the relationship between the two institutions was at an all-time low. So, in 1979, Erling Johansen accepted the post of dean of the Tufts University School of Dental Medicine. With the departure of Johansen, McHugh appointed Dr. Helmut Zander as interim chair of the Department of Dental Research. Zander soon retired, and the department languished for several years. Had McHugh recognized this opportunity at this critical juncture to fully integrate academic dentistry at the university and Eastman through organizational structure changes, the relationship of the Eastman Dental Center with the School of Medicine and Dentistry might have unfolded differently. But the opportunities that existed during the three years after Johansen's departure in 1979 were not seized.

Moreover, some thought that McHugh never attempted to involve himself seriously in the affairs and activities of the medical school, such as being an active member of its committees. Initially, he was given an office in the medical school and an administrative assistant. She was soon let go for lack of anything to do, and the office was closed. "The role of associate dean of dental affairs atrophied because it wasn't properly structured," Cyril Meyerowitz commented later, "and when Bill McHugh left [in 1993], it disappeared."[6]

In March of 1981, the School of Medicine and Dentistry dental faculty, most of whom were primarily faculty of Eastman Dental Center, proposed in a letter to university president Robert L. Sproull "a dental administrative reorganization intended to enhance and secure advancement of dental education and research in our university." The proposal, intended to address the weakness of the associate dean position under the medical dean, was "for establishing a position of dean of dentistry and possibly a graduate school of dentistry at the University of Rochester."[7] The letter was answered in May, not by President Sproull but by Dr. Frank E. Young, MD, PhD, dean of the School of Medicine and Dentistry since 1978. Young mentioned that "two major developments currently underway . . . a review of governance . . . [and] search for chair of the department of dental research" needed to be completed first. Young was also unhappy that the request, since it directly involved the School of Medicine and Dentistry, was not directed in the first instance to him as dean.[8] Once again, structural stalemates and personality clashes were undermining attempts to realize a merger. Yet the desire for unitary leadership, first articulated in 1920 by Eastman and Flexner, did not go away but remained a dream deferred.

As noted earlier, Eastman had described his hope in a letter to the dispensary trustees, written on June 25, 1920. Although the dispensary was founded to provide clinical dental care for indigent children, when the opportunity for it to become "part of a greater project for a higher grade of dental education than had before been attempted," he jumped at the prospect. Burkhart had been referred to in early publications as the "dean of dentistry," but there was no actual structure behind that short-lived title. It was Eastman who proposed that dentistry as well as medicine should be taught in the projected school, and Flexner who accepted the proposal with alacrity by saying at the announcement dinner in 1920 that the new School of Medicine and Dentistry would attempt to place dental education on the same academic and scientific plane as medicine.[9]

Fifty years later, we see Dr. Bibby, who after retirement took a temporary appointment at the National Institute of Dental Research in Bethesda before returning to the Eastman Dental Center to conduct research on dental caries, note that the affiliation between the university and the dental center was an attempt to close the gap between dental school education and new research developments so that dentists would have the most up-to-date knowledge of the field when they began to practice. "We are paralleling what was done in medicine thirty or forty years ago," Bibby said. He explained that it was recognition that the scientifically oriented clinician can bring new methods to teaching.

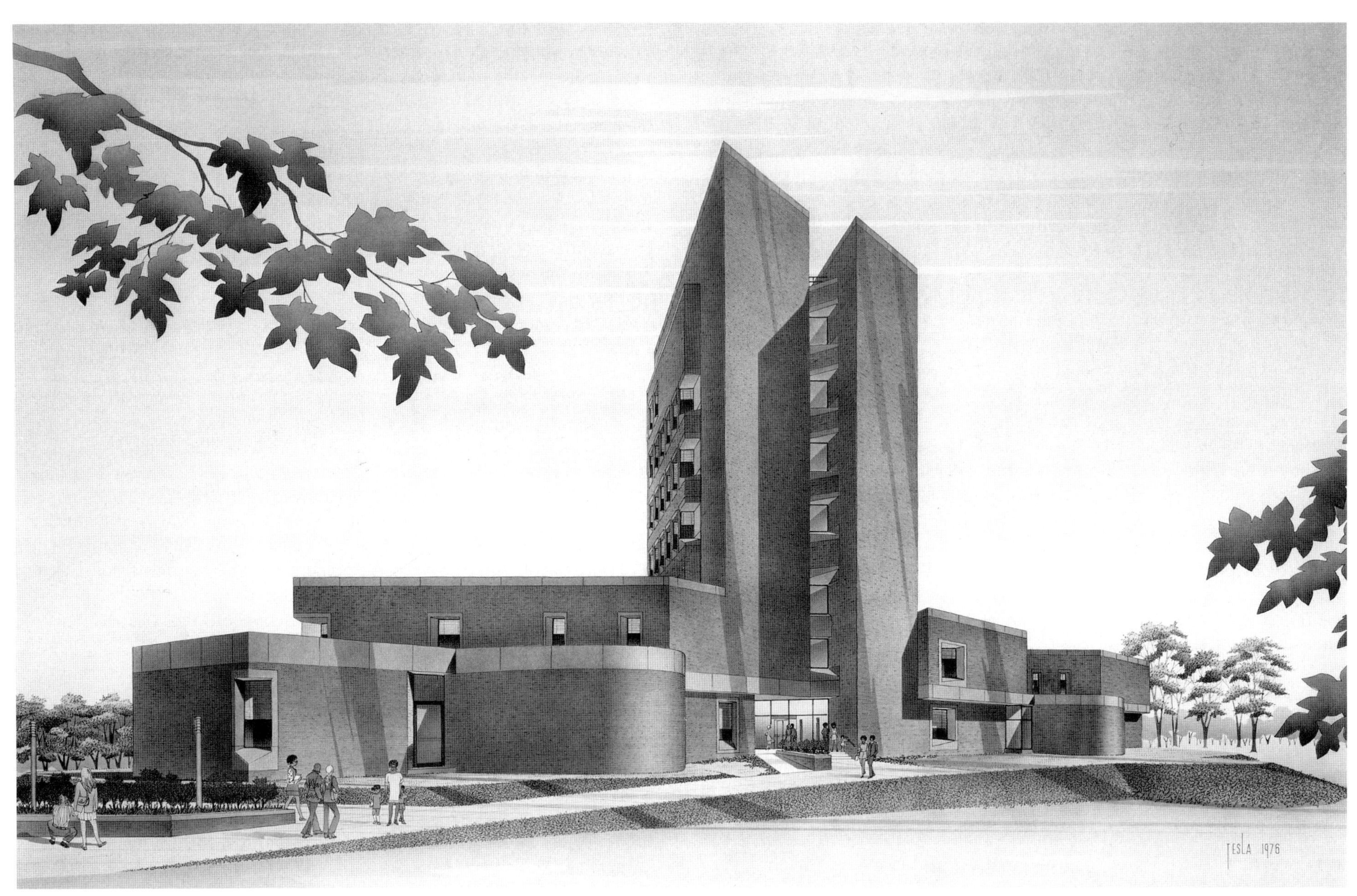

Rendering of the proposed new building for Elmwood Avenue adjacent to the University of Rochester Medical Center

Despite persistent difficulties in achieving a merger at the administrative level, a joint clinical teacher-training program was initiated with the objective of training the highest quality dental teachers and researchers. Training in a dental specialty area was integrated with studies and research in an appropriate basic science leading to a PhD. The program involved close cooperation between clinical faculty, who were mostly based at the Eastman Dental Center, and basic science faculty under Dr. Bowen's leadership, who were mostly based at the University of Rochester Medical Center. Program combinations included periodontology/microbiology, oral surgery/ pathology, periodontology/ biochemistry, and pedodontics/pathology. The number of students in the program remained small, but the impact on dental education, practice, and research was substantial.[10] The first graduates of the new Dentist Scientist Program completed their program in 1991. This joint program was expected to produce tomorrow's leaders in dental education and research.

TO MOVE OR TO STAY?

There are mentions in the board minutes during the Bibby years about moving the Eastman Dental Dispensary closer to the School of Medicine and Dentistry. But, four considerations weighed against the move:

1. Most trustees were against the move.

2. The sentimental attachment to the existing building on Main Street was strong.

3. Concern for the dental hygiene school was strong (Note: board minutes span 1948 to 1970, and the hygienists didn't depart for Monroe Community College until 1965.)

4. Concern for patient convenience was strong.

Bibby decided to let the subject lapse in favor of the status quo. Why? He needed more time to evaluate the situation. He also felt that the challenge of bringing a dead institution back to life was daunting enough. He postponed major decisions about replacing antiquated dental equipment and what to do with a building constructed to last for hundreds of years but which at the time of his retirement was grossly inadequate for delivering modern dental services and conducting research. In the later Bibby years, research activity at the Eastman Dental Center was widely regarded as significantly exceeding what the School of Medicine and Dentistry dental fellows were doing. There was a kind of shadow boxing going on between Bibby and Johansen, but for the most part the interactions between the staffs at the Eastman Dental Center and School of Medicine and Dentistry were like parallel play among children in a nursery school, with occasional bumping into each other. Bibby decided that close physical proximity would not stimulate cooperative effort.

The new director had to deal with whether to move or renovate the dental center, the increasing complexity of modern organizations, inadequate faculty salaries, increasing costs of clinical care, the unresolved conflicts between the dental center and the university, and increasing governmental regulations. In the sixties, the dynamics of recruiting, funding, and maintaining a research faculty was changing. Research required more sophisticated laboratories, support personnel, and investigator training. The days of the single investigator working independently was gone. All of this required closer management and carried the potential for increasing costs and conflicts between researchers and the administration.

In 1972, a careful and critical appraisal of Eastman Dental Center facilities concluded that major remodeling or rebuilding was needed. Remodeling was feasible, less expensive, and would have certain benefits, but the potential advantages of locating a facility near the medical center were substantial. In November 1973, the Eastman Dental Center Board of Trustees announced that it had been contemplating a move for almost a year and would decide within two months whether to move or renovate the Eastman Dental Center at 800 East Main Street. The move would be to a site on Elmwood Avenue obtained through a long-term lease by the University of Rochester. The university provided a choice of sites because of the mutual value of closer cooperation.

One month later, in December 1973, a three-member doctor/dentist panel proposed that the center move. The committee reaffirmed that the Eastman Dental Center should continue its activities in graduate dental education, research, and patient care—thus eschewing the path of the Forsyth Institute, which dropped patient care to concentrate on research. While strongly recommending that the center relocate to a site close to the medical center, the committee stressed that the dental center should continue to maintain independence and autonomy.[11]

Sterling Weaver, president of the board of trustees, cited the reason the panel gave for a move: "Their belief is that dentistry is in the process of change as most health care is. Dentistry is a specialty in the medical field. Its isolation from medicine should be terminated." This could happen only if the Eastman Dental Center moved to a location closer to the University of Rochester Medical Center. Closeness to the medical center was the main reason cited by all for the move. "Many patients are being medically treated as well as dentally," said a spokesperson for the Eastman Dental Center. "Having the hospital close will be good for them."[12]

The committee made five other recommendations relating to long-range planning. These included an agreement that the center retains its fiscal independence. It was recommended that a liaison committee from both boards of trustees (university and dental center) be set up "for achieving and maintaining an orderly and proper coordination of effort and planning for the future." In the interim before the move (four or five years) the continuing updating of essential equipment should be maintained and flexible programming should continue. The factors considered centered on the needs of faculty, students, patients, and the city of Rochester. McHugh said, "Many of our students are also enrolled in programs at the University of Rochester School of Medicine and Dentistry. It would be really advantageous for them, as well as our students enrolled only in clinical programs, to have the stimulation of the academic atmosphere that exists in the School of Medicine and Dentistry."

One controversial aspect of the proposed move was that the center might be moving further away from the population that it had served for fifty-five years. After that amount of time, the Eastman Dental Center had a well-established downtown identity. However, McHugh noted that a study showed that 70 percent of the patients came to the center by car (and parking was difficult on East Main Street), only 21 percent came by bus, and the percentage of patients living within five miles of the center would not change if the center were moved. Many patients could use the university bus. "We came to the conclusion that the site is not critical," McHugh said.

After fifty-six years of use, even with some additions and renovations, the Eastman Dental Center building was being called "outdated and inadequate" for present and future needs. One of the biggest drawbacks, Dr. McHugh said, was lack of air-conditioning. The center could only be used eight or nine

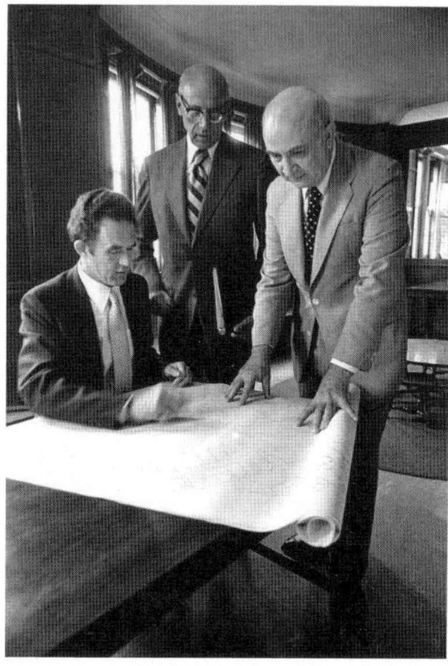

Planning the new building

months of the year without adequate temperature and humidity controls.[13] Buildings from the era before central air-conditioning are never completely satisfactorily converted. But renovation of the present building would cost less than building a new one. Estimates found that the original Main Street center could be renovated at a cost of approximately 60 percent of that of constructing a new building. However, the board concluded as it voted unanimously to move, "If we are going to spend a lot of money to renovate it, we may as well build a new one."[14]

THE NEW EASTMAN DENTAL CENTER

After several years of planning, the Eastman Dental Center received final City Council approval to build at 625 Elmwood Avenue. Ground was broken and construction began in January 1976. As the project was underway, Dr. McHugh made some tooth-related jokes. In a bulletin announcing the beginning of test borings, he referred to the work as "drilling." However, he called the excavation "a large hole filled with concrete"[15] rather than a "cavity."

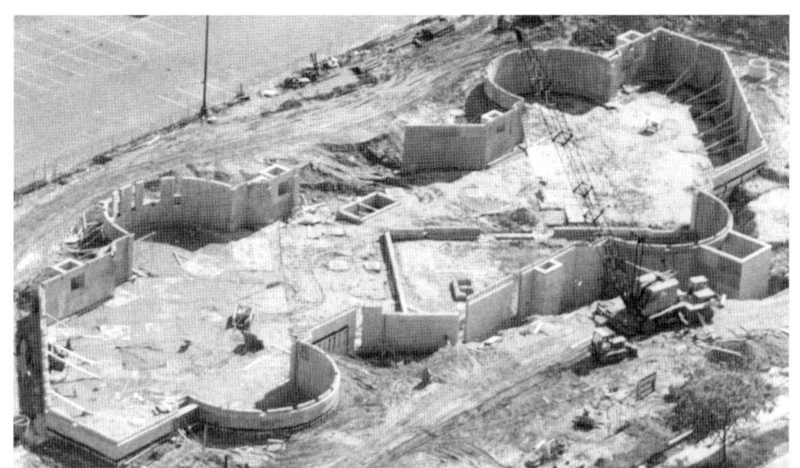
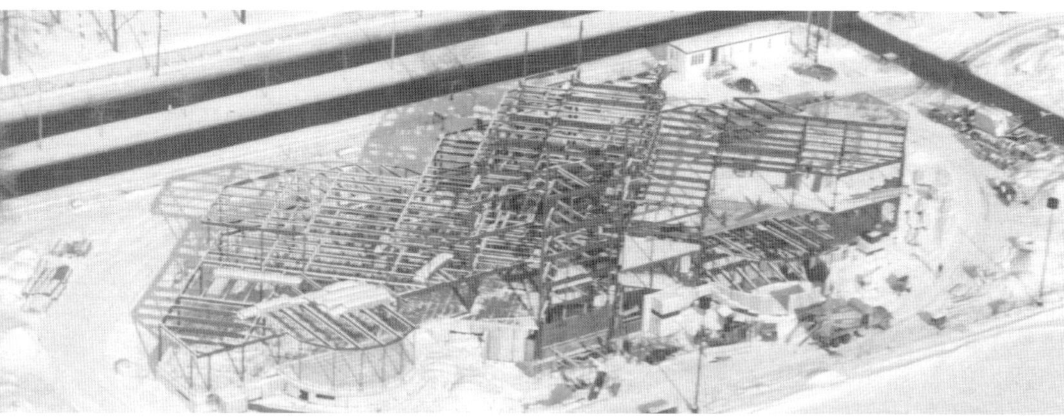
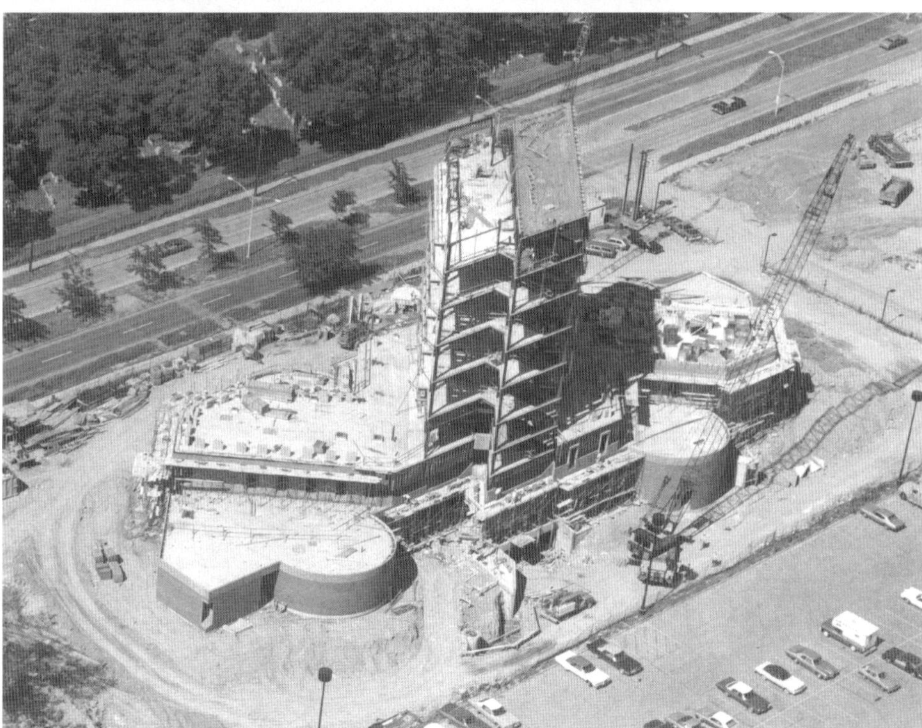
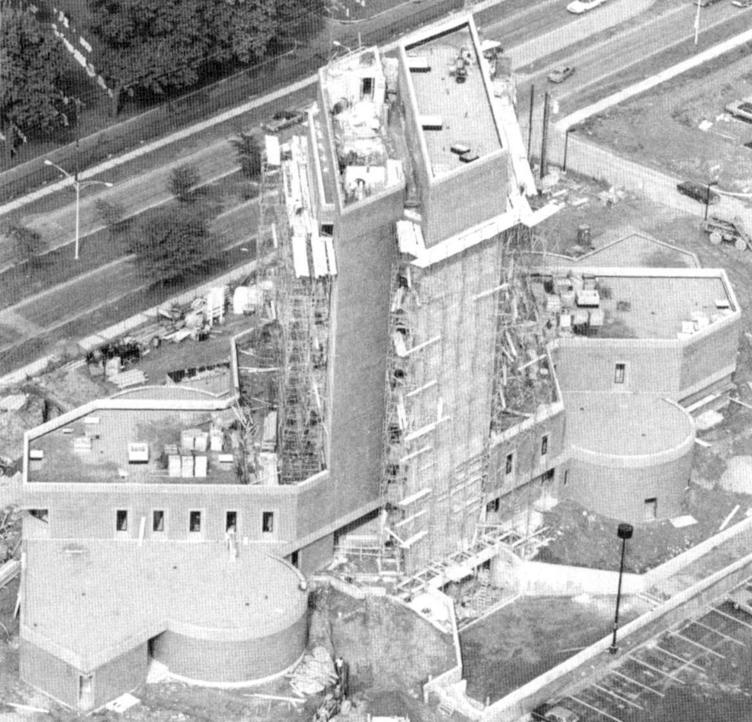

The new Eastman Dental Center goes up.

Nor, as newspaper columnist Peter Taub wrote, did anyone suggest that the tooth fairy would pay for the project.[16]

The cost was originally estimated at $6.7 million but inevitably rose, with a final cost of $7.2 million. Max Farash, who was on the board of trustees and a major real estate developer, played an important role in securing favorable subcontractors. To stay within the original budget, the cost of the auditorium was removed and then Farash made a personal donation to cover the cost of its construction. Richard Foster, who had designed the New York State Theater at Lincoln Center and buildings at Yale, was the architect for the project. The design of the new building, which would be faced with brick to match the nearby Strong Memorial Hospital, emphasized the independent nature of the dental center without conflicting with neighboring buildings. The basic rotunda-shaped building houses teaching and patient care areas on the first two floors. The third floor is a mechanical area, and research laboratories are in the seven-story tower. Half of the tower rises to eight stories.

After the decision was made to move, the Eastman Dental Center immediately launched, under J. Wallace Ely, a $350,000 capital campaign to build and equip the new center. Ely had declined to lead a more ambitious effort originally pegged at two to three million dollars. In May 1978, the new building opened to patients. The physical size of the clinic was increased slightly, but there was no increase in the 250-member staff. "We need it," McHugh said, "but there is no money." Research money came mostly from federal and state grants. Educational money came from student tuition, with the Eastman endowment filling gaps. The greatest amount of funds went to patient care. While the goals of the center were becoming more inclusive, children still represented more than half of the patients.[17]

STATUS OF DENTISTRY, 1970–1993

Cyril Meyerowitz has some impressions from the early 1970s that others echo:

> When you're a student, you get sort of a worm's-eye view of the world. Things are a little different than when you're looking at it from either a distance or from internally having been there for a while. Eastman seemed like a pretty interesting place. The teaching was good. Stan Handelman was trying to build a program, and he was very involved and engaged and an interesting guy. . . .

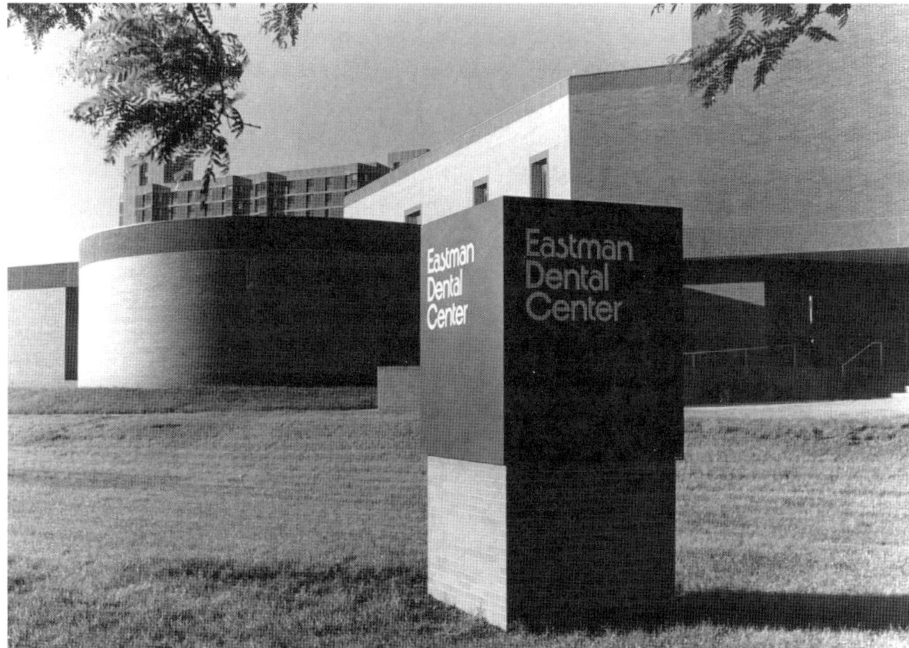

Signage identifying the Eastman Dental Center on Elmwood Avenue after its move to the University of Rochester Medical Center campus

> I met with Johansen. It was a diffident, distant kind [of relationship]. . . . I don't remember him with any of the emotion that I subsequently heard people from Eastman had about him. He was helpful in terms of setting up the Master's program for me. "He also ran the dental research seminar. . . . Most of the people who were doing Ph.D.s or Masters programs used to come there [the School of Medicine and Dentistry] and participate in the activities. And the Masters program was very rigorous . . . a very intense research, thesis-oriented program.[18]

Despite the ongoing and unresolved organizational and status issues, with approximately 100 postdoctoral trainees in dental research, specialty, and academic education, the combined resources of the Eastman Dental Center and the School of Medicine and Dentistry made Rochester in the early 1980s the world's largest graduate dental training center. However, after Erling Johansen left in 1979 to become dean of the Tufts University School of Dental Medicine, the position of chair of the Department of Dental Research remained vacant for at least three years. A contemporary document written by the faculty of dentistry requesting the trustees of the university to approve the creation of the position of dean of dentistry had this to say about the interregnum: "Delay in appointment of a successor [to Johansen] has resulted in the collapse of the unique graduate program whose success in producing teachers and investigators is unquestioned." That these years became a low point is confirmed by one staff member who came back to the Department of Dental Research at the School of Medicine and Dentistry as it was then known: "There was no real action going on. In fact, dental research was about to disappear off the face of the earth and people were very concerned about it."[19] Looking back, this participant-observer, a graduate student at the time, had these impressions of the Eastman Dental Dispensary/School of Medicine and Dentistry relations in the 1950s:

> Even at that stage I could see—even as a lowly resident—relations between the Eastman staff and the dental staff at the university were not good, quite a lot of antipathy. But, the program nevertheless was marvelous. We had meetings, seminar every Friday afternoon, and we all traveled from the Eastman up here [to the School of Medicine and Dentistry] and the dental fellows here gave their presentations and we gave ours on alternate weeks. We had the entire big-time faculty here in the university: Harold Hodge, Bill Neuman . . . at the seminars [along with] the senior faculty of Eastman. . . . So, the training and participation by faculty was outstandingly good. The expectations were very, very high. It was a good experience.[20]

In citing the classic example of the "University of Dentistry" suffering because of extended conflicts between the Eastman Dental Center and School of Medicine and Dentistry, the observer said of the most significant incident that occurred:

> An opportunity appeared [in the 1970s] for a Research Center to be formed and everybody in the United States in the dental scene thought that Rochester should have been a shoe-in to get one. And that would have called for mega collaboration between Eastman and the University dental group. And you hear different versions of it, but at the end of the day a proposal didn't even go in. So, there were four centers formed and they went to four places other than Rochester. And Rochester most emphatically should have had one of those. No question of it. And it set back the whole arena here enormously. It was a disaster.[21]

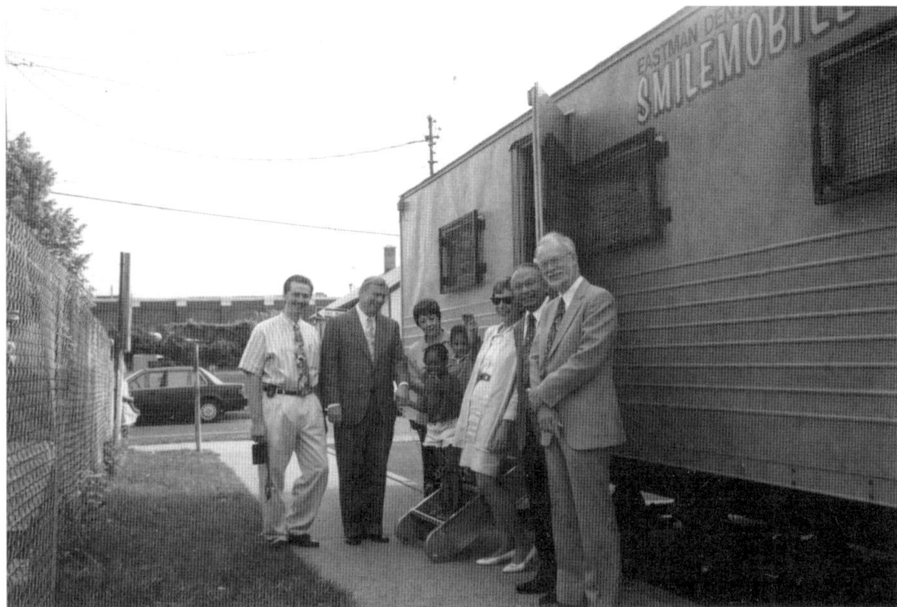

Smilemobile

COMMUNITY DENTISTRY FOR CHILDREN

Despite continuing conflicts with the School of Medicine and Dentistry, the Eastman Dental Center continued in its mission to serve the children of Rochester. The Smilemobile is a mobile dental unit. It captured the spirit of George Eastman's original intention of making dentistry available to the underserved. The traditional hygienic services provided by the clinic—screening examinations and dental prophylaxis—continued, and where there was need for treatment, referrals were made by the Eastman or family dentists. The Smilemobile was designed to reach specifically targeted underserved minority populations. In the case of traditional hygienic services, a parent was responsible for making an appointment and taking the child out of school. With the Smilemobile, minimal school time was lost and there were not canceled or broken appointments. Jack Howitt was the driving force in establishing the Smilemobile. He conceived the project and convinced Sybron Corporation to fund it. He secured additional financial aid as well as approval from the local dental society, which frequently resisted federal, state, and institutional initiatives as impinging on their domain and incomes.

Smilemobile I was donated by Sybron Corporation in 1968. The equipment was furnished by the Ritter division of Sybron and the outfitting was completed by Wegman's. The program began service in 1970 with one trailer. Dr. Dennis Leverett took over the unit in 1980, and Dr. Ronald J. S. Billings took it over in 1984. A second customized trailer, Smilemobile II, was pressed into service in September 1990, again made possible by gifts from local foundations, organizations, companies, and individual benefactors. Similarly, through donations, two additional Smilemobiles were secured in the late 1990s and in 2007, and currently Eastman has four Smilemobiles serving Rochester's children and underserved adults. The center continues to operate the Smilemobiles as part of its community school dental health program. The trailers, equipped with full-service, state-of-the-art operatory equipment, travel to inner city schools in the area and service hundreds of children who qualify for Medicaid.[22] The need among these children is great, and sometimes a Smilemobile is at a school for two or three months at a time. The appointments take place during school hours; students are escorted to the trailer parked on school property. Each child is seen by a certified pediatric dentist, a dental hygienist, an assistant, and a clinical coordinator.

Services range among simple hygiene procedures, radiographs, fluoride treatments, and extractions. Cases the Smilemobile cannot handle are referred to the Eastman Dental Center's pediatric department. The Smilemobile eliminates the need for parents to take time off from work for their children's dental care, and the children spend less time away from school. Children not on Medicaid are seen on an as-needed basis and are never denied service because of finances. Each Smilemobile can treat more than 4,000 children a year, and the program serves fifteen of the thirty-eight city elementary schools as part of Eastman's outreach program, which currently provides over 29,000 patient visits per year. The program does speak to Eastman's premise that all children not only need but also deserve preventive dental care from an early age.

During the summer, the Smilemobiles visit inner-city day care centers and provide care in Mt. Morris to children living in nearby Livingston County. Care is preferentially given to children eligible for Medicaid because they have no discretionary income or private insurance and generally do not have easy access to private care.[23]

CLINICAL CHANGES

In addition to developing the Smilemobile program, the dental profession was monitoring major changes in disease patterns. Fluoride treatments had dramatically reduced caries in children and teens, and there was an increased interest in dental health in general. In sharp contrast to the young patients Burkhart had dealt with, one half of the population aged five to eighteen that might have come to the Eastman Dental Center in the 1980s had never experienced *any* dental decay. There was thus a reduced demand for care, except, as both McHugh and Billings noted, in pockets of minorities in underserved urban areas. Physically and developmentally disabled young people also had major problems with caries. This group was seeking care more actively than in the past. One example was a contract with the Monroe Developmental Center through which postdoctoral students had opportunities to obtain training and experience in caring for the profoundly handicapped.

In addition to the reduction in the incidence of dental caries in children, the other major change in dental health was that adults were keeping their teeth longer. Only 15 percent of adults aged fifty to sixty-four had lost all their teeth compared to 35 percent in 1960. (George Eastman would have welcomed this change, but he was born too soon.) The search for quality care for these adults was increasing. Periodontal disease had become the major problem, and great strides had been made in diagnosing and controlling it. Periodontal disease had always been a problem, but as training for dentists improved, there was more recognition that periodontal disease could be treated. Effective treatment was being sought more frequently. But the net effect of the increasing demand for care among older Americans and a declining need for care among children was an overall increase in the need for dental care. As the 1989 annual report noted, "The Eastman Dental Center treats fewer healthy young patients but sees a greater number of physically and developmentally disabled young people and older patients with multiple medical problems or disabilities that complicate oral health care. It also sees more patients with infectious diseases." This was at the height of the HIV/AIDS crisis as it developed. New policies in response to the crisis significantly increased the cost of care.

Annual patient care visits at the Eastman Dental Center rose to 50,000 by the end of the twenty-three year McHugh directorate. Since then it has risen to close to 100,000. A large number of these visits can be accounted for by

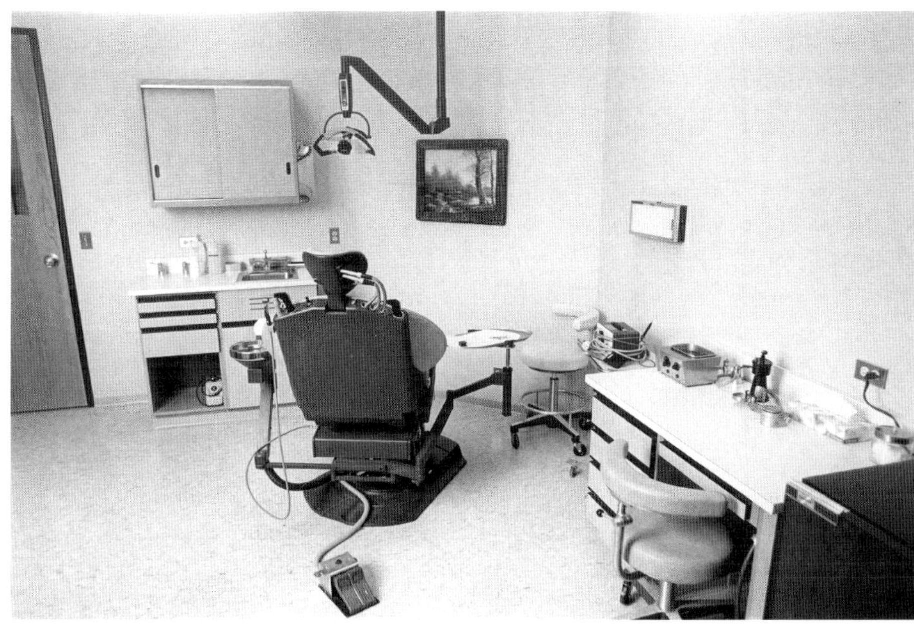

Dental operatory

care to adults. This had a positive effect on the budget, particularly in the growth of income in general dentistry.

A monumental change went almost unnoticed. In 1989, the Monroe County Dental Health Program that had existed since 1915 was terminated. The blame was placed on "budgetary pressure on the county and changes in oral disease patterns." This was certainly true, as was the assertion that "many of the children were seen by the Smilemobile."

New contracts were made to provide dental services to residents of several local nursing homes. These outreach efforts fit with the Eastman Dental Center's increasing emphasis on geriatric dentistry. An office of clinical affairs was established in 1989, and after a national search, Dr. Ronald Billings, who had been a member of the staff since 1983, was appointed associate director for clinical affairs. Patient care at the Eastman Dental Center reached an all-time record of 56,246 patient visits in 1991, surpassing the previous totals of the 1930s and 1940s. Sixty-five publications were listed that year too. It should be noted that while the tripartite division of community

service, education, and research remained throughout the McHugh years, different people favored emphasis on one or the other. Some thought the Eastman Dental Center should go the way of Forsyth and drop patient care. Others, such as Billings, thought it should concentrate on patient care for children. McHugh seemed to favor education as most important; his mission statements reflect this and in this he was strongly supported by the clinical department chairs. As noted, Bibby's main interest had been research. He opted for adult patients and would have been happy if community children's dentistry was deemphasized.

DENTAL EDUCATION

McHugh would write of the revolutionary role education had played during the earliest days of the Rochester Dental Dispensary, a role that he wanted to continue:

> The educational advantages of working in the dispensary were substantial, since the dental schools of the time were in the same state as the medical schools when the Flexner survey was made, and children's dentistry was not part of the dental school curriculum. These advantages greatly facilitated recruitment of staff dentists and many young dental school graduates worked a year or two before setting up their own practice.[24]

Beginning under Bibby, the Eastman Dental Center became recognized as the premier graduate clinical training center in the country. This began with the appointment in 1955 of Dr. J. Daniel Subtelny, professor in the Department of Dentistry and program director and chair in the Orthodontics and Dentofacial Orthopedics Division. The center's graduate training program started out as a service program, Dr. Billings says, and "very quickly orthodontics became a training program, and then pediatric dentistry, subsequently general dentistry, prosthodontics and periodontics and community dentistry was the last of the programs to be accredited by the Council of Dental Education. We became a full-fledged clinical training center. You could find Eastman people in every school in the country."[25] Under Dr. McHugh's leadership the postdoctoral graduate programs gained further distinction and research continued.

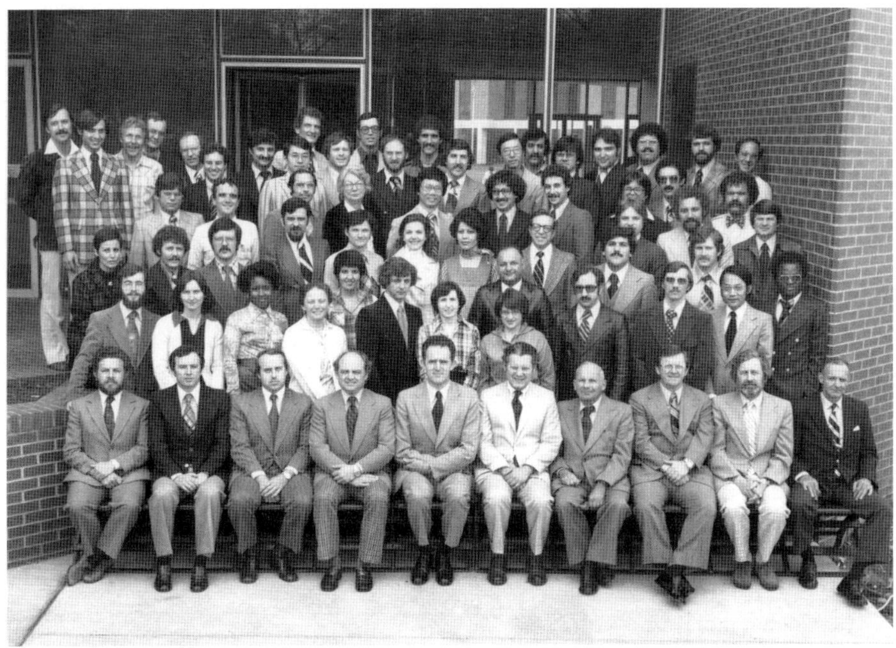

Group shot of EDC staff on Elmwood Avenue

RESEARCH YEARS UNDER McHUGH

Stanley Handelman

When McHugh became director of Eastman Dental Center, he inherited a loose confederation of dental research groups whose organizational structure could best be described as laissez faire. He did not have a radical plan to reorganize research activity, but natural changes in research staff, changing interest with new advances and funding opportunities, the management style and the perspective of the director, and the physical design of the laboratory space in the new building resulted in major changes in research activity at the Eastman Dental Center. Bibby absented himself physically by accepting a six-month appointment at the National Institute of Dental Research in Washington when McHugh arrived. He stated that the institution did not need two directors. On his return, Bibby continued to supervise a research effort on the cariogenic potential of food stuffs.

Buonocore continued to work on further clinical applications in adhesive dentistry, which had gained him and the institution international recognition, but ill health slowed him down. His friends and colleagues mourned his untimely death in 1981. Marion Gilmour was recognized for her work on the production and role of organic acids in dental plaque related to dental caries. Marguerite "Peg" Little, who had inherited the mantle of Brudevold, continued to work on the structure of enamel using nuclear magnetic resonance (NMR) to determine the role of fluoride. With declining financial support, both Little and Gilmour eventually retired. Fred Losee, recruited by Dr. Bibby from the United States Navy, was working on the histology of the early carious lesion and the role of trace elements in the initiation, progress, or prevention of such caries. With the move to the new building, McHugh established Losee as the leader of the group working in cariology. The research on trace elements required extensive field research, and Dr. Martin Curzon, a former pediatric postgraduate research and pediatric student was recruited as an assistant investigator.

The heads of clinical departments—periodontology, orthodontics, and prosthodontics—had their own research groups and their research activity is described in the history of their respective divisions.

When these clinical divisions required their students to participate in a research project, the students' mentor generally was from their division unless the student was in a PhD program. In that case a mentor in the basic sciences from the Medical School was chosen. In contrast, postdoctoral students in general dentistry and pediatric dentistry utilized investigators from the cariology group as their mentors. The laboratory group led by Handelman continued to be associated with the cariology group of investigators.

The major new thrust in cariology research became trace elements. This was initially led by Fred Losee, and subsequent to his early retirement, by Martin Curzon. During the 1970s there was great interest in identifying trace elements that could be used along with or enhancing the action of fluoride. Losee had been actively involved in early studies on trace elements and dental caries in Western Samoa and New Zealand as a dental researcher with the United States Navy. On retirement he was appointed to the EDC research staff by Dr. Bibby. In the late 1960s, working with Dr. Tom Ludwig, who was supported by the New Zealand Medical Research Council, they mapped the

United States for soil composition, trace elements, and dental caries prevalence. During the 1970s the work had progressed, and Dr. Losee was awarded a large grant from NIDR to continue to study trace elements in tooth enamel related to dental caries.

This study required extensive field research, and Dr. Martin Curzon was recruited as an assistant investigator. Teeth were collected from many areas of the Unites States and analyzed by spark source mass spectrometry through collaboration with the Eastman Kodak chemistry department. The work eventually identified a number of trace elements in addition to fluoride, such as strontium, molybdenum, and lithium as potential preventive anticaries agents.

On the retirement of Losee, Dr. McHugh created a new department of caries research under the direction of Dr. Curzon. It was structured as a loose group; senior researchers were largely left to pursue their own lines of research but with overall encouragement for cooperation.

The early work of Losee and Ludwig had noted a group of communities in northwest Ohio with exceptionally low incidence, if not complete absence, of dental caries. An epidemiological study carried out by Curzon in 1967 showed that this was the case. In the mid-1970s Curzon obtained significant funding for the continued study of the trace element strontium, identified as very significant in northwest Ohio. This research grant on strontium required more detailed studies involving animal studies, enamel chemistry, and later bacteriology. A preliminary animal study to check if strontium was anticaries was conducted by Curzon's first postgraduate research student, Dr. Cyril Meyerowitz. These studies showed that strontium had indeed a major effect on preventing dental caries and worked synergistically with fluoride to almost completely prevent dental caries. The ideal strontium salt, strontium chloride, was also identified. A series of laboratory and animal studies showed that a combination of fluoride with strontium as topical solutions were potentially beneficial as preventive agents.

Concurrently, Handelman and Losee demonstrated a significant inhibition in enamel solubility of oral bacteria using the highly mineralized water from northwest Ohio. Herbison and Handelman extended these studies by measuring the effect of the major trace elements in this water, molybdenum lithium and strontium, on dissolution of hydroxyapatite in cariogenic streptococci. A contract was awarded to Curzon and Handelman to study the microbiological effects of the elements fluoride, strontium, and lithium. This work occupied the latter years of the decade and showed that while fluoride had a major effect on oral bacteria, the two other elements had only very minor effects.

The work on strontium was very promising, but more work was needed on the mechanism of action of strontium. For this Curzon recruited a New Zealand physical chemist, Dr. John Featherstone. The work of the department expanded, and this line of research continued into the 1980s and 1990s under the direction of Dr. Featherstone, who took over the leadership of the department when Curzon left to assume the professorship of child dental health at the University of Leeds. These studies showed that the incorporation of strontium at key points in the enamel crystallite structure, along with fluoride, produced a large crystal that had great resistance to enamel dissolution. Moves were made though collaboration with industry to develop a marketable product, such as a toothpaste or mouthwash, based on the fluoride-strontium combination. However, this was to come to no avail because of the public perception of strontium 90 as a dangerous radioactive material. Though many anticipated a major breakthrough similar to that of adhesive dentistry and fluoride, the studies on trace elements can be characterized as a promise that was not fulfilled.

At the end of the 1970s the expertise in animal testing and bacteriology enabled the research department at the EDC to win a major research grant from NIDR to investigate the cariogenicity of twenty-two common snack foods. This extensive study not only identified those snack foods that were or were not cariogenic, but also which food components were more likely to foster dental caries.

The expertise in epidemiology gained in the early trace element studies enabled a collaboration to develop between Leverett (Community Dentistry) and Curzon. The combined expertise was instrumental in gaining grants and contracts from both NIDR and industry to study mouth rinses, prophylaxis pastes, and toothpastes. Later in the 1980s this collaboration continued with Adair (Pediatric Dentistry) and Featherstone on studies concerning fluoride in saliva in high-risk children, prenatal fluoride, and toothpaste fluoride and saliva concentrations.

Plaque plays a role in both dental caries and periodontology. Dominick Zero carried on a combined study concerning plaque acids in tooth biofilms.

From 1980 to 1995, Featherstone and his collaborators focused on mechanisms of demineralization and remineralization of enamel. Laboratory models were used to create carious lesions in the enamel and tooth roots and to study the effect of fluoride on initiation, progression, and reversal of these lesions. The work demonstrated that fluoride inhibits demineralization and enhances remineralization, the latter being the natural repair process for noncavitated lesions in the enamel. This work, together with that of other groups around the world, clarified the role of fluoride applied to the surface of the tooth through water and fluoridated products.

A laboratory pH-cycling model was developed to mimic the early states of dental caries found around orthodontic brackets in human mouths, and this model has been used extensively ever since in several laboratories to unlock the secrets of fluoride action. Other so-called "in situ" models were developed in collaboration with Domenick Zero to study aspects of the caries process in the mouth. For example, a model where partial denture wearers carried enamel blocks with preformed lesions showed the positive role of cheese in inhibiting or reversing dental caries. In parallel with studies on teeth, Featherstone and his collaborators synthesized carbonated hydroxyapatite, the mineral of teeth and bones, and demonstrated how fluoride attached to the surface of the mineral was much more effective in inhibiting demineralization than fluoride incorporated into crystal at levels found in enamel and dentin.

Featherstone teamed up with Dennis Leverett and Ron Billings to conduct laboratory-supported clinical research in the area of caries prediction and risk assessment. In collaboration with scientists from the Laboratory for Laser Energetics at the University of Rochester, Featherstone studied "Laser Interactions on Hard Tissue" and provided the scientific basis for understanding the use of lasers on teeth. The early work was done before lasers were used clinically for dentistry. At the time of the writing of this chapter, Featherstone was interim dean of the dental school at the University of California at San Francisco. One aspect of this work that is still ongoing is the potential to use specific lasers for treating occlusal surfaces of the teeth to make them resistant to dental caries.

The decade of the 1970s was a transition period, with many of the internationally known EDC researchers, such as Bibby, Buonocore, Subtelny, and Zander, winding down and retiring. A younger group of dental researchers, including Billings, Caton, Curzon, Featherstone, Handelman, Leverett, and Zero, gradually developed to maintain the EDC's reputation as one of the leading worldwide dental research institutes.

EDUCATION

A new component in the Eastman Dental Center education curriculum under McHugh was postdoctoral teaching in clinical subjects such as oral surgery, pedodontics, periodontics, prosthodontics, and orthodontics. The subjects were taught in cooperation with the School of Medicine and Dentistry. "The program represents a fundamental change in curriculum," said J. Wallace Ely, acting chair of the newly created Dental Clinical Teaching Program. "The university has had an exceptionally productive program in basic dental sciences for many years and plans to continue to strengthen the program. At the same time the need to train clinical teachers is recognized."

By 1989, McHugh was stating in annual reports that dental education was being downsized. Five dental schools, all affiliated with private universities, had closed during the previous five years. Dental graduates nationwide had reached a high in the early 1980s but dropped by 1989. Despite the smaller pool, McHugh wrote, there was no overall decrease in the number of applicants or the quality of students seeking admission to the Rochester program.

IMPACT OF MEDICAID

Under Title XIX of the Social Security Act, Medicaid dental services were optional for individuals aged twenty-one and older and required for Medicaid-eligible individuals under age twenty-one as a component of the Early and Periodic Screening, Diagnostic, and Treatment benefit. Dental services were generally excluded from Medicare coverage; however, there were a few minor exceptions.

Medicaid support appears to have peaked in 1991, and McHugh's annual report of that year mentions facing "the prospect of significant cuts in the Medicaid program as the state tries to balance its budget and the ever-increasing costs of regulation and infection control."[26] Specifically, cutbacks were expected to eliminate funding for adult dental services except for emergencies. Fortunately, this did not occur. The reimbursement per visit was capped, but the total number of Medicaid visits continued to increase and with them, Medicaid revenue.

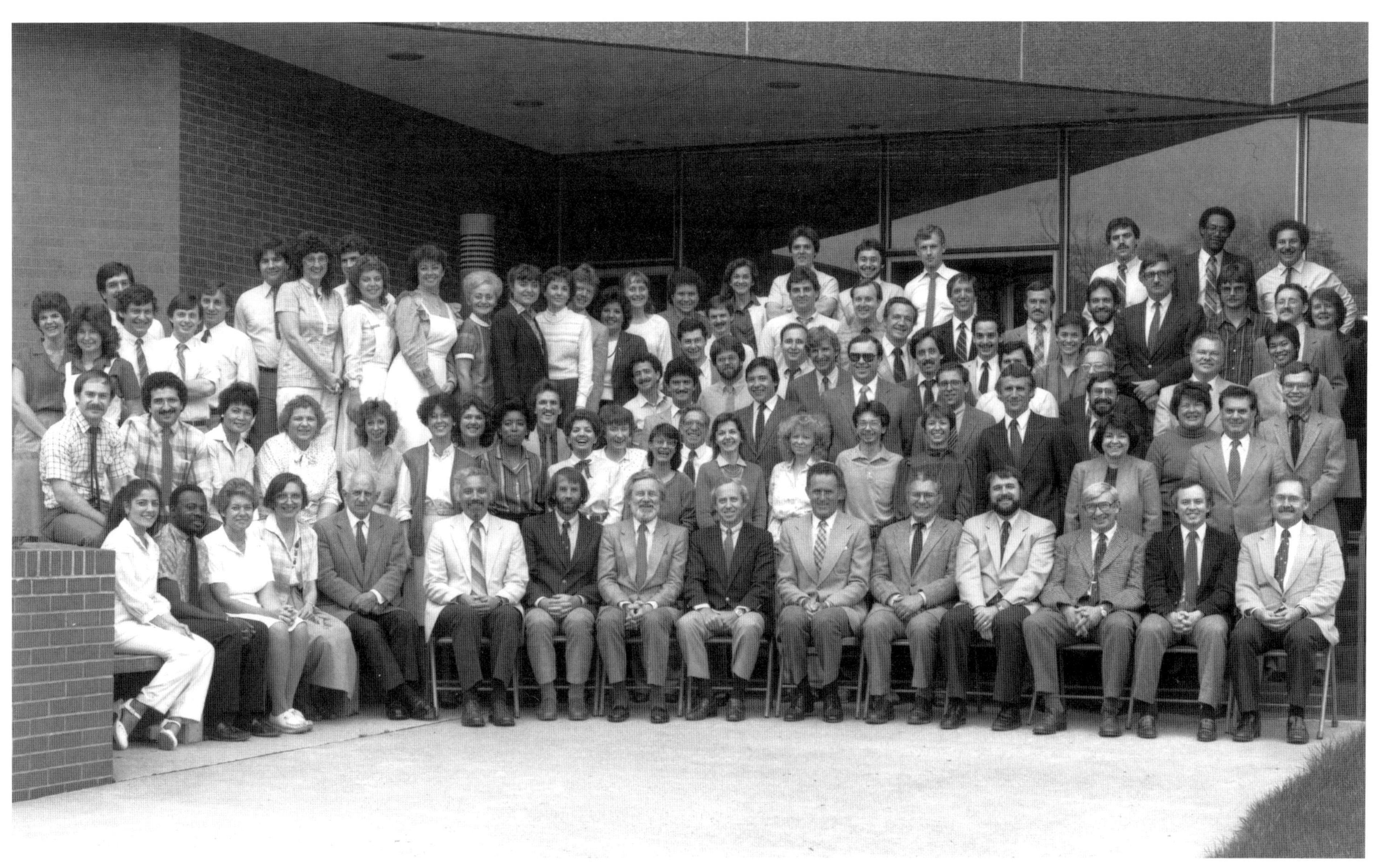

Group shot of EDC staff in 1979

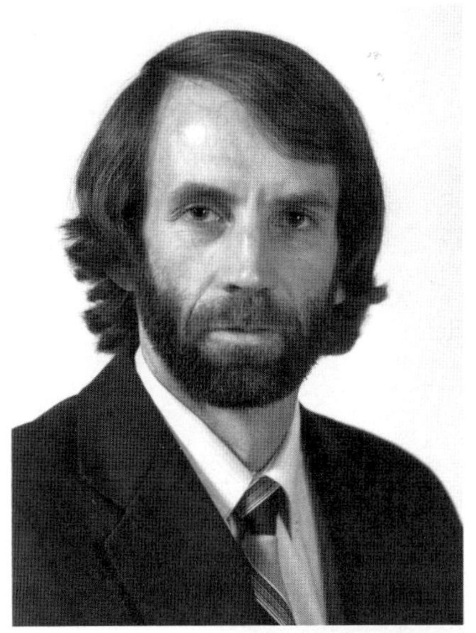

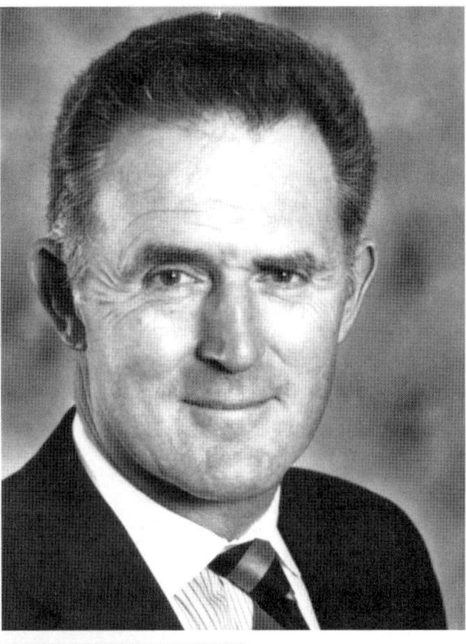

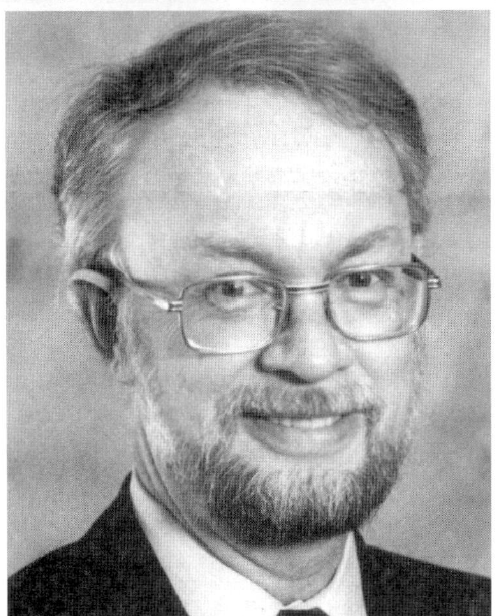

Clockwise from top, left: Drs. John D. B. Featherstone, William McHugh, and Ronald Billings

Medicaid is the lifeline for very poor people to access dentistry, Dr. Billings says. "On the whole, in most states in the country, care is provided by public clinics and places like Eastman. In New York, very few [private] dentists actually participate in the Medicaid program." Billings explained:

If Medicaid went away tomorrow, the five dental schools [including Eastman Dental Center] in New York State would be reduced to practically nothing because we depend extraordinarily heavily on Medicaid to support our training programs. As does NYU, as does Columbia, Buffalo—Stony Brook less so. Cyril has data to show that the academic institutions provide the bulk of non-reimbursed care for people who do not have Medicaid or are not Medicaid eligible. So Medicaid is extremely important to the academic centers of the state, and particularly to Eastman. Certainly our community dentistry programs would go away. Through the mobile units and the school-based programs, over 5,000 children are served. That would just disappear overnight. There would simply be no way to provide that service. We rely on paid professionals—dental hygienists, dental assistants, clerical support staff. There would be a huge hole.[27]

There was a time when Medicaid covered everything. By the 1990s, the Eastman Dental Center was still being reimbursed at the same rate that it was when the program began. And costs continued to rise. Some of this was made up from interest on the endowment, and at one point, the Eastman Dental Center was dipping heavily into the endowment at about 9 or 10 percent. The board insisted that that be reduced to 5 or 6 percent, and it was. One motivation for the merger was to cut costs.

THE BOARD STEPS IN

Robert Witmer, president of the Eastman Dental Center board in the 1990s, says that in that time period, "The activities and primarily the research of the dental center were not as strong as they once had been. The dental center had the reputation of training most of the dental leadership in the country. [Yet] when we tried to replace some of the chairs of the departments, we came to learn that we were not as attractive as we once had been, and realized we needed to focus on that. It was difficult to recruit those high-level people from outside to be department chairs because the reputation had diminished."[28] Witmer focused on the need for a strategic plan, and when McHugh did not come up with what the board considered a satisfactory plan with the correct goals and objectives, it caused Witmer to think that other leadership was needed in the center.

Witmer saw "indications that we weren't as good as we once had been. When North Carolina gave to a candidate the Eastman Dental Center was interested in "a package offer that he had not been able to get in probably two months of negotiating separately here at Rochester," it drew Witmer's "attention to our problem." Unfortunately, there was a dearth of qualified candidates nationally, and many institutions would be faced with a similar problem.

As had happened in earlier generations, Witmer decided "we needed to look carefully at how to bring these two organizations together. We started to negotiate an affiliation agreement with the university." He also concluded, "This was a time of turmoil." And then, "the State Department of Health came down on the dental center with both feet and found us in violations in the clinical area. We discovered that we had an entire culture that needed to be changed. Most of the people we had just thought that these rules were for other people, not for them. And so, we pushed Bill McHugh very hard. He got Ron Billings involved. We also discovered that the center had not been complying with the federal rules regarding scholarship aid to students—record keeping more than anything else. It's hard to tell if there were any other violations if we had no records to look at. That caused a lot of concern as well."

The dental center overdrew the Eastman endowment for at least two years from 1992 to 1994, Witmer states. A 5 1/2 percent, draw would have produced $3.2 million, but $6 million had been drawn. There was no real strategic plan in place that would justify an enhanced draw.

In the fall of 1992, the board met with McHugh and indicated that it was unhappy with communication and planning and needed to look for a new executive director. His retirement would be accelerated by a year. The board began reorganizing the center as well. "Each of the departments was a fiefdom unto itself. . . . We had to put in place an organization that would have one person responsible for the center and not seven different chairs, each responsible only for his or her department."[29]

One of the major issues surrounding McHugh's dismissal was budgetary. A majority of the board was convinced that it was never profitable to support research, even when the research was successful. Interestingly, although

Jay Stein, as senior vice president and vice provost for health affairs beginning in 1995, would be a controversial figure (as discussed in chapter 8), his legacy of emphasis on research has established the university as the largest employer in the greater Rochester area. One could argue that McHugh's leadership in investing heavily in research was ahead of its time. Furthermore, the concept of emphasizing clinical service at the expense of teaching and research would ultimately have had greater negative impact. As Stanley Handelman has noted, "No matter what the justification there is fulfilling social needs, you don't make money treating the poor."

Nonetheless. McHugh achieved a good deal of recognition nationally by the American Association of Dental Research, the International Association of Dental Research, and the American Association of Dental Schools. He led an important committee at the National Institute of Dental and Craniofacial Research (NIDCR; formerly NIDR) that reviewed the role of dental amalgam in clinical practice. It was well received as a consensus document. During McHugh's administration, the clinical educational programs were consistently given commendations for excellence by accreditation committees. Also during McHugh's time as director, the postdoctoral programs came to be as widely recognized as leaders in their respective fields, and this has continued up to the present time. McHugh's leadership role in the construction of the new building on the medical center campus was clearly a major achievement.

TRANSITION: LEVERETT AND SPRINGER

In November 1992, Dr. William McHugh retired and Dr. Dennis H. Leverett was named acting director of Eastman Dental Center. Leverett had been chair of Community Dentistry since 1973. A graduate of Ohio State and Harvard universities, he became a senior scientist and senior clinician at the Eastman Dental Center and was appointed to the faculty of the University of Rochester in 1973, rising to the rank of professor in 1984. In the community, Leverett was dental director of the Monroe County Health Department from 1973 to 1989; editor-in-chief of the *Journal of Public Health Dentistry,* and author of more than fifty articles in scientific and professional journals. He had had a distinguished career in public health dentistry, notably serving on the board and committees of the National Institute of Dental Research and as diplomat of the American Board of Dental Public Health.

During Leverett's year as acting director, faculty, staff, and trustees hammered out a mission statement.

The mission of the Eastman Dental Center is to be preeminent in the education of dentistry's future academic leaders through patient-centered, research-based, post-doctoral programs.

Dr. Wilfred A. Springer followed Leverett and served as acting director from January to March 1994.

BILLINGS

While the center was under interim leadership, a search committee was formed to select a permanent director. In early 1994, Ronald J. S. Billings, DDS, MSD, became the fourth director of the Eastman Dental Center and served a five-year term. He immediately appointed four associate directors to spearhead a leadership team and provide direction in four core areas: patient care (clinical affairs), education, research, and administration. "Our institutional philosophy emphasizes teamwork," Billings wrote, and "developing a fiscally responsible team-driven organizational culture must be a priority." Leading the team were Dov M. Almog, DMD, associate director of clinical affairs; Jack G. Caton, DDS, MS, associate director for educational programs; Domenick T. Zero, DDS, MS, associate director for research; and Thomas P. Riley, associate director for administrative affairs. The diverse, active, and community-oriented board of trustees of the period met twelve times in 1994.

The Eastman Dental Center and School of Medicine and Dentistry signed yet another affiliation agreement in February 1994. Two joint committees were formed—one for educational affairs and the other for oversight of ways the two entities could work together in the future.

Research highlights of 1994 included studies on how lasers affect hard tissue, how wounds heal, and how to test pain-control drugs. Billings led the center through a time of significant change. During that period, Billings says, the center concentrated on meeting its strategic goals regarding "patient-centered care, quality educational programs, and a new research structure" through a team-centered approach to problem solving.[30] A new and simpler

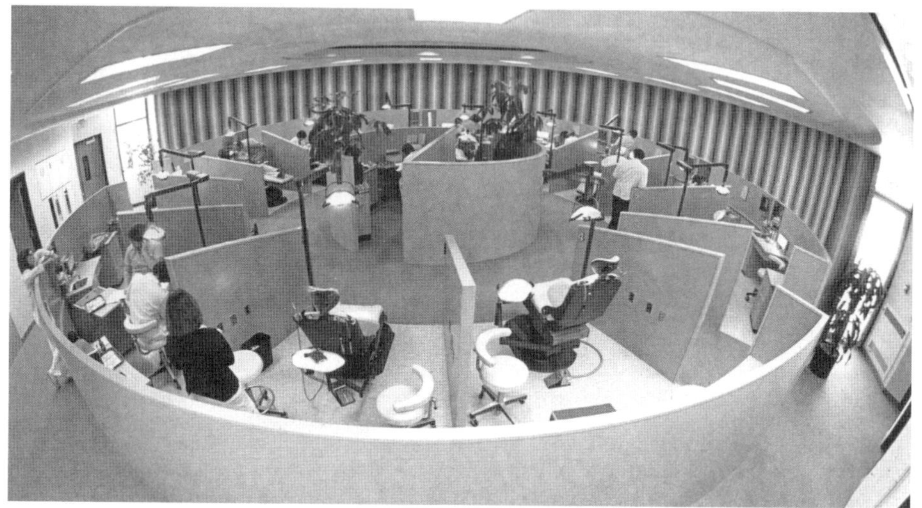

General Dentistry oval

patient-friendly reception system was installed to improve care. As a not-for-profit organization, the emphasis was on making dental care available for socially and economically disadvantaged children in both rural and urban areas. This involved working with other institutions, such as Strong Memorial Hospital's Social Work Division. More than 20,000 patients were seen and 65,000 patient visits recorded in 1995, a record number for the Eastman Dental Center. A pilot program serving the developmentally disabled population of greater Rochester was established in August 1995. Twenty-eight local organizations, including United Cerebral Palsy, utilized the Eastman Dental Center's expertise in oral health care for people with special needs.

More than fifty dental residents were enrolled each year in the postdoctoral training programs. Eastman Dental Center faculty remained leaders within the dental profession and the center's advanced training programs continued to thrive under the faculty's leadership.

The research program's structure of a peer-driven review effort fostered collaboration among researchers. Quality management and a team-centered approach to problem solving were hallmarks. Data continued to show an increasing need for dental treatment in primary teeth among inner-city children. All residents in the general dentistry program were conducting research projects and were exposed to research through workshops, seminars, literature, and courses. The two main areas of ongoing research were diagnostic imaging and studies evaluating the efficacy of over-the-counter medications. Research projects by members of the oral science program under Dr. Domenick Zero included studies to improve the understanding of dental caries and to identify new ways to prevent them. By 1995, Billings's study of microbiological and chemical analysis of saliva was completing its fifth year.

Planning for managed care began with an alliance with New York's four dental schools and a joint project with the University of Rochester's William E. Simon Graduate School of Business Administration. Billings would also be instrumental in the merger between the Eastman Dental Center and the School of Medicine and Dentistry that would be formalized on July 1, 1997. Indeed, it would be during his tenure that a merger actually happened.[31]

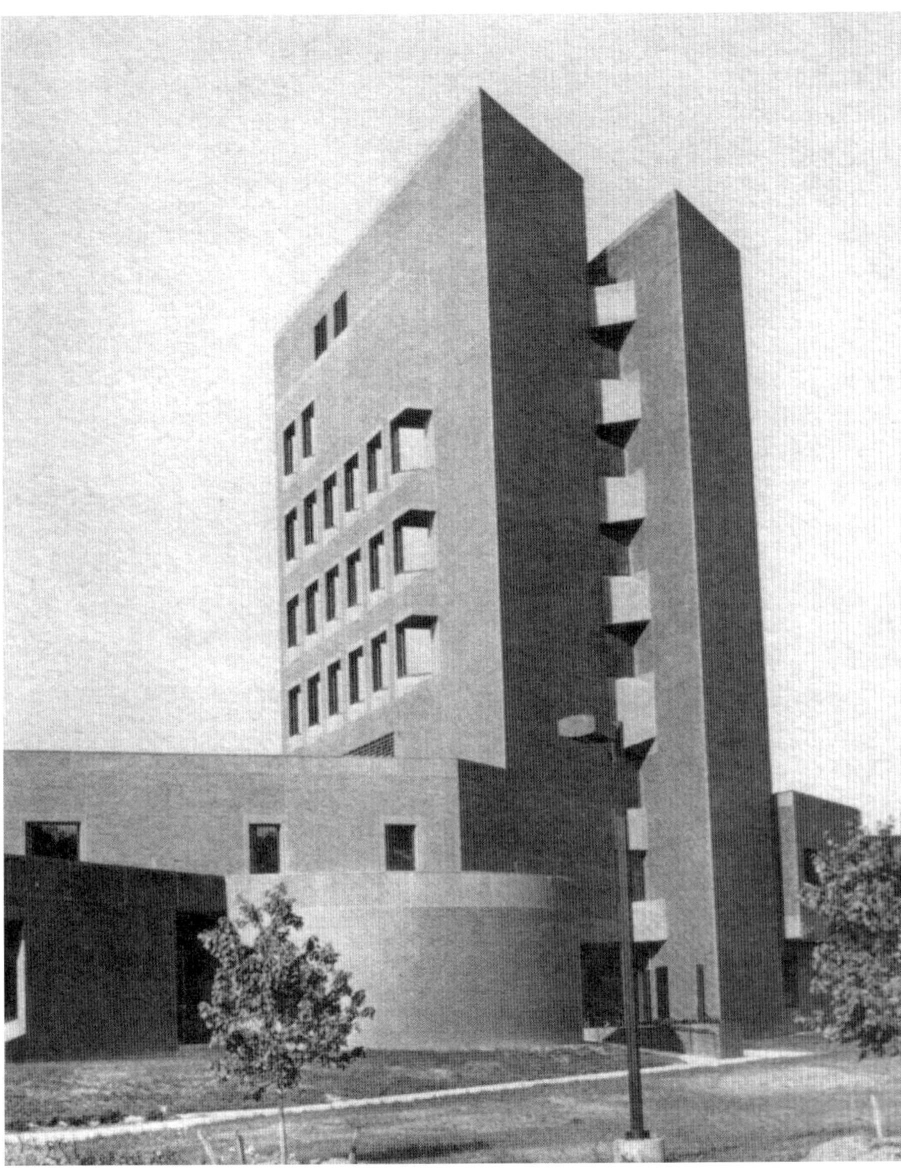

The Eastman Dental Center facility built on
Elmwood Avenue in Rochester, New York, that opened in 1976

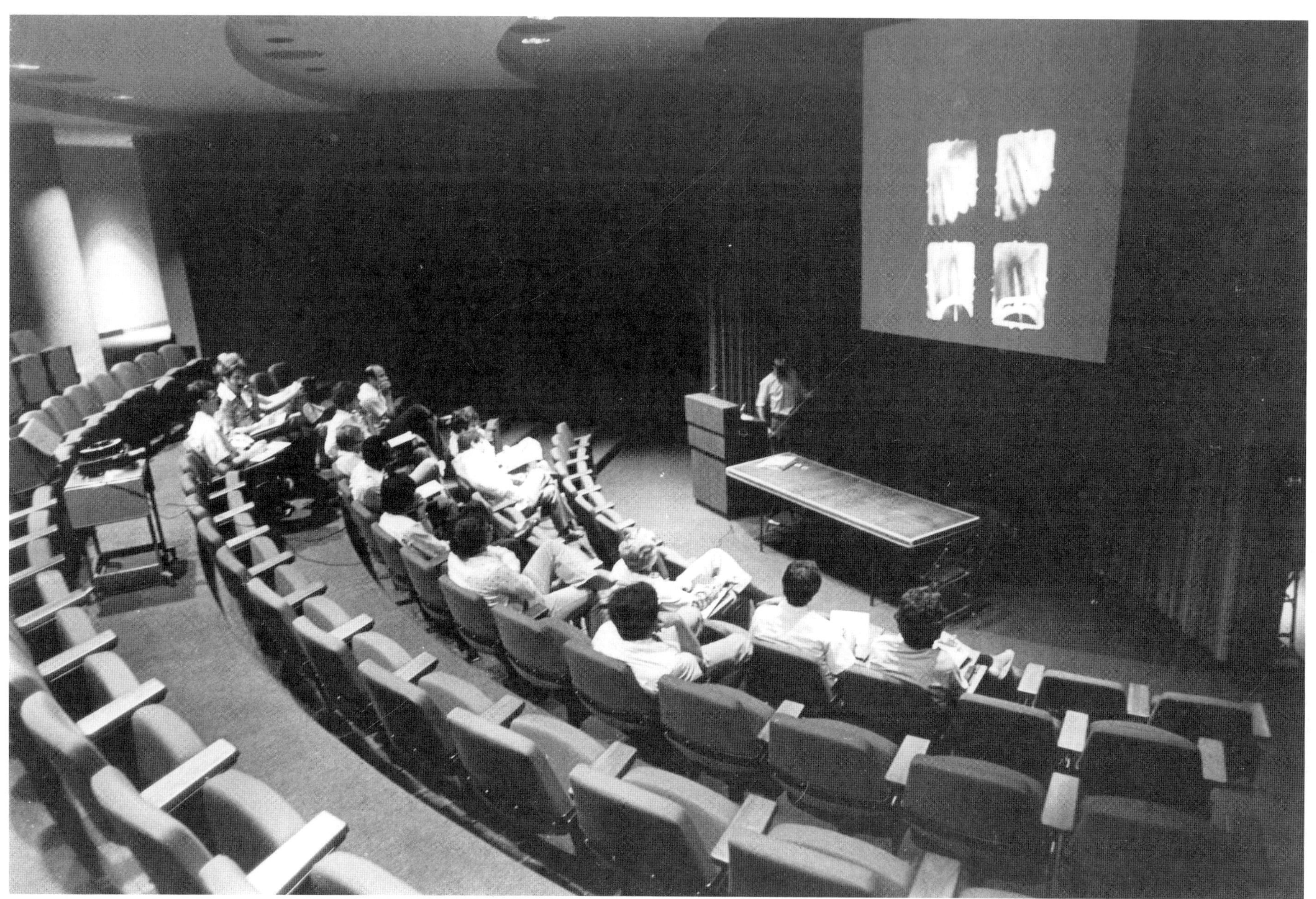

Farash Auditorium and Classroom

Chapter Eight

AT LONG LAST

THE EASTMAN INSTITUTE

The question is not why the merger happened but why it took seventy years.
Thomas H. Jackson, University of Rochester president, 1994–2005

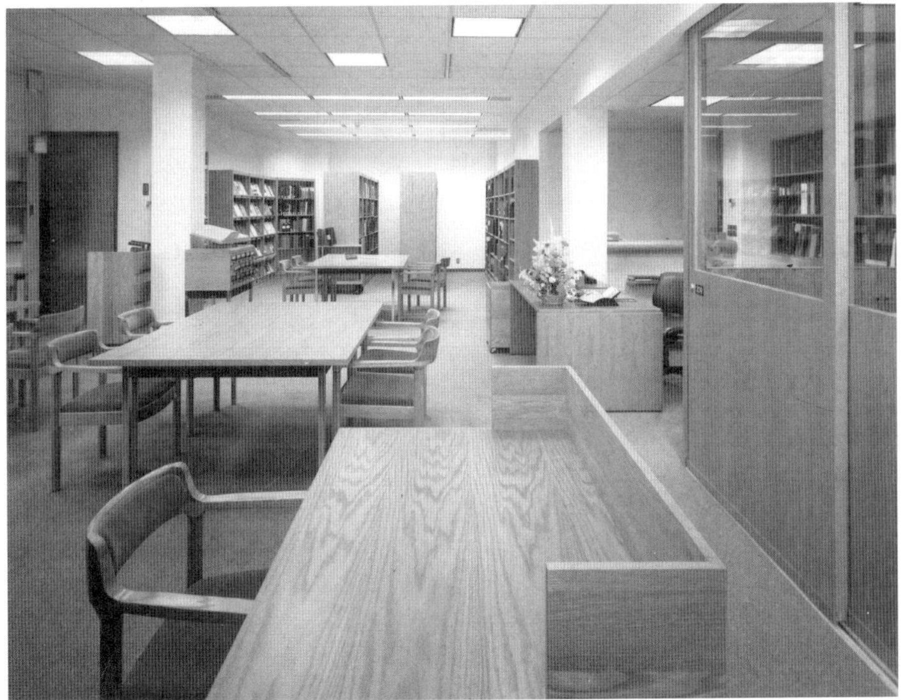

Bibby Library

TALKS OF A MERGER BETWEEN THE UNIVERSITY AND THE DENTAL CENTER commenced during the Bibby years, but there was always the conundrum of who would control the Eastman endowment, which in the Bibby years was worth about $38 million. Nonetheless, there was general agreement among dental center trustees on the desirability of developing clinical research and furthering postgraduate education as well as working toward a closer relationship with the university. Despite partially supporting the School of Medicine and Dentistry fellowship program at the behest of Eastman Dental Dispensary trustees such as Charles Hutchison, the dispensary's endowment income remained greater than its annual budgeted expenses. Basil Bibby was not unhappy at Tufts, but felt challenged to do something for dentistry with the resources that the Eastman Dental Dispensary offered.

During the Bibby years, there were many drawbacks to being an independent institution and not part of a dental school or university. It was not possible to offer appointments with tax exemptions to graduate students. Nor could veterans' benefits be used to supplement or replace salaries of dental trainees. Since the Eastman Dental Dispensary was not part of a hospital, it could not develop a dental internship that would be approved by the American Dental Association. A merger with the School of Medicine and Dentistry offered the possibility of overcoming all of these disadvantages. Bibby saw disadvantages to a merger, too, particularly while Johansen headed the dental program at School of Medicine and Dentistry. Bibby's planned to first bring a moribund facility back to optimal working order and then take advantage of the Eastman Dental Dispensary's strength as an independent institution. An independent institution, Bibby said, could "develop training programs in pedodontics, orthodontics, or general dentistry that other institutions could not offer."[1] In order to achieve this, for example, junior staff member Dr. Roland Hawes qualified for the specialty board in pedodontics and the specialty board in orthodontics approved Dr. Daniel Subtelny, thus reactivating the orthodontia department. Dr. Daniel Subtelny was recruited from the National Institute of Dental Research to reactivate the orthodontia program to meet accreditation standards. And Dr. Roland Hawes developed a two-year pediatric dentistry program to meet the accreditation standards.

Why didn't the merger take place during Bibby's tenure from 1947 to 1970? One answer is the ongoing antipathy between the senior administrators at each institution. Another reason would be that the physical separation of the Eastman Dental Center and the School of Medicine and Dentistry remained until 1978. Degrees were conferred by the School of Medicine and Dentistry, but most of the work was done at the Eastman Dental Center.

THE DREAM DELAYED

The antipathy between the Eastman Dental Center and the School of Medicine and Dentistry can best be understood in terms of certain larger background and historical issues. First, there was the underlying and persistent parity of esteem problem between dentistry and medicine that has to do with the particular way each of them moved from being a craft to a scientific profession at the end of the nineteenth and beginning of the twentieth century. Early on, medicine took a different path, including more basic science and research that led it to perceive itself as enjoying superior legitimacy.

Second, despite the importance of Eastman's patronage and influence, his vision for a school of medicine *and dentistry* was never really bought into existence by the physician leaders and administrators, such as George Whipple and Donald Anderson, who designed and ran the School of Medicine and Dentistry. As John Hein noted, Whipple eschewed setting up a dental school as Eastman and Rhees had directed him to do in favor of establishing a research project with outside funding from the Carnegie and Rockefeller foundations.

Third, there was money. The School of Medicine and Dentistry, despite Eastman's hopes and intention, never consistently used the funding allegedly set aside for dentistry. Dr. Hein laid this out chapter and verse and as the messenger, was "shot" for his trouble. Nevertheless, the Eastman Dental Center with its handsome endowment and other resources was a perennial temptation for the School of Medicine and Dentistry despite the prospect of having to "marry dentists." At the same time, the Eastman Dental Center

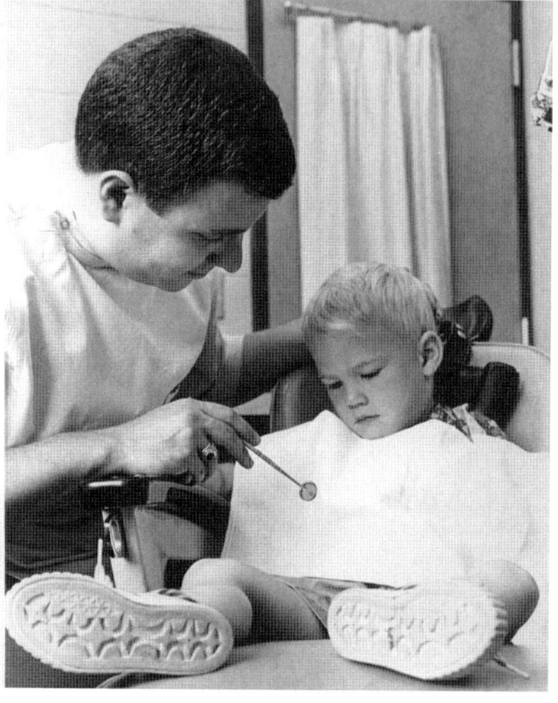

The reluctant patient

worried about being plundered by the School of Medicine and Dentistry if the relationship grew too close.

Throughout a largely unsatisfactory relationship at the institution-to-institution level between dental center and school, there had been positive connections as well. The Dental Fellows program was the most visible. Under the radar, there were many cooperative programs in which Eastman Dental Center faculty members utilized the basic science departments at the School of Medicine and Dentistry, as well as positive research projects between individual staff members at each institution.

Organizational and structural issues stood in the way of closer cooperation. Despite the close proximity of their buildings after the dental center moved next to the University of Rochester Medical Center in 1978, the relationship between the dental center and the university's medical center was at this point tense, ambiguous, and unclear. Cyril Meyerowitz remembers that in this period, "a lot of energy [was being] spent resolving tribal conflicts versus moving ahead in ways that were positive. It just was energy wasted in many different domains."[2]

The tension became apparent to students when they came into the system. "People on both sides either trumped up [the tense state of affairs between the institutions] or described it in a way that made it very difficult for new entries into the system to negotiate this territory easily."[3] The competitive relationships that always exist in an institution, and that might be considered healthy under normal circumstances, were exacerbated by the Eastman Dental Center's unresolved relationship with the university.

The ideological differences were never profound. Everybody agreed that the goals were to train the best academics and leaders of the world in dentistry, provide the best clinical care, and do the best research. But people's perceptions about what that meant were different. The tension could be regarded as tribal rather than ideological. Innate tribal feelings masked broader, more important issues about what should be created and the best way to do it.[4]

JOINT EDC/UR AFFILIATION COMMITTEE

In 1992, yet another joint EDC/UR Affiliation Committee was formed, inching once again toward a clearer affiliation or even a merger of the two organizations. This time the committee was headed by dental trustee Louis Langie Jr., a Rochester banker and Community Chest volunteer. The frustrated desire for an affiliation or merger was still lurking even after seventy-two years had gone without it being realized.

There were "lots of small stumbling blocks that tend[ed] to interfere with a harmonious relationship."[5] For example, conflicting philosophies about the relative importance of basic research and clinical research was an impediment. Drs. Edward Wentworth and Wilfred Springer and several other trustees expressed concern about the potential loss of the center's independence should the center merge with the university. Those who favored the formation of a graduate school of dentistry felt that careful planning could protect the center's autonomy and endowment. Janet Forbes, the first female member of the board of trustees, suggested that in the event of a merger, use of the Eastman Dental Center endowment could be restricted to use by the center. This would be similar to the arrangements between the university and the Eastman School of Music, Memorial Art Gallery, and Simon School. In addition, there was concern over the dental center trustees' level of comfort with university endowment management.[6]

Supervision of graduate students by dental center faculty who had part-time or adjunct appointments at the university surfaced as an important issue. This was a unique situation, very much against university practice, which did not allow for outside supervision by any other entity. However, it was "a very important issue to Eastman Dental Center adjunct faculty because it [was] where they [derived] the most intellectual pleasure," i.e. from the affiliation with the university. The dental center faculty felt strongly that this arrangement should continue.[7]

Also, from the dental center standpoint, major problems existed in the university's master of science degree programs due to severe scheduling conflicts. (In a sense, dentistry was repeating what happened to the university when the men left the women undergraduates at Prince Street and moved to the River Campus. Faculty had to drive back and forth between campuses until President Cornelis W. de Kiewiet finally united students on one campus.)

"Personality conflicts have prevented to a great extent a harmonious and mutually beneficial working relationship," one anonymous report from this period maintained. But then the nameless writer concluded, "Much more can be done to use the combined talents of the two institutions to their fullest potential. I have every confidence that this can be accomplished if people of good will can sit down together and spend the time and effort that is needed to make things happen."

COLLABORATIVE PROGRAMS AND PROJECTS

Notwithstanding the ongoing conflicts between administrative entities and physicians and dentists, many good things and collaborative activities did develop over the years—going back in some cases to the 1960s. An anonymous, undated text, probably from the early 1990s, documents numerous examples.

In periodontology, the relationship between the two entities was on the two major levels of clinical services and research. This included joint grant proposals and active research collaborations. Periodontics residents were pursuing degrees in university departments. There was active participation in Surgical Pathology, Clinical Dentistry, and Research in Progress Seminars (RIPS) in the Cancer Center.

In general dentistry, Dr. Stanley Handelman reported joint didactic programs with the university's Department of Clinical Dentistry, dental center courses carrying university credits, clinical research and educational projects, and the Salivary Dysfunction Clinic. Pediatric dentistry at the dental center had a joint project with the university's Department of Clinical Dentistry and the Strong Center for Developmental Disabilities. The Basil G. Bibby Library in the dental center was the only dental library available to the university. Librarian June E. Glasser put the EDC collection into the Carlson Science and Engineering Library catalog at the request of the School of Medicine and Dentistry.

Dr. John D. B. Featherstone in oral sciences, in addition to his collaboration on the Cariology Center with the Department of Dental Research, collaborated with the university's Department of Chemistry. He conducted a university course entitled "Chemical Aspects of Dental Caries" and prepared a pilot study with the university's Department of Orthopedics on implant materials and biological reactions to them. Featherstone also had a joint grant with the Laboratory for Laser Energetics to study laser effects on dental hard tissues.

Dr. Ronald Billings was a co-investigator with Dr. Larry Tabak on the Cariology Center project entitled "Salivary Mediated Base Production in Humans," designed to investigate a possible genetic factor in caries-free older adults. He was also a consultant to Dr. Cyril Meyerowitz on a Cariology Center project entitled "Caries Experience in Renal Dialysis Patients." Billings was the principal investigator on a project to develop and clinically assess fluoride-releasing systems for which Dr. William Bowen was the technical consultant. Bowen was the principal investigator and driving force behind the creation of the Cariology Center. His research, internationally recognized, was focused on the etiology, pathogenesis, and prevention of dental caries.

In orthodontics, Dr. J. Daniel Subtelny reported on "a long-standing cooperative program in congenital developmental problems of the head and neck." Since 1960, there had been a cleft palate team in cooperation with the university's Department of Plastic Surgery and in concert with speech pathologists from the Department of Otolaryngology. Certain university professors were also on the dental center faculty. There was joint training of dentist scientist

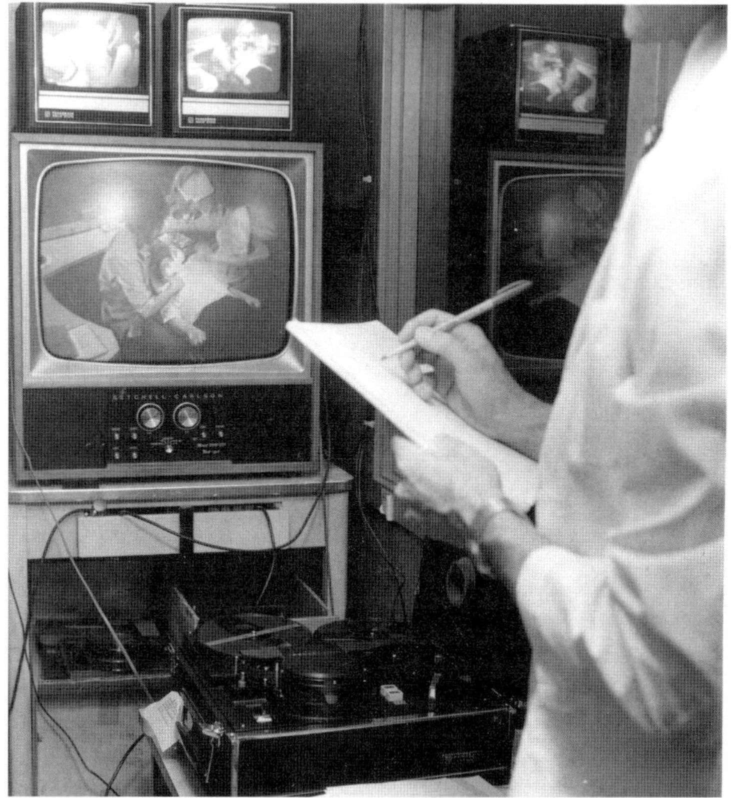

Technician with television view of dental procedure

awardees with the university's Department of Dental Research. Long-term, ongoing cooperative activity with the university's Department of Radiology included joint diagnosis and treatment and the use of CAT scans to evaluate and research anatomic relationships in craniofacial birth defects. Subtelny noted that the "project on orthopedic and dental implants is tremendously exciting and unique. I firmly believe that if this project is allowed to reach its potential it could lead to a world renowned center of medical and dental implantology."[8]

Because of ongoing collaborative activities like these at the ground level, the idea that the Eastman Dental Center and School of Medicine and Dentistry should be more closely affiliated, perhaps even merge, was kept alive.

THE MERGER

Cyril Meyerowitz, who came to the Eastman Dental Center as a postgraduate student in the general dentistry program under Dr. Stanley Handelman in the 1970s and then went on to become chair of clinical dentistry at the School of Medicine and Dentistry in 1991, commented about the affiliation meetings between the Eastman Dental Center and the School of Medicine and Dentistry in the nineties: "The affiliation agreement was a thorny, difficult discussion," Meyerowitz says, because the academic staff at Eastman felt that it was already part of the university, but it really wasn't. The dental center was on the medical campus, having moved there in 1978. The dental center had created its own professorial ranks, but technically, it still wasn't a New York State accredited educational institution. Professorial titles created at Eastman and adjunct appointments at the clinical dentistry and dental research departments did not change this. In addition, difficulties arose with collaborative grant applications because one entity, either the Eastman Dental Center or the School of Medicine and Dentistry, had to be actually in control of each application. Positive results of these early affiliation meetings included improved communications, closer relations, better cooperation, reduced expenses, shared services, and improved organizational operations.[9]

By 1993, the affiliation group (a joint committee) and in-house support groups were meeting regularly in addition to the monthly board of trustees meetings. After each joint committee meeting, the in-house groups at the dental center and university met internally to see where they would go next and to see if there was any disagreement that had come out of the joint meetings. At the next joint meeting they attempted to surface anything that had resulted. Both groups were satisfied with the arrangement. Defining the appointment process for Eastman Dental Center faculty at the university was an early project of the joint committee.[10] A separate joint committee on educational issues was also formed to oversee the admission process and curriculum to avoid overlap. Also discussed were legal issues such as whether dental students were "students" or "residents" and whether dental residents working at Strong Memorial Hospital had to be licensed.[11]

These committees and subcommittees were seen as "primarily a means for sitting and discussing issues . . . but not having any kind of police power or any kind of authority to implement policy. . . . [However,] interactions between the two institutions could take place without having to go through the usual bureaucracy." Some saw the affiliation agreement as downgrading the dental center to the extent that it became an adjunct reality rather than an equal entity, all because the university needed to protect its own dental department and programs.[12] The draft of the affiliation agreement, presented in December 1993, called for the director of Eastman Dental Center and the senior associate dean for academic affairs and research at the university to work together.

JAY STEIN

Jay H. Stein, MD, came on board in August 1995 as senior vice president and vice provost for health affairs at the University of Rochester Medical Center. With that, the inching along approach of the informal committees that characterized the relationship between the university and the dental center came to an abrupt end. As one observer recalls, "Jay Stein was an energizer who created opportunities and possibilities, whereas a stodgy move ahead didn't do that. He was one of those people who when he got hold of something like this, he would just go to it. He was like a bulldog, very fast moving and also a student of history. He also had read some of the history of what had happened. And he took this as sort of a personal mission."[13] Stein would have the background, personality, and larger objectives to become the instrument in breaking the Gordian knot that had kept the Eastman Dental Center and School of Medicine and Dentistry on separate tracks since 1920. He would ultimately be the catalyst that brought about the culmination of seventy-five years of an on-again/off-again relationship.

In 1975, Jay Stein began his administrative career as chair of medicine at the newly established University of Texas Health Science Center, and he developing his department into a nationally recognized program. In 1992, he gave up his research grants to run the University of Oklahoma Health Sciences Center. (He was there to pick up the pieces when the federal building in Oklahoma City was blown up in 1995.) At a time of flat state funding, Stein prioritized programs and freed $6.3 million to recruit researchers who boosted Oklahoma's reputation, and he also went to private foundations for additional funds.

Stein was brought to the University of Rochester because it needed the same kind of leadership to focus its medical school and move it into the future, President Thomas Jackson said at the time (1995). His strategic plan was designed to integrate the medical center's research and clinical sides, boost the health system's profitability so it could compete effectively, and focus the medical center's growth. This would also lead to the dental merger that had eluded his predecessors for seventy-five years. When the merger was on its way to completion, Stein shrugged and remarked: "Eastman said in a letter in 1920 that he thought it should happen. So, it took a few years. I think it will lead to one of the best research dental programs in the country, if not the best." Stein attended the dental center's board of trustees meeting in November 1995, where he emphasized that "in the tradition of what George Eastman started, the university and the center must become known nationally as a training site for graduates and researchers. Key to this was the relationship between the university and the center," and Stein stated that he wanted to enhance that relationship over the next several years.[14]

When Stein arrived, he interviewed department heads, asking what each of them thought was "the single most important thing to do here . . . over the next number of years." Many answered that the issue of the Eastman Dental Center and its anomalous position within the university needed to be resolved.[15] Dr. Ronald Billings, then the director of the Eastman Dental Center, was in favor of a merger. Billings, Louis Langie, chairman of the board, and Stein met for lunch at Oak Hill Country Club. Stein was initially interested in just a closer relationship between the two institutions, but over the course of two or three hours the discussion shifted toward an actual merger. "Jay asked Lou Langie and myself what we would require," Billings recalls. The major issue on the table was that the endowment be protected. Stein quickly and willingly agreed to that. He also agreed that all Eastman Dental Center faculty and staff be absorbed into the university at their current salaries and ranks and that there would be no net job loss as a consequence.[16]

"It took more than a Jay Stein to accomplish the merger," Billings says. "It took a change in leadership in both institutions. When Marshall Lichtman became dean of the University of Rochester School of Medicine and Dentistry in 1990, the rank of associate dean that McHugh held was withdrawn and along with it the salary support for the position. The attitude of the university at that time was that the position was largely ceremonial and that the university was not interested in maintaining it."

Serious effort to forge a permanent merger began when an ad hoc Work Group was convened in February 1996.[17] Building upon the academic

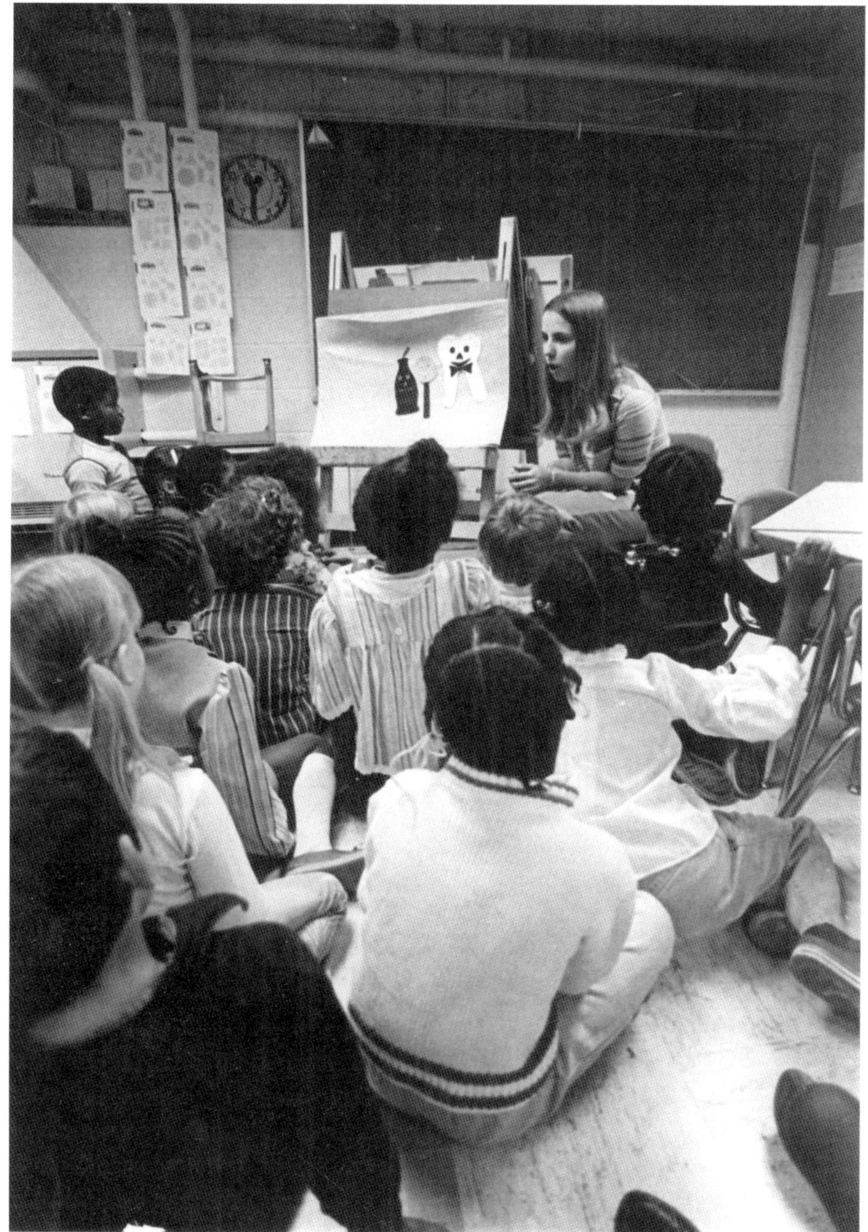

Teaching kids

relationship between the Eastman Dental Center and University of Rochester Medical Center and working with a facilitator, the group embarked on defining goals and future plans. Jay Stein led the retreats in which each participant had to describe his vision of what was going to happen in the future. The Work Group, with members drawn from the dental center and the medical center, reviewed the current strategic goals of each and formulated concrete and pragmatically stated objectives for the proposed affiliation. It further conducted high-level cost-benefit analyses for the primary activities and initiatives identified, developed a structural configuration for the proposed affiliation, and prepared and presented a final Phase I report of findings and recommendations. The Work Group cautioned, "Before proceeding, it is critical to determine Eastman Dental Center board support for the proposed affiliation approach." The historic university/dental center agreement of April 14, 1997, described the merging entities as becoming "partners in the provision of oral health care, graduate education, and research." Furthermore, the entire dental center faculty was to become university faculty.

The agreement listed the reasons for the merger in legalese: Nine paragraphs each beginning "WHEREAS . . ." listed the reasons for the merger:

- The UR is authorized to operate the URMC comprising Strong Memorial Hospital, the School of Medicine and Dentistry, the School of Nursing, and the University of Rochester Faculty Medical Group

- The EDC operates a dental diagnostic and treatment center

- The EDC's graduate dental education programs are co-registered by the NYS Education Department

- The EDC is located adjacent to the URMC on land leased from the UR

- The SMD and EDC having participated in a mutually advantageous academic affiliation for many years, jointly convened the Work Group

- The Affiliation Plan envisioned that the combined energy and resources of the URMC and EDC would result in a single entity dedicated to becoming the premier institution for oral health care, graduate dental education and dental research

- The Affiliation Plan identifies goals as expanding dental education, research and education funding, link clinical services within the dental community to advance oral health care and succeed under managed care

- The Affiliation Plan identified that the EDC shall maintain a separate identity within the URMC membership and that the EDC endowment shall be transferred to a new foundation corporation under the continued control of an initial board of directors selected by the current EDC trustees.

- The boards of trustees of both the university and the dental center had each approved the Affiliation Plan prior to April 14, 1997.

"Once the merger happened," Meyerowitz recalls, "it was quite clear that the kind of structure we had to set up was to create a much more unitary leadership. We were having retreats as a group, bringing people together—it was Larry Tabak and Meyerowitz from the university and the Eastman leadership at the time—Ron Billings, Dom Zero, Jack Caton, Dov Almog, and some planning and marketing people, plus Jay Stein, Peter Robinson, and Dean Lowell Goldsmith from The Medical Center's leadership. The organizational outcome was to create one department within SMD that would house all the dental faculty, establish the Center for Oral Biology as the extension of the Department of Dental Research, and leave Eastman Dental Center as the Clinical arm of the Medical Center. There was some discussion about creating a post-graduate school, but, there was not enough support for the idea," Meyerowitz says.[18] As a result of the merger, the Eastman Department of Dentistry was created within the School of Medicine and Dentistry, and the Eastman Dental Center remained as the oral health clinical arm of the medical center.

The vision statement the group developed said, "The combined energy and resources of EDC and URMC will result in one organization dedicated to becoming the number one institution for oral health care, dental postgraduate education, and dental research." Specifically, the collective organization would expand dental education, research, and clinical capabilities; respond to and withstand reductions in research and education funding; link clinical services with the dental community to advance oral health and

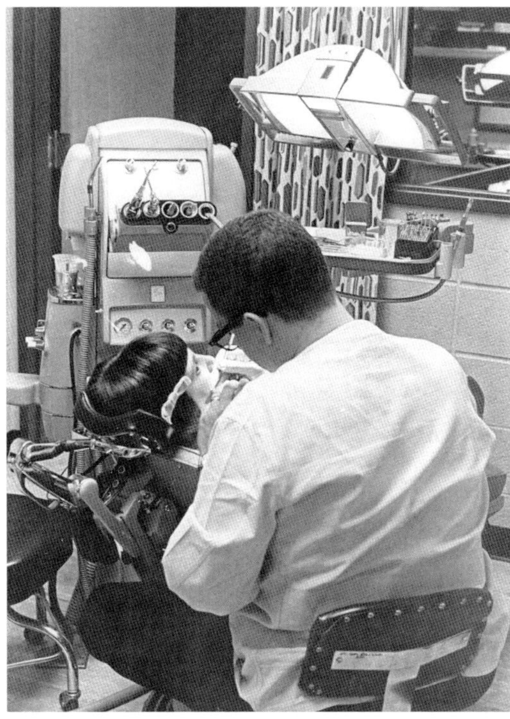

Dentist and child

succeed under managed care; and selectively reduce unnecessary duplication and operating cost.

In working out the vision, the Work Group considered a variety of options and identified four affiliation principles, two of which were of particular importance. First, Eastman Dental Center would continue to have a prominent identity as a member entity of URMC. Second, and most important since this was the sticking point in earlier talks of merger, "EDC's endowment will be placed in a separate foundation and preserved exclusively for the advancement of oral health." The new foundation was created to hold the endowment that began with George Eastman's gifts of 1915, 1920, and 1932. The dental center board determined who would serve on the foundation board. The foundation proceeds were to be used to support oral health, education, and research needs identified by the dental management team chaired by Jay Stein. A nine-member board of directors would provide oversight of the endowment, then valued at $41 million. Wilfred A. Springer, DDS, president of the dental center's board of trustees at the time of the merger, said in July 1997:

> Our combined resources in dental education, research, and patient care will not only expand Rochester's role locally, but also in the national and international dental arenas. By working in partnership, the Eastman Dental Center and the university's departments of Clinical Dentistry and Dental Research will make a difference in ways that we could not do alone.

With the merger, the Eastman Dental Center joined with Strong Memorial Hospital, the School of Medicine and Dentistry, the School of Nursing, and the Medical Faculty Practice Group to become an integral part of the University of Rochester Medical Center. The URMC's board, which included a six-member subcommittee of dental board members, was delegated authority from the university board for matters related compliance with state regulations.[19]

Cyril Meyerowitz became the chair of the newly created Eastman Department of Dentistry within the SMD and succeeded Billings as fifth director of the Eastman Dental Center on January 1, 1999. Billings would write, "This coalescence of leadership provides a unique opportunity for academic dentistry to flourish in ways envisioned for so long by so many."[20]

EASTMAN'S VISION ON THE WAY TO BECOMING A REALITY

Following seventy-seven years of negotiations, the actual merger took place after six months of preparation on July 1, 1997, earlier than the three years that had been projected before Stein's arrival. Henceforth, the Eastman Dental Center would be known as the University of Rochester Eastman Dental Center, a division of the University of Rochester Medical Center. With the merger, a press release read, "The resources and energies of EDC and URMC are now combined into one organization dedicated to becoming the foremost institution worldwide for oral health care, dental post-graduate education, and dental research."[21]

The next year, 1998, the dental faculty from the Eastman Dental Center and School of Medicine and Dentistry's departments of Clinical Dentistry and Dental Research were integrated into a new department, the Eastman Department of Dentistry. Cyril Meyerowitz, DDS, MS, was appointed chair of the Eastman Department of Dentistry of the School of Medicine and Dentistry. At the same time, the Center for Oral Biology (COB) was formed to pursue basic research in oral health under the direction of Lawrence A. Tabak, DDS, PhD, who also assumed the role of senior associate dean for research in the School of Medicine and Dentistry. The Center for Oral Biology was the first of the basic science research centers in the university's new Aab Institute of Biomedical Sciences. However, in 2000, Dr. Tabak left to become director of the National Institute of Dental and Craniofacial Research. In 2001, Dr. James Melvin was named director of the Center for Oral Biology.

The mission statement of the new Eastman Department of Dentistry was as follows: "We improve oral health through caring, discovery, teaching, and learning."

The vision statement of the new Eastman Department of Dentistry was as follows:

1. To be the premier dental postgraduate training environment for the education of dentistry's future academic leaders.

2. To develop a service/education system which is a national model for the integration of dentistry with medicine and the health care system at all levels of education, research, and clinical service.

3. To be a local and national leader of high quality oral health care which is evidence-based with an emphasis on prevention.

4. In close cooperation with the Center for Oral Biology (COB) of the Rochester Institute of Biomedical Science, to move into the top three ranking in NIDCR funding, the primary focus in the Eastman Department of Dentistry being clinical and translational research.

With the merger, three entities were created: the Eastman Dental Center (EDC), which became the oral health arm of the medical center; the Eastman

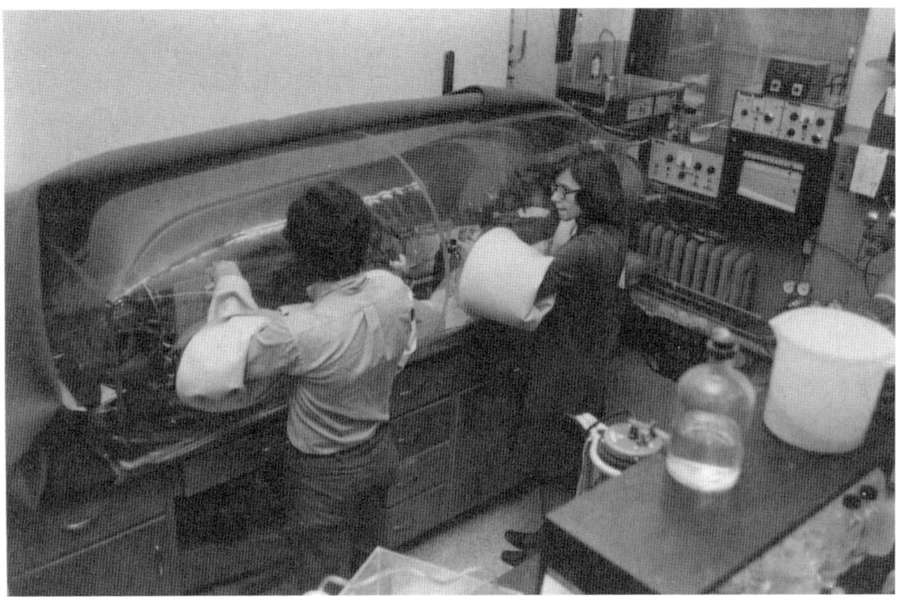

Microbiology laboratory

Department of Dentistry (EDD), the academic department of dentistry within the School of Medicine and Dentistry; and the Center for Oral Biology (COB), the basic science unit within the Research Institute of the URMC. Together these three entities became known as "Dentistry, University of Rochester Medical Center."

Among other dental schools across the United States, some are called "school of dentistry," others are named "school of dental medicine." A few are even described as a "college of dentistry" or a "college of dental medicine." The latter are separate institutions within academic health centers or stand-alone schools. Harvard has a "school of dentistry," but uniquely, the faculty is part of a department in its school of medicine. In Canada, some dental schools have become departments in medicine or are a part of an academic health science faculty. The dental institutions at the University of Rochester have their own distinct organization, hammered out over many years of competition and cooperation between the Eastman Dental Center and the School of Medicine and Dentistry.

STEIN RESIGNS

Jay Stein was credited with being the catalyst of the merger and was seen to be beginning to transform the medical center into a major research institution. Stein's aim had been to put it in the top fifteen schools funded by the National Institutes of Health. It was an ambitious goal and one he did not meet despite a 74 percent growth in grant revenue between 1997 and 2002. In 1997, the URMC was rated twenty-sixth in NIH grant funding, but by 2002 it had fallen to twenty-eighth. (In 2006, three years after Stein's departure, it was twenty-fourth.)

In May 2003, *Democrat and Chronicle* headlines shocked the Rochester community by announcing Stein's resignation. The statement by university president Thomas Jackson and the board of trustees specified without further explanation "serious concerns about issues and methods of coordination involving the medical center and the university." Many interpretations held that Stein had wanted to make the medical center independent of the university, an outcome that university officials could not allow to happen.[22]

DENTAL HEALTH AT THE UNIVERSITY OF ROCHESTER

With Dr. Cyril Meyerowitz, professor and chair of the Eastman Department of Dentistry since 1998 and director of the Eastman Dental Center since 1999, dentistry at the university entered a new era. Meyerowitz had a history here. He was an alumnus of Eastman Dental Center, had received his MS degree at the School of Medicine and Dentistry, and at the time of the merger in 1996, he was a department chairman.

Upon graduation from the University of Witwatersrand School of Dentistry in South Africa in 1973, Meyerowitz was recruited to be part of the General Dentistry Program by Dr. Stanley Handelman, who was interested in offering a position to someone in South Africa. After a year in Handelman's program, Meyerowitz was offered a research project that could result in a master's degree in dental science. He became Dr. Martin Curzon's first graduate student, doing "a research project on trace elements, on the effects of strontium and fluoride on dental caries—an animal study in rats." Meyerowitz experienced the master's program as rigorous—"a very intense

research, thesis-oriented program. It probably should have been a PhD program . . . given the quality of the research product you had to produce." His major in experimental pathology was taken at the medical center.[23]

In his role as chair of the Eastman Department of Dentistry, Meyerowitz moved to secure the retention of academic and clinical faculty at Eastman Dental Center, to recruit translational researchers, and to ensure the transition of the leadership of Eastman's divisions. These translational researchers, which included Stephanos Kyrkanides, who went on to become the chair of orthodontics, Michel Koo, Gene Watson, and Andy Teng, were successful at attracting NIH and other research funding. The Center for Oral Biology (COB) recruited several basic science researchers, including Rulang Yang and Wei Tsu, both successful, well-funded developmental biologists.

In addition to the other two NIH research training grants in infectious diseases and molecular biology in the COB, Rochester was awarded a Clinical Research Training grant from NIDCR, with Meyerowitz as the principal investigator. This grant closely linked to URMC's Clinical Research Curriculum award, which was the educational basis for the Clinical and Translational Research Science Award (CTSA) that the URMC received in 2006.

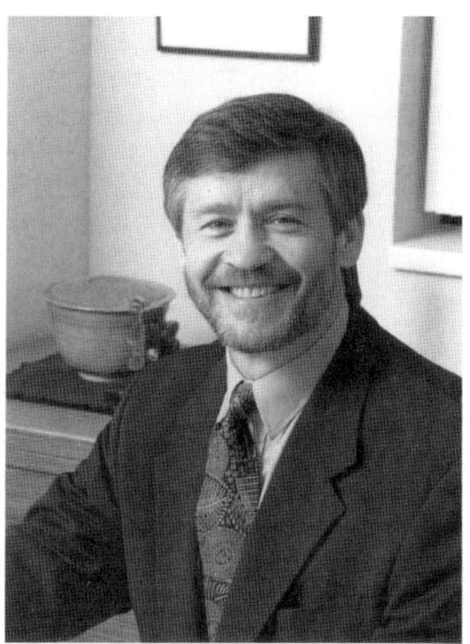

Cyril Meyerowitz

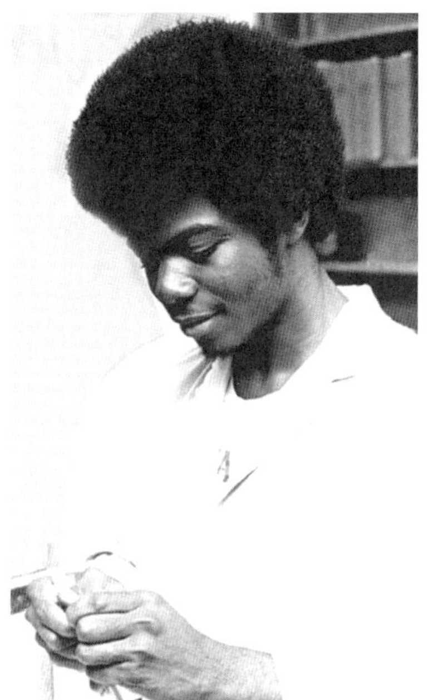

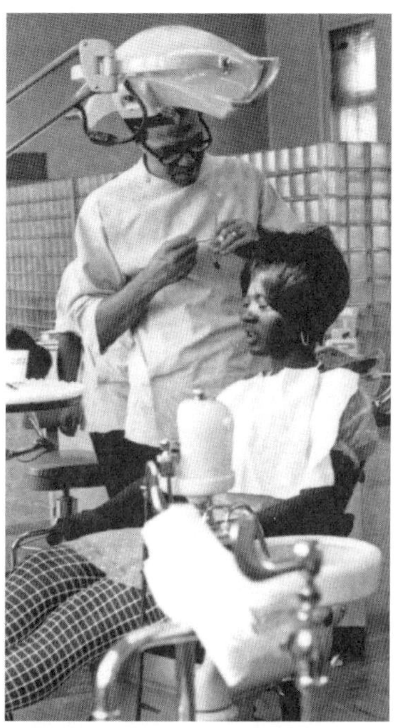

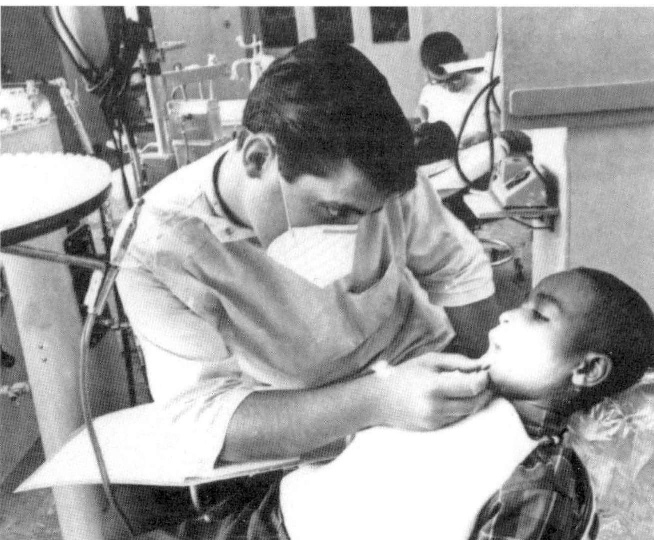

Dentists and children

Eight students were recruited into the program, all of whom completed their master's programs in clinical investigation. Two of them, Yanfang Ren and Dorota Kopychka Kedzierawski, later became faculty members and were successful in securing NIH research career development awards.

By 2003, dentistry at the University of Rochester had moved up to fifth place in NIDCR funding. A significant part of this was from the COB, which maintained and grew its support while the research funding at Eastman increased its NIH and other funding from $600,000 in 2000 to $2.9 million in 2008.

In 2003, the first EDC/UR Dentistry All-Alumni and Friends Alumni Conference was held in Naples, Florida, with more than 300 people attending.

Advanced education programs grew following the merger. The Eastman Department of Dentistry's advanced education programs at the dental center received full accreditation status in 2004 from the Commission on Dental Accreditation (CODA), the body that accredits all dental education programs and is recognized by the United States Department of Education. A CODA committee conducted an evaluation of the advanced dental education programs in orthodontics and dentofacial orthopedics, pediatric dentistry, periodontics, prosthodontics, and advanced education in general dentistry. The visiting committee focused on a number of areas, including institutional commitment and program effectiveness, the program director and teaching staff, the curriculum and program duration, and the quality and quantity of resident research.

At its meeting in January 2005, CODA considered the visiting committee's reports on the postdoctoral programs at Eastman. The programs were granted the accreditation status of "approval without any reporting requirements" and there were a number of commendations. Meyerowitz noted at the time that it was "significant that we received full approval from CODA and there were no citations. It's most unusual that all elements in five programs are approved and it reflects the hard work of the program directors, faculty, residents, and staff." The next accreditation site visit will occur in 2011. Full accreditation of the oral and maxillofacial surgery and the general practice residency programs at Strong Memorial Hospital was ongoing.

Among the commendations from CODA are the following:

- In the orthodontic program, "The quality and quantity of the residents' research meets or exceeds the level of a masters degree program at other institutions."

- The pediatric dentistry program "incorporated an outstanding clinical outreach program in community dentistry at School 17 as part of their extramural experience. In additional to providing the residents outstanding experiences in community dentistry, the outreach program also provides a necessary service to the community."

- The periodontic program "documents 100 percent board eligibility or board certification of recent graduates from 1997–2003 with the majority being fully certified." The program was commended for its "strong preparation and uniform encouragement of graduates to seek and complete the board certification process."

- The newly renovated prosthodontic laboratory "provides excellent space for the projected number of residents. The institution is commended for providing the necessary facilities and resources to ensure an outstanding educational environment."

- The Advanced Education in General Dentistry program "provides the largest number of patient visits per year with 83,865 at the Dental Center, 18,487 at the Community Dentistry satellite clinics, 1,270 visits at the Monroe Community Hospital Developmental Disabled Clinic, 500 visits at the Jewish Home in Rochester."

Dental education accreditation, initiated in the early 1900s, is conducted today by the Commission on Dental Accreditation, which operates under the auspices of the American Dental Association. This peer review mechanism involves members of the discipline, the broad educational community, employers, practitioners, the dental licensing community, and public members. All of these groups participate in a process designed to ensure educational quality.

By 2008 the clinical programs of dentistry at the URMC had grown to more than 140,000 patient visits a year. Notable, in accordance with Eastman's original mission, was an increase in patient visits in the outreach program to more than 29,000 per annum by 2008. This growth came about with the establishment of clinics in high poverty areas, including at School 17 (Franklin) and in the downtown Sibley building, as well as an enlargement of the Smilemobile program.

In August 2005, the cornerstone of the community outreach activities, the Smilemobile program, was honored with the Healthcare Association of New York State's prestigious Community Health Improvement Award. This award is given annually to recognize outstanding initiatives that improve community health and patient well-being in the state.

The almost forty-year-old dental office on wheels continues to bring oral health services year-round to children who would otherwise not have access to much-needed dental care. Eastman Dental Center dentists, hygienists, and dental residents provide comprehensive oral healthcare services through the Smilemobile program. There are now four fully equipped dental vans. By 2005, the program had served an estimated 39,000 children and teens at fifteen inner-city schools, eight Head Start programs, and three remote rural locations.

The international tradition begun by George Eastman is being renewed. Alliances were established with the Eastman Institutes in London and in Rome, with the Dental Schools of the University of Rome and the University of Sienna in Italy, and with the dental school in Jerusalem, Israel. In 2005, an alliance was established between the University of Rochester Eastman Dental Center and faculty of dentistry of Piracicaba University of Campinas in Brazil to promote innovative research ideas and cooperation on scientific projects. The Brazilian alliance, spearheaded by Michel Koo, is the result of an intensive collaboration among scientists from these two renowned institutions. The alliance began in 1995 and has resulted in over twenty-five scientific papers, two pending patent applications, and other cooperative ventures.

RESEARCH

Research continues to win recognition nationally and internationally. Oral biologist Hyun (Michel) Koo, DDS, PhD, and microbiologist Robert Marquis, PhD, received Distinguished Scientist Awards at a meeting in Australia of the International Association of Dental Research (IADR), the largest organization of dental researchers in the world. Koo became interested in food science and used his knowledge to try to stop bacteria such as *Streptococcus mutans* that cause cavities. With the university since 1999, Koo was honored four times previously by IADR. He identified compounds in propolis (a sticky substance made by honeybees to protect their hives) that inhibit the activity of a key enzyme that forms dental plaque. Another team led by Koo discovered that the same traits that make cranberry juice a powerful weapon against urinary tract infections also hold promise for protecting teeth against

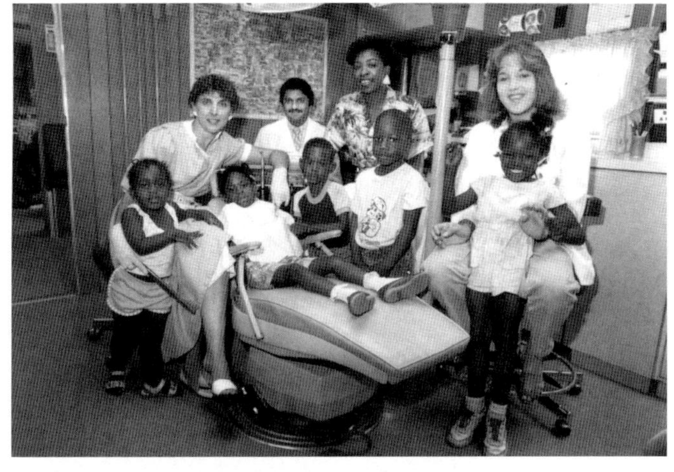
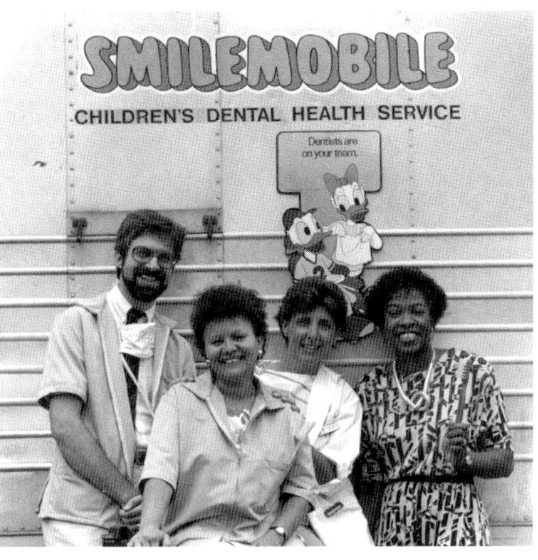

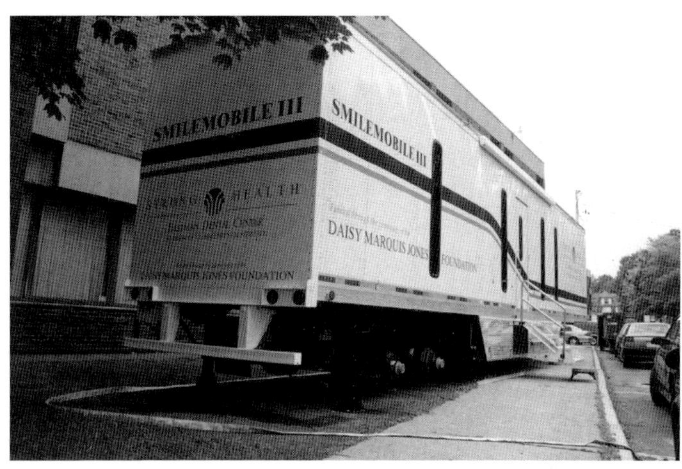

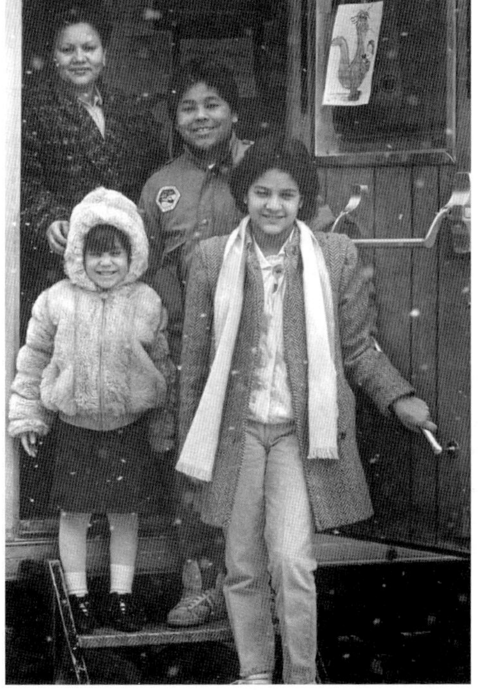
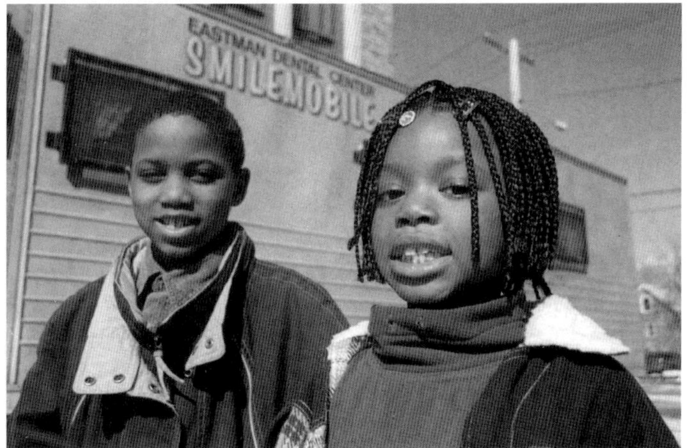

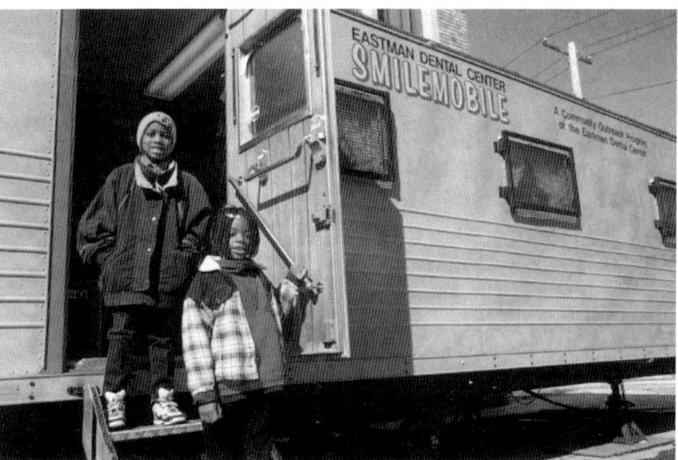

Smilemobile

cavities. "Scientists believe that one of the main ways that cranberries prevent urinary tract infections is by inhibiting the adherence of pathogens on the surface of the bladder. Perhaps the same is true in the mouth, where bacteria use adhesion molecules to hold onto teeth," Koo said. Koo's work with cranberry juice is one of nine projects funded through a special program by the National Institutes of Health to test the berry's reputed health-enhancing effects.

Dr. Marquis is a microbial physiologist who studies how bacteria get the nutrients they need to stay alive. During the last two decades he has focused on the bacteria in our mouth, such as *S. mutans,* the number one cause of tooth decay around the world. He discovered how such bacteria are able to stay alive amid the acidic environment in our mouths. He showed how preservatives commonly found in diet soda, frozen foods, juices, and other foods can inhibit this defense mechanism, helping to prevent cavities by mimicking the cavity-preventing action of fluoride. Marquis, who has been on the faculty since 1963, also has discovered a new way to kill bacterial spores, a method now used in the canning industry.

The American Academy of Periodontology (AAP) Gold Medal Award was presented to Jack G. Caton, DDS, MS, in recognition of his outstanding contributions in the field of periodontal research, education, and service. Caton's earlier honors include the William J. Gies Award in 1993 and an AAP Fellowship in 1995. He is a past president of the AAP and past chair of the American Board of Periodontology. Caton received his periodontal specialty certificate from EDC in 1973 and earned his MS degree from the University of Rochester in 1973. He has been on the Eastman faculty since 1973 and has served as division chair and program director since 1990. He and his graduate students have conducted research in periodontal wound healing, animal models, diagnosis, and human clinical trials. He has authored more than eighty publications; given more than 190 major presentations worldwide; and served as principal investigator on many research grants. Caton also serves as associate editor of the *Journal of Periodontology;* commissioner on the Commission on Dental Accreditation (CODA); chair of the Periodontics Advisory Committee of CODA; and director of the American Academy of Periodontology Foundation Board. Recently Caton was informed that he is the recipient of the ADA 2008 Norton Ross award for excellence in clinical research. This is a high honor indeed.

These awards showcase the university's role as one of the leading institutions in the world for dental research. As noted in earlier chapters, university dentists were the first to demonstrate the protective role that saliva plays in preventing cavity formation, and they were the first to understand how fluoride works in the body, a significant contribution to its widespread use to protect against tooth decay. Its dental researchers also discovered how to make dental sealants better adhere to tooth enamel, leading to their widespread use to prevent dental decay.

Robert Quivey Jr., PhD, a microbiologist and currently professor and director of the Center for Oral Biology, heads a group studying how to force bacteria in our mouths to "choke on their own acids." The microbiologists have discovered a chink in the armor that bacteria use to survive the hostile environment of the human mouth. *S. mutans,* the dominant mouth bacterium, latches onto teeth, eats sugar, and then rearranges its cell membranes to make itself impervious to the acid assault that it lets loose. Quivley's team found that a gene known as *fabM* is responsible for changing the membrane's composition and enables *S. mutans* to become more resistant to acid. When the team knocked out this gene in *S. mutans,* the bacteria's defenses fell; the cell membrane was no longer able to protect against the acid the bacteria churn out. Researchers have thus "identified a potentially useful and novel pathway," says Quivey, who is also on the faculty of the Eastman Department of Dentistry and the Department of Microbiology and Immunology, but researchers still "have a very long road to go to identifying and isolating a compound that stops the process in bacteria." They are "cautiously optimistic" about the eventual identification. The National Institute of Dental and Craniofacial Research funded the prize-winning research.

Notable research contribution have come from other faculty at the institution. Stephanos Kyrkanides, who completed his PhD at the University of Rochester and became chair of orthodonics in 2005, has, together with Ross Tallents, identified an interesting association between arthritis and pain, located centrally in the brain and peripherally in joints and muscle. This work, which has received NIH funding, has substantial potential for translation. Kyrkanides, who has received a number of patents, has been successful in developing translational partnerships and venues for his work in this area and in craniofacial development. He is also working on developing novel treatment regimes for the management of disabling or fatal disorders, with an emphasis on the face and the cranial skeleton.

James Melvin, an internationally known salivary biologist, recipient of a merit award from NIDCR, former director of the COB, and recipient of the 2008 Salivary Research award from the IADR, has focused on exocrine gland dysfunction. His laboratory has focused on determining the molecular identity, including structure and function, of transport proteins that regulate fluid secretion. Melvin's work will provide important insights necessary to develop treatment strategies for salivary gland dysfunction. Rulang Jiang's laboratory has worked on gaining a better understanding of the molecular mechanisms underlying normal craniofacial development and the pathogenic processes leading to congenital craniofacial malformations. He has used a combination of genetic, biochemical, and embryological approaches to analyze craniofacial development, delineate the molecular pathways, and identify novel genes that interact with known critical regulators of craniofacial development. These studies are providing new insights into the molecular genetic mechanisms underlying human craniofacial development and birth defects.

William Bowen, an internationally recognized dental caries researcher, former director of the COB, and recipient of the ADA Gold Medal, focuses on the molecular mechanisms involved in the colonization of surfaces by microorganisms. His recent investigations have provided valuable information on a group of enzymes, the glucosyltransferases, formed by oral streptococci, which form glucan from sucrose. This work has significant translational potential in the prevention of dental caries, and Bowen and Robert Berkowitz have been funded to explore this in clinical studies. Bowen is also exploring the influence of common food preservatives on the development of caries.

EPILOGUE: THE END OF THE BEGINNING

The saga of dentistry in Rochester does not end with the elusive but long-sought merger of the Eastman Dental Center and the university's School of Medicine and Dentistry. But the merger does mark some climactic closing stages of a significant chapter in that historical saga. Beginning in 1915, George Eastman and Harvey Burkhart wanted a dental school to be associated with their new dispensary for indigent children. Burkhart contacting Abraham Flexner in 1919 was meant to be the first step in establishing that school. Instead, it led to a new medical school—with the word "dentistry" tacked on in part to placate the donor.

The search for unitary leadership has been present from the beginning too. Burkhart thought that his appointment as dean of dentistry at the School of Medicine and Dentistry would lead to a real school of dentistry under his

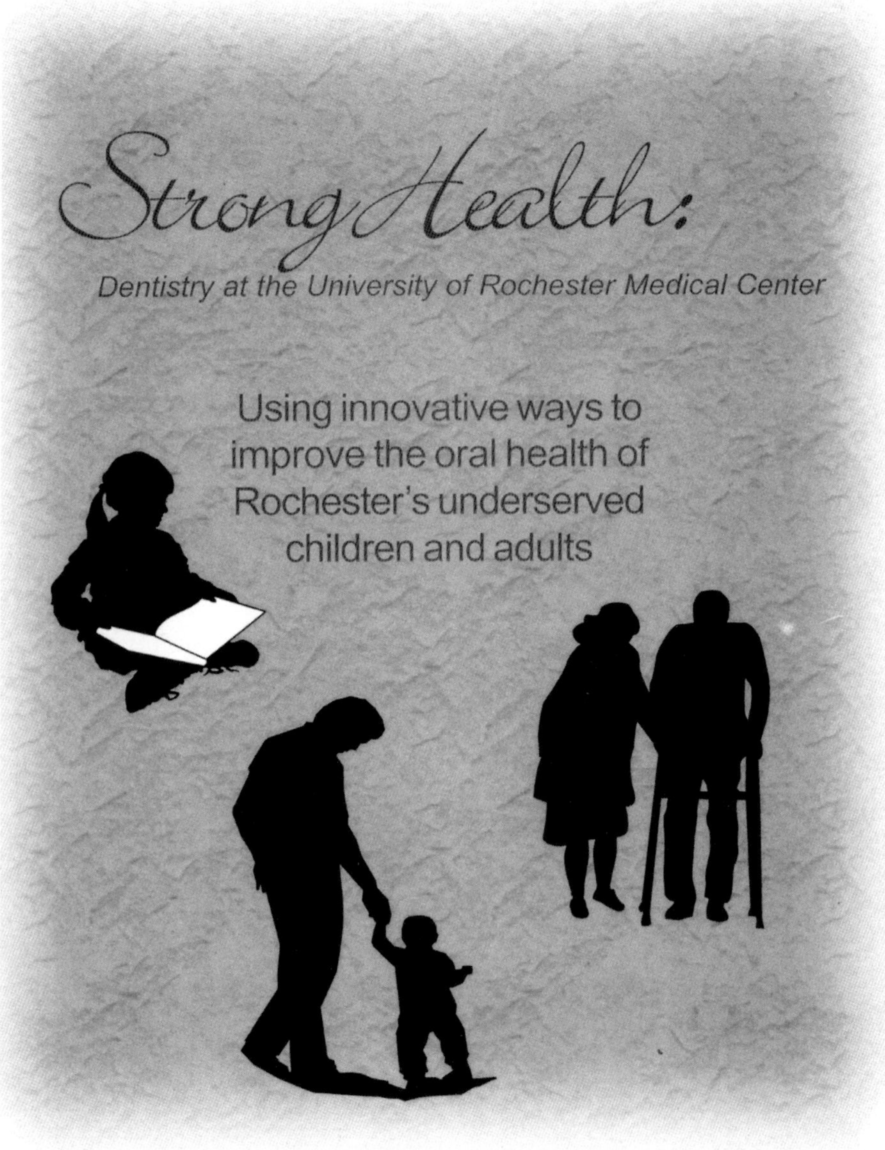

Cover of brochure published in 2001 explaining the scope and programs of dentistry at the University of Rochester

Prevention and Treatment

Dentistry at the University of Rochester Medical Center has a substantial commitment to the oral health care of children in our community.

Our experience and data strongly suggest that a well-planned collaborative school-based dental program can dramatically reduce dental access disparity and enhance utilization of oral health care for the difficult-to-reach child population.

Three full-time SMILEmobile units, two part-time portable school/rural clinics, three partnership, part-time satellite clinics, and eight year-round part-time satellite clinics provide over 18,500 treatment visits and 2,500 screening and referral visits.

SMILEmobile Program

Three fully-equipped dental vans provide comprehensive dental care to thousands of local children. During the school year, the SMILEmobiles serve Rochester's inner-city school children.

The three units treat 6,500 children in day care settings and rural communities.

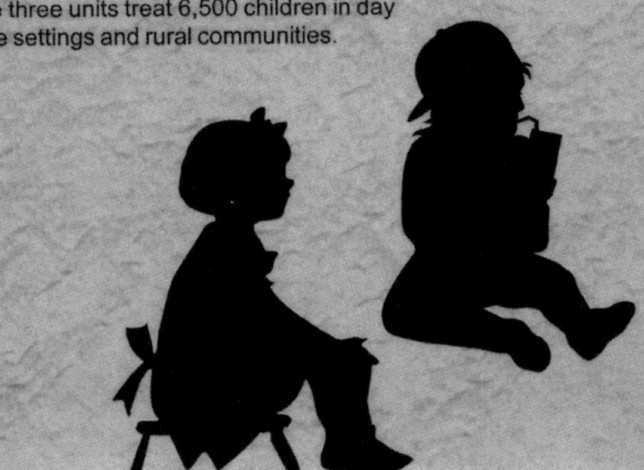

Education
for dental postdoctoral candidates

FUNDED TRAINING PROJECTS add to the educational programs and are targeted at sensitizing the residents to the plight of the underserved.

Enhancing Oral Health Care to Underserved Children

This is a training grant from Health Resources Service Administration (HRSA), which is under the US Department of Health and Human Services.

It's purpose is to expand the number of pediatric dentists who are sensitive to the oral health care needs of our nation's underserved children.

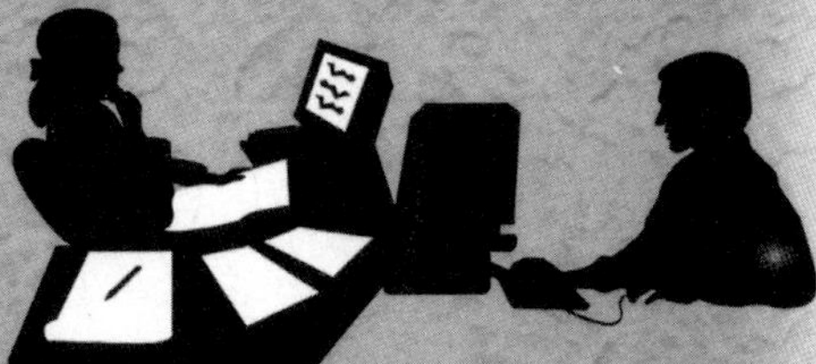

The Rochester Collaborative to Reduce Oral Health Disparities

The goal of this project is to develop intervention strategies that will prevent or reduce disparities in both the levels of oral diseases as well as in access to and effective utilizations of the oral health care system.

The project's principal investigator will partner this award with the HRSA grant entitled *Enhancing Oral Health care to Underserved Children.*

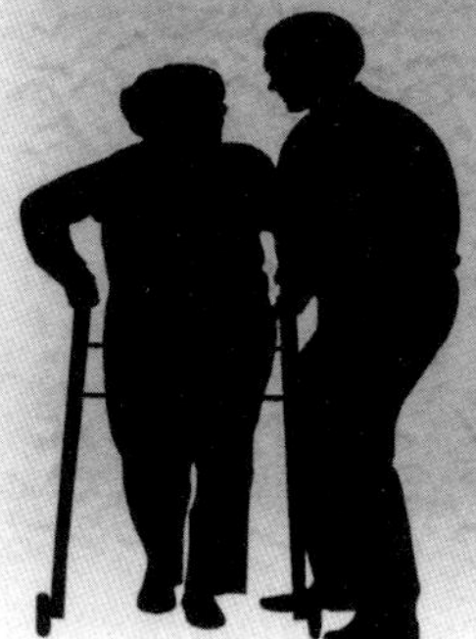

Interdisciplinary Geriatric Fellowship Program

This is a two-year fellowship that is intended to train those who will become leaders in geriatric dentistry.

The program is interdisciplinary with geriatric medicine and psychiatry and includes training in clinical care, education, research, and administration relative to care of older adults.

Pages from brochure explaining the center's prevention and education programs in the twenty-first century

Research

Research is a vital part of Dentistry at the University of Rochester Medical Center. Whether it's basic science research or the translational research that brings it from the laboratory into the clinic, the emphasis is on discovery.

Examples of Translational Research Projects

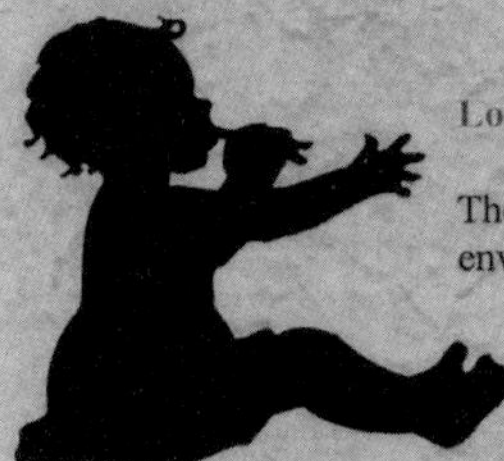

Longitudinal Study of Lead Exposure and Dental Caries

The major goal of this project is to assess the role of environmental lead exposure as a risk factor for dental caries in children.

Oral Health Disparities Grant

An oral health survey of elementary school children to compare the prevalence of oral disease and craniofacial dysmorphology among Latino children with African-American and Caucasian children.

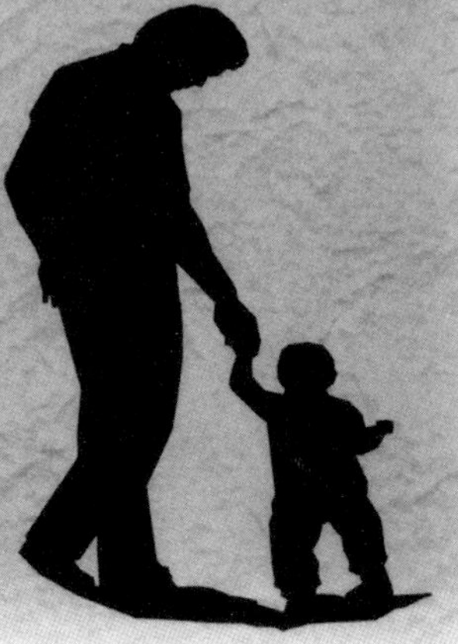

Developmentally Disabled Clinic at Monroe Community Hospital

Eastman Dental Center provides oral health care for developmentally disabled patients at the Monroe Community Hospital. Our staff is specially trained to work with children and adults who have special needs.

Eastman Dental Center's Developmentally Disabled Dental (DD) Clinic is located at the Monroe Community Hospital (MCH) site for easier patient access.

There were over 1500 visits to the clinic. Seven care providers specialize in care to the DD population at both the Monroe Community Hospital and Strong Memorial Hospital sites, and the Finger Lakes Developmentally Disabled Service Organization's Geneseo site.

About 170 DD operating room cases were done at Strong Memorial Hospital last year.

David has cerebral palsy and lived with his parents for the first 39 years of his life. He visited a dentist regularly and had good oral hygiene habits and followed a nutritional diet. As his physical health deteriorated, his parents could no longer provide care at home and he now lives in a group home. He developed a number of oral health problems and was enrolled in the clinic for the develomentally disabled.

His new dentist understands David's health problems and has developed a treatment plan that provides care in a easily accessible facility.

Geriatric Clinic at Monroe Community Hospital

The geriatric in-patient clinic is located at Monroe Community Hospital to take care of the hospital's aging patients.

A large senior citizen population is also treated at Eastman Dental Center and Strong Memorial Hospital.

Mrs. Donaldson is 83, had lost a number of teeth, and has a number of severe health problems.

She recently moved into Monroe Community Hospital and her new dentist has patiently worked with her in fitting dentures that allow her to smile and enjoy her meals.

Pages from brochure explaining some of the center's research projects and clinical sites leadership. When it didn't, Burkhart dug in his heels, keeping the Rochester Dental Dispensary on track as the nation's poster child of preventive clinical dentistry for children. He also picked up the gauntlet of worldwide preventive clinical dentistry for children that George Eastman had posited in founding the pioneering original clinic.

George Eastman's role in founding the School of Medicine and Dentistry in 1920, with his emphasis on dentistry as part of the school's mix, kept the dream of a real school of dentistry alive. But when, for various reasons, no one applied to be a dental student, Dean George Whipple, a research man to the bone, sought to found a dental fellows program that would introduce dental research into the university mix. Whipple was highly successful, but the program always relied on outside funding (including stipends from the dental endowment at the behest of trustee Charles Hutchison).

Dr. Basil Bibby was an original dental fellow who, among other early university researchers, targeted fluoride in the 1930s as the next step in the war against dental caries, the world's most prevalent disease. When Bibby left the university in 1940 to become the dean of the Tufts dental school, university president Alan Valentine assured him that he would be invited back as soon as the university took over the dental dispensary. This merger by acquisition never happened, partly because Burkhart refused to retire—dying instead at his post at age eighty-one in 1946—and partly because the dispensary trustees were opposed to a merger that they always considered a takeover.

Bibby's tenure from 1947 to 1970 was marked by research rising to the fore. In 1965, Bibby built a research wing to the original dispensary building and renamed the dispensary the Eastman Dental Center. He considered moving the dental center closer to the medical center but found little support for the move. His postgraduate students revered Bibby as mentor.

Dr. William McHugh became the third director in 1970. He was also named the associate dean for dental affairs. McHugh initiated and completed the center's move to a new building adjacent to the medical center campus, a move designed to strengthen the affiliation and enhance interaction between the entities.

Dr. Ronald Billings was appointed fourth director of the EDC in the spring of 1994 and served for the next five years. He led the center through a period of significant change and was instrumental in the merger, formalized on July 1, 1997, that joined all the resources and energies of each institution into one organization dedicated to becoming the foremost institution worldwide for oral health care, dental postgraduate education, and dental research.

In 1998, dental faculty from the Eastman Dental Center and the School of Medicine and Dentistry's departments of Clinical Dentistry and Dental Research were integrated into a new department, the Eastman Department of Dentistry. Cyril Meyerowitz was named chair of the new department. At the same time, the Center for Oral Biology came under the leadership of Lawrence Tabak. Cyril Meyerowitz succeeded Billings as the fifth Eastman Dental Center director in January 1999, a leadership post he continued to hold along with chair of the Eastman Department of Dentistry. This coalescence of leadership would provide a unique opportunity for dentistry to flourish in ways long envisioned by so many for so long. The themes of clinical service, education, and research present since the Eastman/Burkhart years will be readdressed. The synergy and conflict among themes and consequentially between institutions (along with personality issues), needs to be highlighted more strongly.

In 2006, the EDC foundation, prompted by interest from McCollister Evarts, the CEO and senior vice president of the Medical Center at that time, funded a feasibility study to establish a School of Dental Medicine and to initiate a unique leadership-oriented predoctoral program leading to a DMD. Although the initial report of the study found general support for the idea and recommended continued exploration of the concept, the feasibility study was shelved, largely due to the strong opposition to it by the faculty of the COB. Nevertheless, that study became the basis for the consideration of a new structure for dentistry at the university, the Eastman Institute for Oral Health.

THE EASTMAN INSTITUTE
FOR ORAL HEALTH

As this book goes to press in 2009, an entity called the Eastman Institute for Oral Health has been proposed. The institute is seen as a natural extension of the merger of the Eastman Dental Center into the university and as a way to ensure effective integration of the administrative, fiscal, and academic functions of the dental elements of the medical center (Center for Oral Biology, Eastman Department of Dentistry, and Eastman Dental Center). The institute would replace the Eastman Dental Center as a division within the University of Rochester Medical Center, functioning as the integrated entity responsible for research, education, and clinical care in oral health. The institute would seek to become the preeminent postgraduate institution of oral health research and training in the United States, building upon continuing excellence in patient care.

Under a new administrative structure for this Eastman Institute, a single individual, reporting directly to the medical center CEO, directs the oral health enterprise at University of Rochester Medical Center. In this manner the Eastman Institute occupies the same position on the medical center organizational chart as the School of Nursing, the School of Medicine and Dentistry, and Strong Memorial Hospital. A critical feature of this plan, which differs from the present structure, is that education in oral health, along with basic, translational, and clinical research, is integrated, thus bringing together the education and research programs of Eastman Department of Dentistry and Center for Oral Biology into one organization under unitary leadership. Characteristics of the director of the Eastman Institute includes significant accomplishment in independent research along with expertise in training (clinical and/or scientific), dental practice, and administration. The director of the Eastman Institute could also be chair of the Eastman Department of Dentistry or the director of COB or delegate those responsibilities.

The proposed organizational structure for the Eastman Institute is shown in the chart. Working under the oversight of the medical center CEO, an endowment and finance committee would be comprised of the director of the Eastman Institute, the dean of the School of Medicine and Dentistry, the medical center CFO, the director of finance and administration of the Eastman Institute, and the SMD CFO. This committee would prepare the financial proposals to be delivered by the director of the Eastman Institute to the Eastman Dental Center Foundation, School of Medicine and Dentistry, and Strong Memorial Hospital regarding allocations between the clinical, research, and education missions. The Eastman Institute budget would require the approval of the medical center CEO. Funds allocated to the oral health sciences enterprise from the Eastman Dental Center Foundation, School of Medicine and Dentistry, and Strong Memorial Hospital would flow directly through the Eastman Institute and would be expensed off the Eastman Institute accounts.

An associate director of clinical services would be appointed for this institute. This individual would work closely with the clinical service management team and would be responsible for coordination and day-to-day operations of the various clinical entities shown in the organizational chart. An associate director of education would be appointed who would be responsible for residency programs and graduate education within the Eastman Institute.

A Research Advisory Committee would be created to provide oversight of the integrated basic, translational, and clinical research of the Eastman Institute. Reporting to this Committee would be the associate director for basic science (formerly director of the Center for Oral Biology) and associate director for clinical and translational science. The Research Advisory Committee would be chaired by the School of Medicine and Dentistry dean and would also include the School of Medicine and Dentistry senior associate deans for basic and clinical research and the two Eastman Institute associate research directors. This committee would make recommendations to the Eastman Institute director and medical center CEO on the strategic directions for research in oral health sciences at University of Rochester Medical Center and on the distribution of funds that had been allocated to research by the endowment and finance committee between basic, clinical, and translational research.

As all Eastman Institute faculty would have academic appointments in the School of Medicine and Dentistry, and the chair of the Eastman Department of Dentistry and director of the Center for Oral Biology would continue to report to the School of Medicine and Dentistry dean on matters that pertain to academic appointments and on the use of School of Medicine and Dentistry core budgets. Faculty in the Eastman Department of Dentistry will report to the chair of Eastman Department of Dentistry, and Center for Oral Biology faculty with primary appointments in School of Medicine and Dentistry departments would report to the Center for Oral Biology director and to their appropriate School of Medicine and Dentistry chairs. Reporting lines within the School of Medicine and Dentistry and their connections to the Eastman Institute, are shown in the accompanying organizational chart.

The establishment of the Eastman Institute would, after ninety-three years of history, create a fully integrated dental enterprise within the University of Rochester Medical Center and establish important linkages to the university while preserving the important historical academic relationships of dental research and education with the School of Medicine and Dentistry. It would establish a fiscal and administrative structure that would foster excellence across the clinical, education, and research missions. The Eastman Institute will be launched on June 9, 2009, with Cyril Meyerowitz as the institute director.

Eastman Institute for Oral Health

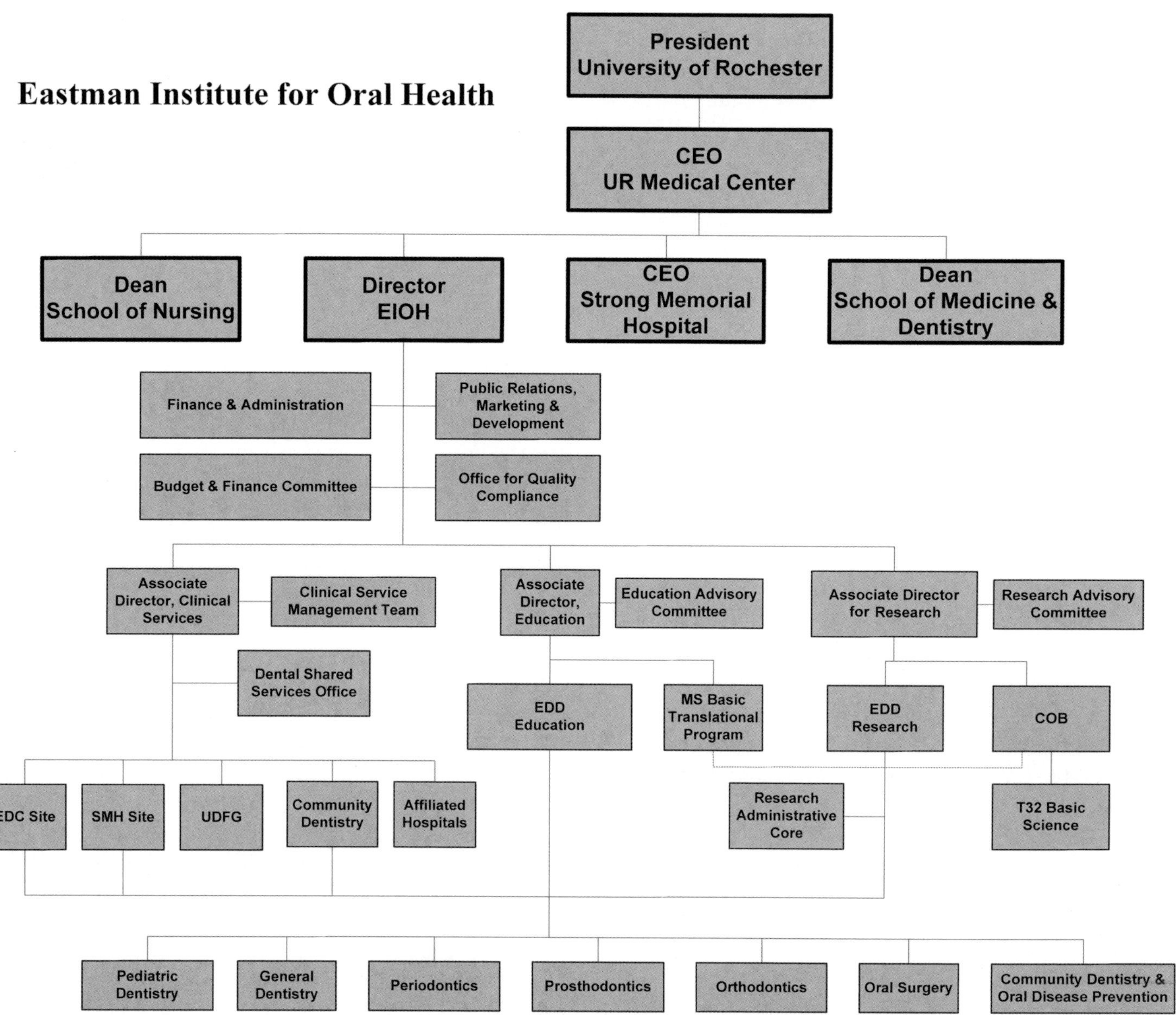

All Faculty in COB and EDD have appointments in SMD. The Director of COB and Chair of EDD report to the Dean of SMD for academic matters.

Chapter Nine

DEPARTMENTS AND DIVISIONS

The history of the Eastman Dental Center and oral health research and training at the University of Rochester School of Medicine and Dentistry would not be complete without digging a little deeper. We wish to thank each of the authors who have provided one of the first-hand accounts of their divisions and departments that make up this chapter. They have been edited for style and length in accordance with University of Rochester Press requirements. Dr. Stanley Handelman initiated this chapter and collected these accounts.

PEDIATRIC DENTISTRY AT THE EASTMAN DENTAL CENTER

Dr. David Levy

THE HISTORY OF THE PEDIATRIC DENTISTRY TRAINING PROGRAMS is closely tied to the origin of and reasons for the Eastman Dental Center. The mission of the dispensary in 1915 was to provide treatment to children whose families could not afford services at a private office. In addition to dental care, children were treated for medical problems of the tonsils and adenoids.

From the time of the founding of the dispensary, prevention of disease was recognized as more important than its treatment. While treatment in the form of reparative work was necessary, the ultimate objective restated in a 1945 report of the dispensary was "the development of methods and practices to prove the value of preventive dentistry." Furthermore, this objective was to be enhanced through the education of parents and children. It was expected that mothers would be taught to bring their babies to the dispensary as soon as the first tooth erupted. The dispensary would then become the child's dental home until age sixteen. Not only would this approach provide continuity of care, but also it would create a base of clinical information from which research activities could be enhanced.

As a provision of the establishment of the dispensary, Mr. Eastman required the City of Rochester to develop dental services in public and parochial schools. The focus of these services was preventive. Teams of dental hygienists provided dental prophylaxis to schoolchildren by utilizing portable chairs and dental equipment. These hygienists also referred those children most in need of dental care to the dispensary.

From its inception in 1917 until the late 1950s, children up to the age of sixteen were treated. Admission to the clinic was based on weekly family income. A Social Service Department was established at the dispensary to see that "none receive treatment in any department of the dispensary, whose circumstances will permit them to employ a regular medical or dental practitioner." It was recognized that complexities in judging eligibility might arise. For any question of eligibility that became too difficult to solve, the benefit of the doubt would always be given to the child.

As we have seen, Mr. Eastman hoped that the dispensary would become not only a place for service but also a place for educational opportunities for dentists. It was envisioned that clinical training would accrue to graduate dentists who participated in long-term formal programs and that the dispensary would become a meeting place for the dental profession to exchange ideas and to participate in what is now termed continuing education. By the 1930s, a formal dental education program was established as a ten-month rotating internship focused on children. In addition to treating children in the dental department, interns rotated into the extraction, orthodontia, x-ray, and surgical departments. Dr. Harvey Burkhart, director from 1916 to 1946, Dr. Elmer Pammenter, the chief of clinics, and other members of the faculty provided educational leadership.

There were a number of factors both external and internal that provided the context for the creation of the two-year pedodontic specialty training program. The history of the establishment of the specialty in pedodontics can be traced back to 1921 when the American Society for the Promotion of Children's Dentistry was begun. Since there was less than a handful of clinicians who were treating children exclusively, Dr. Burkhart suggested at a meeting in Milwaukee that the organization should be set up to include all those who were interested in the practice of dentistry for children. In 1922, the name of the group was changed to the American Society of Dentistry for Children and included dentists who limited their practices to children, public health nurses, dentists working in school clinics, and others in general practice interested in dentistry for children. This small group had difficulty keeping interest, and it was reconstituted in 1928, keeping the same name. The American Society of Dentistry for Children slowly but steadily flourished. In 1938, in response to the American Dental Association's specialty initiative, the American Society of Dentistry for Children agreed to sponsor an independent organization, the American Board of Pedodontics, to establish criteria and guidelines for designating a dentist as a specialist in pedodontics. During this early developmental period of the American Board of Pedodontics, the American Dental Association formally recognized pedodontics in 1942 as its third dental specialty; the other two were orthodontics and oral surgery. The American Board of Pedodontics began in 1940, but due to World War II, it did not finalize the process to certify pedodontists until 1947. The first certified dentists were charter founders of the board, and the criteria were based on years of exclusive treatment of children; no examination was required. In 1957, the board began promoting the requirement that a candidate for specialty status should have two years of graduate or postgraduate training in the specialty of pedodontics taken at a dental school, hospital, or institution recognized by the Council on Dental Education (now the Commission on Dental Accreditation). That criterion became a requirement in 1962. Eventually, the board established criteria that included a two-year post-dental school education program, submission of case histories, and clinical, written, and oral examinations.

In 1947, Dr. Basil Bibby brought with him a strong desire to enhance the educational and research programs of the dispensary. In 1948, Dr. Bibby encouraged Dr. Roland Hawes, a recent graduate of Tufts School of Dental Medicine, to join the teaching and supervising staff of the dispensary. Hawes eventually became head of clinical services in the pedodontics division. After Dr. Hawes completed an active tour of duty in the U.S. Air Force, he successfully passed the 1954 examination of the American Board of Pedodontics, becoming one the first fifty certified American pedodontists.

A two-year educational program in pedodontics was realized at the Eastman Dental Dispensary in 1958. The establishment of the program was a result of the external requirements by the American Dental Association, its Council on Dental Education, the American Board of Pedodontics, and internal forces, particularly the vision of Dr. Bibby and the professional maturation of Dr. Hawes. A certificate of completion to one candidate, Dr. Roger Coe of Great Britain, was awarded that first year. The development of the two-year educational program in pedodontics parallels the development of similar two-year educational programs at Eastman in periodontics, orthodontics, and prosthodontics. Soon thereafter, the one-year pedodontic rotating internship was eliminated and incorporated into the newly established general dentistry internship. Since 1958, there have been approximately 250 individuals who have received certificates in pedodontics or, as a result of a 1984 specialty name change by the American Dental Association, pediatric dentistry. Most of these individuals are from the United States and Canada. Approximately forty people from twenty-three other countries have also earned certificates and returned to their respective homelands.

Dr. Hawes remained chair and program director of pedodontics until 1969, when he left the Eastman Dental Center to become chair of pedodontics at Case Western Reserve School of Dental Medicine. The acting chair and program director in pedodontics from 1969 to 1970 was Dr. Jack Howitt, a 1962 graduate of the two-year pedodontic training program. Although his tenure was short, Dr. Howitt established the Smilemobile. A fully equipped mobile dental unit was sent to various schools to provide comprehensive dental services for children who had particularly difficult access to dental care. Another graduate of the two-year program, Dr. Louis Ripa, who had been chair of general dentistry from 1967 to 1970, became chair and program director of pedodontics from 1970 to 1973. Yet another graduate of the two-year pedodontic training program, Dr. Odd Sveen, who had earned his PhD at the University of Minnesota, followed Ripa. Dr. Sveen was chair and program director for ten years, from 1973 to 1983. Dr. Steven Adair, who had completed his pedodontic and master's degree programs at the University of Iowa, succeeded Dr. Sveen. Dr. Adair had been an Eastman faculty member since 1978 and in 1983 was promoted to chair and program director, a position he held until his departure in 1990. At this point, the dual responsibility of chair and program director was split between two individuals. On an interim basis, Dr. Ronald Billings was named acting chair, and Dr. David Levy was named acting program director from 1990 to 1992.

This model of departmental organization continued with the appointment of Dr. Pamela DenBesten as chair and Dr. Robert Berkowitz as program director, from 1992 to 1995. Dr. Berkowitz's recruitment was, in part, to establish a major hospital component to the program. In 1993, the Division of Pediatric Dentistry was established at Strong Memorial Hospital in the Departments of Clinical Dentistry and Pediatrics, and Dr. Berkowitz served as division chief. Upon the departure of Dr. DenBesten in 1995, Dr. Berkowitz was appointed as chair and program director, positions that he holds until the present. The hospital component of the program was solidified over the next decade, with the pediatric dental residents at Eastman Dental Center being credentialed as Strong Memorial Hospital residents. The curriculum changed significantly during that period, as did the clinical service. Pediatric dental residents had tutorials in pediatric physical diagnosis and rotations in pediatric medicine, pediatric anesthesia, and pediatric emergency medicine. The clinical services expanded to include coverage of the Strong Memorial Hospital Emergency Department, a large consultative inpatient service at Strong Memorial Hospital for medically compromised children, and a Strong Memorial Hospital operating room service that currently attends to approximately 400 children per year.

The community service vision of George Eastman was also expanded. With the help of federal funding, Dr. Berkowitz expanded the program from six residents in 2000 to fourteen residents in 2007. Pediatric dental residents not only provide clinical service at Eastman Dental Center but also in the Eastman Dental Center outreach program via school-based clinics and Smilemobiles. The program has been funded by graduate medical education and received 142 applications for the class matriculating in July of 2007. The traditions of George Eastman's clinical service vision are in place, and the program maintains a cutting-edge stature in context of the evolution of graduate pediatric dental education.

COMMUNITY DENTISTRY AND ORAL DISEASE PREVENTION AT THE EASTMAN DENTAL CENTER, 1915–2008

Dr. Ronald Billings

One condition of George Eastman's gift establishing the Rochester Dental Dispensary was that the city must finance a dental prophylaxis program in city schools. Thus, even before the doors to the dispensary were officially opened, community dentistry was firmly entrenched as a core mission. Between 1916 and 1947, dental hygienists and dental hygiene students provided dental prophylaxes and dental health education free of charge to public and parochial school children through this unique and far-reaching community program. Shortly after Dr. Bibby's arrival, the first studies on caries prevention were initiated and overseen by staff in the Department of Dental Health, the forerunner of today's Division of Community Dentistry and Oral Disease Prevention.

The initial milestone was provision of the first topically applied sodium fluoride to children attending Public School No. 14. Between 1947 and 1951, emphasis on dental prophylaxes began to shift to classroom lectures on dental health, a pivotal change marking the beginning of the end of an era in dental public health. Although dental prophylaxes were provided in the schools for many more years, this service was gradually phased out in favor of classroom education and a tilt toward screening and referral for care of children found in need by dental hygienists permanently assigned to public and parochial schools.

The next major events in community dental health were the introduction of fluoride into city water in 1952 and the first school-based epidemiologic surveys of children's oral health in 1954 to estimate the impact of water fluoridation on dental caries. In 1955, Dr. Hugh Averill, prominent Rochester dentist and dental public health advocate, following completion of his MPH at Harvard, was appointed dental public health officer and soon expanded existing surveys on children's oral health. He studied the social aspects of providing dental care for poor children, and published his paper on school dental health services in 1958 and a five-year study of the impact of water fluoridation on dental caries on city school children. He expanded research to include studies in Brazil on the effect of supplemental dietary phosphates on the prevention of caries and studies of suburban Rochester school children on the effect of promising new topical fluoride treatments on dental caries. From 1965 to 1967, Dr. Averill was director of the dispensary's dental health department before accepting a faculty position at the University of Georgia School of Dentistry. While at the dispensary, his administrative duties included oversight for the State Aid Orthodontic Screening Program and consultant to the Monroe County Department of Health and the Monroe County Department of Social Welfare. It was in these areas that he made exceptionally noteworthy contributions to the future direction of the school health program. His proposals to emphasize oral health education, early case-finding, referral for high-risk cases, and follow-up were landmarks that shaped the course of community dentistry well into the 1980s.

Partly a result of reorganization of the school program and increased emphasis on oral health education, in 1966 Dr. Elbert Powell was appointed assistant director of the dental health department. Department staff now comprised Drs. Averill and Powell, Ms. Germaine Schleuter, a dental hygienist with a college degree who acted as a consultant in dental health education, and fifty-nine practicing dental hygienists who provided oral health instruction and prophylaxes for 160,000 Monroe County school children. Dr. Powell's first major contribution was to organize and put into service two dental clinics within the Neighborhood Service Information Centers, the first such outreach activities outside of the schools. He also oversaw preventive oral health services to Head Start children and nursery school children under the Work Education Training Program. Following Dr. Averill's departure, Dr. Powell was appointed director of the renamed Department of Community Dental Health. Dr. Powell also planned a more comprehensive dental facility in what became the Jordon Health Center, the first such facility in northeast Rochester. These clinics plus the Head Start and Work Education Training Center programs continued to grow and in 1967 recorded over 6,000 patient visits. As the staff of practicing dental hygienists grew to sixty-three, the number of children served grew to 171,000.

In 1967, the state Medicaid program was launched, and Dr. Powell and Dr. Jack Howitt assessed the feasibility of mobile dental units. Powell worked closely with the Monroe County Dental Society in the development and implementation of the Indigent Children's Dental Health Care program. Ominously, 1969 marked the first major reduction in funding of the school-based prophylaxis program from $500,000 to $260,000 by the Monroe County legislature, forcing a substantial reorganization of the program. Although a unified city/county school oral health program continued on a reduced level, the reduction in funding signaled changing priorities. The change in emphasis was influenced by the declining caries prevalence from water fluoridation.

In 1970, Dr. Gavriloff and Dr. Howitt initiated the first mobile dental unit to deliver comprehensive oral health services in New York State, a program that was made possible by support from the Sybron Corporation, the Ritter Corporation, and the Monroe County Dental Society. The children of Rochester named it the Smilemobile.

In 1973, Dr. Dennis Leverett, executive director of the Portland, ME, Center for Community Dental Health, was appointed chair of the Department of Community Dentistry, a post he held until his appointment as interim director of the Eastman Dental Center in 1992. Dr. Leverett held a conjoint appointment in the Department of Community and Preventive Medicine in the School of Medicine and Dentistry and he served as the dental director for the Monroe County Department of Health from 1973 to 1989. Dr. Leverett also collaborated with the Monroe County Dental Society in the operation of the Smilemobile and became the director of the program when ownership of the Smilemobile was transferred from the dental society to the dental center in 1973. Although a full-time staff composed of a program coordinator, a dental hygienist, and a dental assistant was hired to operate the unit on a daily basis, dental care was still provided by volunteer dentists until 1985. The Smilemobile also served as the venue for groundbreaking research conducted by Drs. Leverett and Stanley Handelman, chair of general dentistry, who collaborated on studies of dental sealants and other significant caries preventive modalities during the 1970s.

As the department's research activities increased, Dr. David Levy was appointed assistant chair in 1979 following completion of his pediatric dentistry residency and his MPH degree. Dr. Levy participated in several of the department's research projects, most notably studies on fluoride rinses and dental fluorosis in fluoride deficient and optimally fluoridated communities. He left the department in 1981 to practice pediatric dentistry privately. Under Dr. Leverett's leadership, the department prospered in both community service and research in the pursuit of George Eastman's vision for the dispensary as a model for community service, education, and research. Dr. Leverett initiated graduate-level courses on social issues in community dentistry and oral epidemiology. He was instrumental in developing the center's biostatistics program and had oversight of the program, including a full-time biostatistian and computer programmer, until his retirement in 1993.

Dr. Leverett had a profound impact on many individuals in the local as well as national and international dental communities. He was the principal investigator of commercial and NIH-funded research grants and contracts and was widely recognized for his clinical research and public health dentistry in sealants, fluorides, and community water fluoridation. He was among the first researchers to recognize the need for a valid, reliable, simple-to-use, and cost-effective multifactorial model to assess the risk of dental caries in children. He was also recognized for his pioneering work on the relationship between prenatal fluoride use and dental caries. He had over 130 abstracts, book chapters, and publications. Dr. Leverett's landmark paper on fluorides was published in the May 1982 issue of the journal *Science*. He served the American Association of Public Health Dentistry as editor of the *Journal of Public Health Dentistry* from 1987 to 1993. He received its Distinguished Service Award in 1993 and served as its president in 1996. As a result of lifetime efforts on behalf of public health dentistry, the Oral Health Section of the American Public Health Association named him the 1996 recipient of the prestigious John W. Knutson Award for Distinguished Service in Dental Public Health.

In 1984, Dr. Ronald Billings was recruited from the University of Texas dental branch to serve as associate director of Community Dentistry, and in 1985 he was appointed director of the Smilemobile program. He served as acting chair of pediatric dentistry from 1990 to 1992 and as the center's associate director for clinical affairs from 1989 to 1994. Between 1984 and 1994, Drs. Leverett and Billings collaborated on commercial and government-funded studies, including studies on dental caries among elementary school children who participated in a supervised fluoride-rinse program, caries risk factors in children, oral health in community-dwelling older adults, and the effect of prenatal fluoride supplements on dental caries in a birth cohort of children from fluoride-deficient communities in Maine. Later, following Dr. Leverett's retirement, Dr. Billings focused on NIH-funded exploratory studies of oral health disparities in Latino children. These studies led to work funded by the New York State Department of Health and the NIH to improve access and utilization of dental care for children, especially minority children. During the mid 1980s, annual caries surveys undertaken on behalf of the Monroe County Department of Health revealed a continuing decline in the prevalence of caries among Monroe County children, but with notable exceptions for inner-city ethnic minority and recent immigrant children.

In 1989, the health department again reduced funding for the school-based screening and referral program as well as for the Brockport, NY, fluoride-rinse program, thus bringing school-based preventive programs one step closer to extinction. Only four dental hygienists were now left to administer the school program. With the increasing prevalence of caries among inner-city children, a drive was initiated and substantial community, private, and philanthropic support led to the acquisition of another full-service Smilemobile. The second unit was dedicated in 1990. Four additional schools in the Rochester city school district were determined to be in greatest need. Both units together provided basic restorative and preventive care for more than 2,000 Rochester school children per year. Four pediatric dentists with faculty appointments in community dentistry (Drs. Manu Thakrar, Thomas Bork, Krista Richey, and Jila Jalali), two dental hygienists, two dental assistants, and two dental aides provided the care. (Dental aides escort children between classrooms and the Smilemobile safely and efficiently.)

Teaching efforts intensified during the late 1980s with a reorganization of the epidemiology course to meet the increasing need of the specialty departments for residents to receive basic training in epidemiology and clinical research study design. A second course in research design and analysis that focused on biostatistics was added and was initially taught by Dr. Howard Proskin, the center's full-time biostatistician. In 1991, the Monroe County Department of Health ceased funding the school-based screening and referral program altogether and, with the exception of modest funding to continue oral health surveillance of county children, this ended an era of unmatched preventive care by the city and county for children in need.

The department recruited Dr. Mark Moss following completion of his PhD in epidemiology at the University of North Carolina in 1994; he would have a conjoint appointment in the Department of Community and Preventive Medicine. He succeeded Dr. Proskin as the course director for research design and analysis and Dr. Leverett as the course director of oral epidemiology. Dr. Moss also continued the department's research activities at a high level, receiving grants from NIH for work on dental caries in both children and adults. He contributed significantly to a better understanding of the relationship between childhood exposure to high lead levels and caries in adulthood. His coauthorship of a paper showing a relationship between childhood exposure to second-hand tobacco smoke and dental caries in the deciduous dentition stimulated several studies by others on the impact of second-hand smoke on children's oral health.

In 1993, Dr. Billings was appointed director of the Eastman Dental Center and Dr. Buddhi Shrestha left Jordan Health Center to join the department as the director of community dentistry. Dr. Shrestha was influential in creating an increasing number of ties to the community at large. Through his efforts, community dentistry began to place greater emphasis on rural oral health care needs. The Monroe County Department of Health surveillance program continued under his direction. In addition to the county surveillance program,

Dr. Shrestha received a grant from the New York State Department of Health to implement a sealant program. Following the dental center's merger with the University of Rochester and the formation of a single dental department that merged the center's departments with the medical school's Department of Clinical Dentistry, the Eastman Department of Dentistry was formed and the Department of Community Dentistry became the Division of Community Dentistry and Oral Disease Prevention. Following Dr. Billings's retirement from the directorship of Eastman Dental Center in 1999, Dr. Cyril Meyerowitz was appointed as center director. In September 2000, the New York State Department of Health changed its focus from intervention through the sealant program to surveillance and provided funds for surveying the oral health of children in Rochester and surrounding counties. The New York State oral health surveillance program was concentrated mostly in rural areas, while the Monroe County Department of Health surveillance efforts were concentrated in city and suburban elementary schools. However, the newly formed linkage to surrounding rural communities created opportunities for community dentistry to expand its services.

Dr. Shrestha emphasized and significantly expanded clinical services. He secured grants from various foundations for capital investments to help with start-up costs for opening satellite and school-based clinics in Rochester and nearby communities. For example, the Rochester Primary Care Network (RPCN) provided start-up funding for the Downtown Dental Center Satellite Clinic. In September 2000, a third Smilemobile was constructed with support provided by the Daisy Marquis Jones Foundation. The third Smilemobile greatly expanded the reach of community dentistry both in the Rochester City School District and surrounding counties. In 1999, the city school district developed a program to place wellness centers in schools to address children's health problems, including oral health. Jefferson Middle School was the first wellness center to provide full-service dental care for middle school children. Dr. Shrestha placed the first of several comprehensive dental health clinics throughout the city and county and was instrumental in the development and construction of the School No. 17 Orchard Street dental clinic, a multifunctional, full-service clinic that served the needs of all of the children and families in the Orchard Street community. In 2003, Dr. Shrestha accepted a position as vice president of oral health services for the Rochester Primary Care Network, and Dr. Meyerowitz assumed overall leadership for community dentistry as the interim chair.

In 2003, Dr. Dorota Kopycka-Kedzierawski joined the division following receipt of her MPH and completion of the NIH-funded training program in oral health clinical research. Dr. Kopycka-Kedzierawski has revived the division's research activities with foundational and NIH-funded support, including a five-year mentored clinical research training grant. Currently, she is exploring teledentistry, a novel approach in reducing oral disease in preschool inner-city children. In 2005, Dr. Sangeeta Gajendra joined the division as associate director for clinical services following the completion of her residency in general dentistry at EDC. Dr. Gajendra also holds an MPH degree and completed her dental public health residency at the New York State Department of Health. With substantial expertise, she has developed a framework for continuous program monitoring and evaluation and played a major role in the smoke-free campaign. She plays a key role in oral health promotion efforts. Dr. Billings has remained engaged in the division's research and teaching activities. He serves as a mentor to young faculty and residents and directs the division's core courses: Research Design and Analysis and Introduction to Oral Epidemiology.

As of 2008, the Division of Community Dentistry and Oral Disease Prevention outreach program, under the direction of Holly Barone, RDH, is the area's largest safety-net provider to the poor and underserved. In the past twelve years, the program has grown from two mobile dental units with 6,000 visits per year to four mobile dental units and four satellite offices with over 25,000 visits per year. While the majority of care is provided to schoolchildren, three offices also provide care to adults.

GENERAL DENTISTRY AT THE EASTMAN DENTAL CENTER

Dr. Stanley Handelman

The University of Rochester School of Medicine and Dentistry and the Eastman Dental Center individually and together have played important roles in the development of general practice residency programs and advanced education in general dentistry programs on a national level. Of specific interest is the genesis of advanced education in general dentistry programs that is attributed to the initiatives taken by the Eastman Dental Center and is the central focus of this review.

Although differences between general practice residency and advanced education in general dentistry programs have been increasingly blurred, the original sponsorship and intent have a significant impact on the historical background and events. General practice residency programs evolved from dental emergency services in hospitals and have enhanced the skills of dentists in the management of the medically compromised patient in the hospital setting and in private practice. Advanced education in general dentistry programs were developed as an alternative to general practice residency programs. The emphasis in clinical training in advanced education in general dentistry programs is comprehensive care in all the major dental clinical disciplines, and these programs are sponsored by dental schools, postdoctoral dental institutions, the military services, and more recently by community health centers. The School of Medicine and Dentistry sponsors both a general practice residency program at Strong Memorial Hospital and an advanced education in general dentistry program at the Eastman Dental Center. Both are linked as part of the Eastman Department of Dentistry of the School of Medicine and Dentistry.

Although the patient base of the ten-month program was primarily children, it had a number of adult dentistry components, including a daytime dental emergency clinic and an oral surgery clinic. Dr. Bibby and Dr. Iranpour, head of the Oral Surgery Clinic, favored its modification into a general dentistry program. In 1968, Dr. Louis Ripa, a graduate of Eastman, was recruited by Dr. Bibby to head the newly designated ten-month general dentistry program. Also in 1968, Dr. Hawes accepted an appointment at Case Western, and Dr. Ripa was appointed the director of the two-year pediatric program. In 1970, Dr. Bibby asked Dr. Stanley Handelman, a general dentist who was on the part-time clinical faculty and engaged in oral bacteriological research, to assume the leadership of the ten-month general intern program. Other than reaffirming his commitment to general dentistry education, Dr. Bibby gave Dr. Handelman no instructions. This was Dr. Bibby's last major act as director. He retired before the general dentistry program started with an enrollment of twelve trainees.

Dr. William McHugh was appointed the new director of the Eastman Dental Center. At the first meeting where Dr. McHugh presided over the executive committee of the senior staff, the suggestion was made that the general dentistry training program be disbanded and the money from the endowment be used for additional support for existing educational and research programs. Dr. McHugh stated that it was premature to make a decision at that time, and discussion was postponed to a future date when the newly created program could be evaluated.

During its first years, the program was extended to twelve months. The stipend was increased but still was significantly less than hospital-based programs. The didactic content was significantly enriched and extended. Examples include seminars in the various dental clinical disciplines, case presentations, lectures by residents based on a thorough review of the literature on selected topics, and a course on how to evaluate the scientific literature. These were in addition to courses open to all graduate students at the Eastman Dental Center, such as courses on dental caries, pharmacology, community dentistry, and oral pathology that were available to general dentistry residents. Enrichment also included many lectures and presentations of faculty and visiting scholars that are part of a leading academic and research institution.

The focus of the main general dentistry clinic was comprehensive care for the adult dental patient. Patients were also treated in an emergency dental clinic and the pediatric dentistry and oral surgery clinics. Elective rotations were developed in nursing homes and community health centers. Trainees were encouraged to participate in dental research under the guidance of faculty mentors. As a result of these changes, there was an increase in the number and quality of its applicants from both the United States and foreign dental schools. However, there was no mechanism available for accreditation by the Council on Dental Accreditation of the American Dental Association, which only recognized hospital general practice residency programs. In an attempt to seek accreditation, the Eastman Dental Center established a combined program with the Genesee Hospital with rotations in general anesthesia, physical diagnosis, and in participation with the after-hours emergency services. Although it secured preliminary approval, the program was denied final accreditation because all of its residents did not participate in all of the hospital rotations.

The denial of accreditation set in motion a concerted effort to establish an alternative accreditation mechanism for the general dentistry programs in 1978. Under the leadership of Dr. William D. McHugh, the American Association of Dental Schools strongly supported a recommendation to the Council on Dental Education for the establishment of an advanced education in general dentistry program based on the educational model developed at Eastman Dental Center. This new type of program also had the support of the military programs, because the majority of military programs were based in outpatient clinics and treated healthy ambulatory patients, and they had difficulty and limited interest in meeting the hospital requirements of general practice residency programs.

The Assembly of the American Dental Association approved the establishment of the proposed advanced education in general dentistry program. The Eastman Dental Center was the first institutional-based program not associated with the military to be recognized under the new requirements and guidelines. At the time of writing (2007), the enrollment and number of advanced education in general dentistry programs exceeds that of general practice residency programs.

At the same time that accreditation was secured for advanced education in general dentistry programs, the federal government through the Health Resources and Services Administration developed grants to support postdoctoral general dentistry training. One of the stated reasons was the concern that dentistry would become over-specialized to the neglect of primary care, especially for the poor and underserved minorities. Programs applied for three-year grants to develop new or expanded accredited programs. With the accreditation of advanced education in general dentistry programs, the Eastman Dental Center was eligible for these grants. The center received a number of grants under this award, and as a result, the total number of residents was increased to twenty-one first-year residents. To further enhance their training and assure continuity of patient care, a two-year residency program was established. In addition, its affiliated general practice residency programs at Strong Memorial Hospital and Genesee Hospital also received grants to expand and enhance their programs. The Genesee Hospital also received a grant from the Robert Wood Johnson Foundation. Additional rotations were developed in nursing homes and community health centers. A successful minority recruitment program was also initiated as part of these grants.

To support its general dentistry grants program, the federal government issued a request for proposals for a major contract to write a manual and conduct national workshops for the development of postgraduate general dentistry programs. Dr. Gerald Gladstein, an educational psychologist at the University of Rochester, was named as a consultant to the grant. The

advanced education in general dentistry program at the Eastman Dental Center and the general practice residency programs at Genesee Hospital and Strong Memorial Hospital were awarded the contract. This was unexpected since the American Association of Dental Schools also submitted competitive proposals.

The workshops conducted in Los Angeles, CA, Augusta, GA, and Rochester, NY, were well received and the publishing of a manual on the development of general practice residencies as a special issue of the *Journal of Dental Education* in 1979 established the general dentistry programs of Rochester as educational leaders in the field. Additional development and evaluation grants, publications, and appointments of faculty from both the Eastman Dental Center and the general practice residency programs to the advisory committee of advanced education programs and general practice residency programs of the Commission on Dental Accreditation further solidified its reputation.

In 1990, both the Eastman Dental Center and the University of Rochester were instrumental in the formation of the Postdoctoral General Dentistry Section of the American Association of Dental Schools. This brought both the advanced education in general dentistry and general practice residency programs under one educational roof, although two accreditation mechanisms still existed.

Over time, the requirement and guidelines for both programs have moved closer together. Although there are still strong advocates on the uniqueness of general practice residency versus advanced education in general dentistry, it is conceivable that some time in the future there may be a single accreditation mechanism. Graduates of both general practice residency and advanced education in general dentistry have used their training experience to define long-term career goals, enhance their credentials in applying for specialty programs, and increase their skills as generalists.

In negotiation with Dr. Martin Rubin, the executive secretary of the New York State Board for Dentistry, an agreement was reached that foreign-trained dentists who had completed two years of training conducted by general dentistry under the sponsorship of the University of Rochester would be eligible to take the State Boards for licensure in the State of New York. As a result, a number of the graduates of the two-year general dentistry program have become licensed and have assumed academic positions in Rochester and elsewhere.

Dr. Handelman retired in 1994 and Dr. Hans Malmström, who was recruited to the program four years previously, assumed his position in 1992. He has continued the development of the program.

The major modifications and accomplishments under Dr. Malmström's leadership are the expansion of the curriculum in aesthetic dentistry and implantology and the inclusion of high-tech equipment and procedures such as lasers, rotary endodontic instruments, and dental implants in the clinical treatment of patients. With the expansion of knowledge and skills required for clinical practice, the program has been extended to two or three years and an increasing number of its graduates have pursued a graduate degree. Dr. Malmström has taken a leadership role in developing continuing education programs for dentists in private clinical practice, including the well-attended Handelman Conference. This conference has been cosponsored with the Monroe County Dental Society and provides residents with additional exposure to national and international speakers on a broad array of clinical topics.

The importance of research in general dentistry is exemplified by the research requirement for the two-year residents and the appointment of Dr. Yan Fang Ren (General Dentistry 1996) as the director of research in the advanced education in general dentistry program. Dr. Ren recently received the prestigious and highly competitive Career Development Award from the National Institute of Dental and Craniofacial Research based on his studies in the dental emergency clinic and correlating these findings with medical health problems.

Graduates of the Division of General Dentistry have successfully competed in the Basil G. Bibby and Buonocore competitions, sponsored by the local chapter of the American Association of Dental Research, and the Edward Hatton Awards Competition of the International Association of Dental Research. Research conducted by faculty and residents in the Division of General Dentistry have included such varied topics as oral bacteriology, trace elements, inhibition of dental caries by sealants, dental team performance, temporomandibular joint syndrome, restorative dentistry, postoperative sequela to third molar extractions, and salivary gland dysfunction.

The general dentistry programs take great pride in the accomplishments of its graduates. In addition to its alumni being recognized for quality of care in private practice, they have assumed leadership roles in organized dentistry at the local, state, and national levels. Graduates of the general dentistry programs of Rochester have assumed leadership roles in education as vice chancellors of medical centers, associate deans, chairs of departments, and full-time faculty in dental schools out of proportion to their numbers. At the Eastman Dental Center, the division chief of the orthodontic program, Dr. Stephanos Kyrkanides (General Dentistry 1999), and the division chief of prosthodontics, Dr. Carlo Ercoli (General Dentistry 1998), completed their eligibility requirements for licensure in the State of New York in the Department of General Dentistry.

ORTHODONTICS AT THE EASTMAN DENTAL CENTER

J. Daniel Subtelny

Orthodontics is the dental specialty dealing with the irregularities of teeth and their correction—especially by mechanical means. At the Eastman Dental Center, this specialty has defined itself more broadly and has incorporated coursework in speech development, physiology, and pathology in its curriculum as well as temporomandibular joint disorders.

The Division of Orthodontics, as we know it today, was initiated in October 1955. Prior to that time the center was a service-oriented clinic with a minimal educational component. With the appointment of J. Daniel Subtelny, efforts were initiated to develop a program that was more academically oriented and literature-based. During the fifty years as the head of the division, Subtelny created an internationally recognized program with an outstanding faculty and extremely dedicated alumni.

Initially, the orthodontic program was twenty-two months in duration, had a well-structured curriculum and an underlying philosophy that training should have a strong biological foundation and that clinical treatment should be based on pertinent clinical research. New and innovative course work was developed and dedicated, and well-trained faculty members were recruited. Seminars rather than lectures became the preferred method of teaching and provided stimulation for both students and faculty in keeping with postdoctoral education. Research by both faculty and students was encouraged.

The first class in the orthodontic program graduated in June of 1957. Two of the four students, Edgar Debbane and Young Ho Kim, continued to earn master of science degrees from the University of Rochester. Dr. Debbane also won second prize in the American Association of Orthodontics and the Milo Hellman Research Award for his histological study on maxillary palatal expansion in cats. In the early years, 1955 to 1960, the teachers were J. Daniel Subtelny, Andy Andronaco, and James Tonery. Some of the new courses that were developed were patterned after the highly regarded orthodontic educational program at the University of Illinois developed by Allan G. Brodie. These included courses in craniofacial anatomy, which required wax bone carving of the skeletal structures of the craniofacial complex; growth and development of the craniofacial skeleton; cephalometric analysis; cephalometric radiography and tracing; and a course in congenital cleft lip and palate and other craniofacial dysmorphologies pertinent to the jaws and functional tissues. A course unique to teaching orthodontic diagnostics and treatment was introduced at Eastman by Subtelny and referred to as the "hot seat." In this course, students defended their approach to diagnosis and treatment of their patients based on the basic sciences and published research rather than unsupported reports.

After being discharged from military service, Dr. Edward Gilda returned to Rochester to teach cephalometric radiography and cephalometric tracing. He eventually became known as "Dr. Cephalometrics." A seminar room is dedicated to his memory. In the 1960s, Drs. Andronaco, Tonery, and Fantaci discontinued their teaching roles. About the same time, Dr. Robert Baker Sr. joined the faculty and drove from Ithaca, New York, every Monday to teach orthodontic diagnosis and treatment and practice administration, areas in which he had gained national recognition. Dr. Joanne Subtelny, PhD, a speech pathologist, joined the orthodontic faculty during these formative years. She led a course in speech development, speech physiology, and speech pathology and also served as a speech diagnostician on the multidisciplinary cleft palate team. In addition to teaching oral care of the patient with cleft palate and lip and other craniofacial congenital dismorphologies, the team included a plastic surgeon, an orthodontist, a restorative dentist, a psychologist, and a social worker. As graduates of the program developed experience and unique skills, they also were asked to join the faculty, oftentimes traveling great distances. For example, in the 1970s, Dr. Marshall Deeney joined our faculty and instituted his course on biomechanics. Graduates of other orthodontic programs were also welcomed as part-time faculty.

After almost fifty years, Dr. J. Daniel Subtelny retired. Dr. Stephanos Kyrkanides was appointed as division chief in 2004. Dr. Marshall Deeney assumed the role of program director. The orthodontic faculty continues to work together as a cohesive group and provide instruction in a smorgasbord of clinical procedures, private practice philosophies, and research experience. Many of them have become board certified and all are actively engaged in private practice that lends credence to their teaching of clinical orthodontics.

Since the inception of the department, research has been valued to stimulate interests on the part of students; to solve problems; and to be able to clinically apply answers derived from research. Clinical application of research information stimulated the interest and excitement on the part of students. For example, during the earlier years, students participated in several first-time ventures. At the time that Dr. J. D. Subtelny came to Eastman, Dr. Michael Buonocore was already a research faculty member at the Eastman Dental Dispensary actively working on developing dental adhesives. In orthodontics he is considered the father of direct bonding, whereby attachments are directly bonded to teeth instead of cementing metal bands that fit around the tooth. An orthodontic supply company fabricated special steel brackets, and with Dr. Buonocore, the orthodontic department was the first to bond a steel bracket on enamel. Dr. E. Queto, who had worked in Buonocore's lab and then matriculated as an orthodontic student, was the first to do so with those specially fabricated brackets. Dr. Lieberman, then an orthodontic student, was the first to retract four incisors with heavy-force closing loops. Both are firsts in the history of orthodontics and direct bonding. Also early in the 1960s, J. Daniel Subtelny, principal investigator, and Joanne D. Subtelny, PhD, a speech pathologist and research associate in the orthodontic department, were the recipients of a Public Health Service research grant to evaluate the efficacy of pharyngeal flap surgery to normalize undesired nasalized speech in cleft palate individuals. Surgery was undertaken at two institutional sites by two plastic surgeons, Dr. Robert McCormick at the University of Rochester and Dr. Jack Curtin at the University of Illinois. Very fine cineradiographic equipment was used to record physiologic events occurring relative to the oral, palatal pharyngeal valving, and pharyngeal structures during speech output to properly modify intra-oral pressure and the direction of airflow for desired speech intelligibility. Engineers Joseph Worth, MS, and James Runyan, MS, became members of the research team and helped to adapt the cineradiograph to record at 240 frames per second and to develop and adapt a specially designed, small, silicone strain gauge pressure transducer to record intra-oral air pressure and another one to simultaneously record nasal air pressures. A special integrated flow meter was also developed and designed to record oral and nasal airflow. Pharyngeal flap surgery was found to result positively in a significant reduction in nasal airflow and significantly improve oralized speech production. Information from the study stimulated additional informative speech studies in our division and at other universities in this country and around the world.

The cineradiographic equipment was also used to study the relationships of speech and deglutition (swallowing) to malocclusion, both as an outcome and a causative problem. Surprisingly, the swallowing processes and functional adaptations as they occurred in the head and neck region were very poorly understood, and there was little or no documented information. Base information in orofacial and cervical deglutition processes were recorded as part of treatment processes, and a more complete understanding of the basic functional vegetative process of swallowing evolved. The cineradiographic equipment was very valuable to departmental diagnostics, treatment, and informative procedures as well.

In the early 1980s, Dr. Ross Tallents, a prosthodontist, became a member of our orthodontic faculty, and the study, diagnosis, and treatment of temporomandibular joint problems was incorporated into our teaching program. Dr. Tallents initiated a fellowship program in the same. Both orthodontic and American Society of Dentistry for Children residents participate in some courses. Joint research studies were undertaken. Many times, orthodontic residents upon graduation elected to undertake the temporomandibular joint fellowship curriculum and vice versa. An interdisciplinary faculty has been developed, which includes Donald Macher, an oral surgeon, and Per-Lennart Westesson, a radiologist.

The history of the orthodontic department is also a history of its students. Most of the present orthodontic faculty are graduates of this department and are recognized for their accomplishments and capabilities. Other graduates teach in other departments around the world as well as in this country. Several have been appointed chairs of orthodontic departments; some have become deans and/or assistant deans at their dental schools.

The establishment of the Eastman Dental Center Alumni Association in the 1960s is illustrative of the loyalty and support of its graduates; the association was developed under the leadership of Dr. Howard Aduss. Initially, alumni meetings were arranged to take place in Rochester frequently at the time of graduation. Alumni would present papers and sponsor a guest presenter, a person well known in the orthodontic world. These speakers were granted honorary alumni Eastman orthodontic status. They included such people as Robert Ricketts, Jaroback, Al Moore, Hal Perry, and Arne Bjork. As the numbers of alumni continued to grow, attendance increased, meetings were held at different areas around the country, and eventually meetings were held in conjunction with the Annual Meeting of the American Association of Orthodontics. In the 1970s, a board of directors was established to develop and oversee the accumulation, investment, and utilization of funds donated by alumni to an orthodontic fund. Initially and still functioning as directors are Po Peterson, Tony Quinn, Al Guay, Bob Bray, and Dr. Robert Baker Sr. A major achievement was the renovation of the orthodontic clinic led by Dr. Baker Sr. and called the "Keep His Dream Alive Campaign." The newly renovated clinic was dedicated on June 20, 1977, and named the J. Daniel Subtelny Orthodontic Clinic. The J. Daniel Subtelny Endowment Fund was established to endow a chair in the orthodontic department, and Dr. Stephanos Kyrkanides was formally appointed as the chair at the second annual alumni meeting in Florida in November of 2007 by the president of the University of Rochester, Dr. Joel Seligman.

The orthodontic alumni continued to contribute to the Subtelny endowment fund, and in the early spring of 2007, they had achieved the $2 million level to fund the endowed chair. The Alumni Association continues to reflect the quality of the education orthodontists received at Eastman and the cohesiveness, caring, and friendship developed in Rochester.

PROSTHODONTICS AT THE EASTMAN DENTAL CENTER

Gerald N. Graser and Carlo Ercoli

A decision was made by Dr. Bibby and the senior faculty in the 1960s to add specialty training in prosthodontics, the restoration and replacement of teeth, through a department. The dental needs of the population and the demands for advanced training had changed dramatically since the establishment of the Rochester Dental Dispensary. The use of fluoride substantially reduced the high dental decay rate among children locally and nationally, and it was determined that it was increasingly important to address the needs of the adult population as long as dental care and dental educational programs in pediatric dentistry continued on a high level. Previous to this, emergency dental service was expanded during the regular work week to include adults. In the 1950s, a department of periodontology, a dental disease that primarily affects adults, was established at Eastman.

In 1967, Dr. Allen A. Brewer was appointed as the first chair and program director of prosthodontics. Dr. Brewer had recently retired from the Air Force. His major interest areas were in removable prosthodontics and research (telemetry studies). Dr. Helmut Zander, who was chair of periodontology at that time, had strongly supported a search for a prosthodontist but saw the major need for a prosthodontist with a strong background in fixed prosthodontics, i.e. crown and bridge. Nationally there was a great deal of interest in the integrated discipline of periodontics-prosthodontics. As the prosthodontic program matured, there was an increasing emphasis on fixed prosthodontics as well as maxillofacial prosthetics.

The first prosthodontic resident accepted into the program in 1968 was Dr. John A. Oster, who was a highly regarded dentist in general practice in Rochester for almost twenty years before enrolling in the program. He received a certificate in prosthodontics in 1970, received his MS at the University of Rochester in the Department of Dentistry, and subsequently became a visiting faculty member with the rank of instructor.

For the first ten years of the prosthodontics program, generally one resident per year participated in the two-year training program. The clinic of the Department of Prosthodontics was on the third floor of the "new wing." It consisted of two dental operatories, a small reception-secretary space, an office for the department chair, and a dental laboratory with five stations for two to three residents, a lab technician, and Dr. Brewer—with an ash tray on top of his bench, as smoking was allowed at that time.

Dr. Gerald N. Graser completed the program in 1972 and was appointed to the part-time faculty in 1975. When Dr. Brewer retired and after an intensive national search, Dr. Graser was appointed chair and program director in 1977. He and Dr. Gary Rogoff, another early graduate of the program, played a major role in the design of the prosthodontic clinic in the new dental center building on Elmwood Avenue.

The new facilities consisted of six operatories, eight laboratory stations with a separate ceramic room, and three offices. The program began accepting two residents per year in 1978. In 1980 the prosthodontic clinic was remodeled, with new dental units to replace the Ritter dental units that had been donated to the center as Ritter was going out of business. The number of operatories expanded to seven. Drs. Oster and Graser started the very successful Allen A. Brewer Upstate New York Prosthodontic Conference in honor of the first division chair. The goal of the conference was the provision of prosthodontic education for dentists in upstate New York, with guest lecturers whose work was "evidence-based," in contrast to lecturers who presented their own personal viewpoints, cases, and techniques. The twenty-ninth annual Brewer Conference was held in June 2007.

In 1983 to 1984, Drs. Bejan Iranpour and Gerald Graser working with Dr. P. I. Branemark established one of the four U.S.-based training centers to promote the dissemination of the concept of osseo-integration of dental implants. This revolutionized the replacement of missing teeth. The other training centers were at the Mayo Clinic in Rochester, Minnesota, the University of Washington in Seattle, Washington, and the University of Texas in San Antonio, Texas. In the training program, Dr. Branemark demonstrated the surgical procedures for five patients and Dr. Bejan Iranpour, who was then head of dentistry at Genesee Hospital, assisted. They then reversed positions and Dr. Iranpour did the surgery. Dr. Graser did the prosthodontic restorations, which were attached to the implants by small gold screws so it was fixed in position and could only be removed by the dentist. The result was a prosthesis entirely supported by five or six implants in the mandible. Hitherto, metal implant frameworks were directly overlaid on cortical bone and screwed into place. The new titanium implant allowed for the successful integration of bone into the interstices of the implant and resulted in a biologic bond and a very predictable high rate of success.

In 2001 Dr. Carlo Ercoli, who completed the program in 1996, was appointed the program director in place of Dr. Graser, who continued as the division chair. In 2001 the prosthodontic laboratory was remodeled and enlarged and dedicated in honor of Dr. Gerald N. Graser. Prosthodontic alumni, friends, and corporate sponsors provided major funding. Recognizing the need for a fellowship to support additional training for prosthodontists interested in advancing their skill in the surgical aspects of dental implants and enhancing their credentials for an academic career, the Graser

Fellowship was established in 2003, again honoring the highly regarded Dr. Gerald N. Graser. The prosthodontic alumni again responded generously and raised over one-half million dollars for this fund with the help of corporate friends, patients, dental laboratories, friends, and family. Continued support of the fellowship was also initiated in 2004 with the "The Pearls of Practice" lectures, presentations primarily by prosthodontic alumni. The lectures are held at Eastman Dental Center in the fall and offer very practical clinical prosthodontic information for general dentists of upstate New York. Dr. Graser retired as division chair in 2006 after serving for thirty years, and Dr. Ercoli was appointed the third chair of the division during the forty years of the existence of the program.

During the past forty years, more than seventy-five prosthodontic residents have completed their specialty training. Over thirty awards have been received related to prosthodontic research conducted while in training. Eleven MS degrees and three PhD degrees were granted to prosthodontic residents during these years. Many have presented their work at national or international meetings, and/or have had their research published in peer-reviewed journals. Many of the graduates of the prosthodontic program have distinguished themselves as national and international authorities and lecturers in the field of prosthodontics. Graduates of the prosthodontic program have continued on as faculty at EDC. These include, among others, Ross Tallents (1979), Charles Oster (1984), and James Soltys (1994). Dr. Ronald Sambaursky, Dr. Julian Kahn, Dr. Theresa Hofstede, and Dr. Majd Almardini are currently part-time alumni faculty. Others have established distinguished careers as full- and part-time faculty at other institutions. Approximately 25 percent of the residents have been involved in full-time academics at various times during their careers. When including part-time faculty involvement, over 60 percent of alumni have been involved in academia.

Research by prosthodontic residents and faculty reflects current clinical practice and interest in the basic sciences. In the early years of the prosthodontic program, research was clinically oriented and led to a master of science awarded by the Department of Dental Research. The Department of Dental Research de-emphasized clinical research and the MS degree and encouraged basic science research leading to a doctorate. There were three PhD degrees awarded to prosthodontic residents. In addition to degree programs, meaningful clinically oriented projects by faculty and residents not necessarily leading to an MS continued along with the basic science research.

As noted previously, osseo-integrated implants as described by Professor Branemark and colleagues have revolutionized how prosthodontics is practiced today. One study conducted by members of the division, Barzilay, Graser and Iranpour, placed implants at the time of extraction in a primate model. The concept of immediate implantation was so successful that it is used routinely in clinical practice today. Other implant studies included evaluation of atraumatic bone-cutting procedures prior to placement of implants, testing of implant components, and animal studies of new implant design using a canine model. In addition, other studies on evaluating products used in clinical practice, such as denture lining materials and biomaterials research, continued. Interestingly, the pendulum may be swinging back as there is increasing awareness and need for translational research.

ORAL AND MAXILLOFACIAL SURGERY

Bejan Iranpour

ORAL SURGERY AT THE EASTMAN DENTAL CENTER

Until the mid-1970s, the large ambulatory patient base, multiple postdoctoral dental training programs, and multitude of research activities of the Eastman Dental Center at 800 Main Street created a need for an oral surgery department. After the retirement of Dr. Pammeter in the early 1960s, Dr. Donald Robinson was appointed chief of the oral surgery department. Two years later he returned to his hometown and was replaced by Dr. Erwin Buck as interim chief. In 1964, Dr. Bejan Iranpour was appointed the chief of the department. Many of Eastman's faculty also had faculty appointments at the University of Rochester. Some were very active in both institutions and fostered various collaborative academic relationships; the department itself was one with a mutually productive collaborative relationship with its university counterpart.

The oral surgery department at Eastman provided ambulatory oral surgery care to adults and children, including sedation when deemed appropriate. General dentistry students rotated through the department and performed surgical procedures under faculty supervision. The oral surgery department also provided consultations to other departments and presented many didactic courses.

Genesee Hospital and Eastman Dental Center were located in close proximity and had a formal affiliation agreement for patient care as well as academic support. Certain patient emergencies and major oral surgical procedures that presented at Eastman were referred to Genesee Hospital. After the Eastman Dental Center moved, it was felt that there was no longer a need for an oral surgery department at Eastman because of the proximity to the oral surgery service at Strong Memorial Hospital.

ORAL SURGERY AT THE UNIVERSITY OF ROCHESTER

The oral and maxillofacial surgery training program in Rochester has been based at the University of Rochester with various levels of collaboration with other local academic instructions since its inception. In the mid-1950s, an internship in oral surgery was established at Strong Memorial Hospital. The internship was located in its dental clinic and was directed by Dr. Elmer Palmeter. One intern a year was enrolled for each of the two years in the oral surgery training program at Strong Memorial Hospital. After the completion of two years of training in Rochester, the interns enrolled in other institutions for a third year of training as required by the accreditation agency.

In the mid-1960s, Dr. James Bryan was appointed program director, and the program received accreditation for three years of residency training. Genesee Hospital, an affiliate of the University of Rochester, became cosponsor of oral surgery training. Dr. Bejan Iranpour, a full-time faculty member of the University of Rochester and chief of the hospital's Department of Dentistry, supervised residents at Genesee Hospital. This collaboration expanded the patient base and faculty resource for the residents.

Recognizing the importance of scientific research for the advancement of the specialty, residents were required to undertake a research project, and a fourth year was added to the program leading to a master of science degree. Residents engaged in a variety of research protocols mentored by experienced researchers in the medical center. Few other oral surgery training programs had a similar research requirement.

In the early 1970s, Dr. H. Langley Page Jr. served as interim director of the program. The didactic program was expanded significantly, off-service rotations were enhanced, and the entire oral surgery volunteer faculty participated in the weekly grand rounds. Later, Dr. Fred Emmings, an oral surgeon, was appointed full-time chair of the Department of Dentistry of the University of Rochester Medical Center. He also directed the oral surgery training program jointly with Dr. Lee Pollan. The Department of Dentistry at Strong Memorial Hospital moved to larger quarters in the hospital to accommodate its growing service and educational needs.

In the mid-1970s, through the efforts of Drs. William McHugh and Helmut Zander, a Dental Teachers Training Program was established, and it was funded by the university and a grant from the National Institute of Dental Research through the Department of Dental Research. The purpose was to train dentists who intend to pursue academic careers. The program required satisfactory completion of an accredited dental specialty and basic science study leading to a PhD degree. The oral surgery training program embraced this opportunity and added a second track, the teachers training track, to its residency training program. It took seven to eight years to complete the program. Dr. Stephen Feinberg was the first graduate of this program. All of the six graduates have been engaged in oral and maxillofacial-related academic and research activities in U.S. dental schools. Only three other oral and maxillofacial training programs in the country offered this teachers training track option.

The term *oral surgery* was changed nationally in the early 1980s to oral and maxillofacial surgery (OMFS) to reflect the scope of the specialty. In 1986, the length of required training increased from three to four years. The University of Rochester's OMFS training program no longer required the completion of a master of science degree, but it did require completion of a publishable research project during the four years of clinical training. As a result of Dr. Fred Emmings establishing an interdisciplinary collaborative relationship with other services in 1987, the management of facial trauma was rotated weekly among oral and maxillofacial surgery, otolaryngology, and plastic surgery services. This protocol included Rochester General Hospital and Genesee Hospital, both affiliates of the University of Rochester. The arrangement was remarkably successful and has continued to date (2008). At the time of initiation, only a few other hospitals nationally had a similar working approach.

In the mid-1990s, after Dr. Emmings moved to private practice, Dr. Lee Pollan assumed the duties of the interim program director and chief of oral and maxillofacial surgery. Dr. Robert Shapiro was recruited as the chief of oral and maxillofacial surgery. The Department of Dentistry relocated to a large, new wing of the hospital that was well equipped for performing ambulatory surgical procedures. The residents' training base was expanded by rotating through the Rochester General Hospital two days a week under the supervision of the OMFS faculty. In addition, a cadre of eight dedicated voluntary faculty members participated regularly in the supervision of residents. The program has been fortunate to have such devoted voluntary faculty throughout the years and highly values their contribution.

In 2001, Dr. Karl deLeeuw became chief of the division. In 2003, the program was granted approval from the Council on Dental Education of the American Dental Association to increase enrollment from one to two residents per each year of training. This was a major achievement, indicative of a significant increase in patient load and the academic strengths of the program. In 2005, Dr. Joseph Fantuzzo joined the Eastman Department of Dentistry. Upon achieving Certification as a Diplomate of the American Board of Oral and Maxillofacial Surgery, Dr. Fantuzzo was named oral and maxillofacial surgery program director. He held that position until leaving the university in June of 2008 for full-time private practice outside of the Rochester area. At this writing in 2008, Dr. Pollan leads the division as interim program director while also serving as the president of the American Association of Oral and Maxillofacial Surgeons.

NOTES

The following abbreviations are used in the notes and photo captions to designate collections of primary source materials:

GEC: George Eastman correspondence. These are letters by Eastman that have been preserved in forty-one outgoing letter press books, dating 1879–1932. These letter books were at the Business Information Center of the Eastman Kodak Company, Rochester, New York, when the author did her research but are now at the George Eastman House, International Museum of Photography and Film.

INC-GEC: Incoming George Eastman correspondence, filed chronologically in boxes, 1890–1932. These, too, were at the Eastman Kodak Company and are now housed at the George Eastman House.

GEH: George Eastman House, International Museum of Photography and Film, Rochester, New York.

UR: Signifies that the collection is in the Department of Rare Books and Special Collections, Rush Rhees Library, University of Rochester. The collections of materials relating to George Eastman are located here.

1. RGE-UR: Recollections of George Eastman at the University of Rochester are 137 interviews recorded in 1939 and 1940 for a proposed biography by AndreMaurois. They were conducted under the direction of Frank Lovejoy, president of the Eastman Kodak Company, and Oscar Solbert of Kodak's Public Relations Department.

2. GEC-UR: George Eastman correspondence at the University of Rochester. The collection consists of over 700 letters written between 1864 and March 11, 1932.

Basil Glover Bibby Library is often shortened to Bibby Library. The bulk of the materials are from the archive room here.

CHAPTER 1

1. Letters from Maria Eastman to Emily Kilbourn Cope, 1840s and 1850s (GEC-UR). Interview with Netta (Mrs. Robert) Ranlet, 1940 (RGE-UR).

2. David Levy, "The Evolution of American Dentistry as an Autonomous Profession" (unpublished paper, 1979).

3. Ibid.

4. Ibid. Gies (1926) Asgis (1941) Cleman's syllabus (1971) as quoted by Levy.

5. Ibid. M. Rogers (1844), a well-known physician-dentist, as quoted in Levy: "To get an idea of the importance of our profession, it is well to inquire who are the subjects of it. It is not with us as with the profession of medicine, where the lame, the blind, the halt, the poor, and the distressed of like, get the largest share of professional labor. Our principal business is performed for the most valued, most useful, and the most beloved members of society."

6. Ibid., 15.

7. Crawford Long, a physician, later claimed that he used ether as an anesthetic in an operation as early as 1842, but he did not publish his work.

8. Beatrice Bibby, interview by Cathy Salibian, April 14, 2004, Eastman Dental Center Interview Project (unpublished manuscript, Bibby Library). Beatrice Bibby grew up in Rochester during the period.

9. The Columbian Chair was so named because 1892 was the 400th anniversary of Columbus's arrival in the Western Hemisphere.

10. "The Early Years: 1887–1919," www.ritterdental.com/Story/TheEarlyYears.htm.

11. Harvey J. Burkhart, "Centennial History of Dentistry in Rochester," vol. 4 in *The Centennial History of Rochester, New York,* vol. 13 in the Rochester Historical Society Publication Fund Series, 1934, 281–320.

12. Carl Ackerman, *George Eastman* (Boston: Houghton Mifflin, 1930), 8.

13. In the 1950s, the Pfaudler, Castle, Ritter, and Taylor companies merged to become the Sybron Company.

14. Marilyn J. Field, ed., *Dental Education at the Crossroads* (Washington, DC: National Academy Press, 1995), 36, 54.

15. George Eastman Dryden, interview with author, 1988.

16. Ackerman, *George Eastman,* 386.

17. Ackerman, *George Eastman,* 385.

18. George Eastman to William Bausch, July 6, 1915 (GEC-GEH).

19. The Rochester Dental Dispensary became the Eastman Dental Dispensary in 1947, when a new director succeeded Harvey Burkhart, who died in 1946. The name was changed to the Eastman Dental Center in 1965, perhaps reflecting the falling-out of favor of the word *dispensary.*

20. Thomas Forsyth, as quoted in Ackerman, *George Eastman,* 388.

21. The dental equipment and furniture was given in memory of its Rochester inventor Frank Ritter by Ritter's daughters Adelina Ritter Shumway and Laura A. Ritter.

22. William D. McHugh, *Upstate Magazine,* Letters, "say aaaah," July 11, 1976.

23. Ackerman, *George Eastman* 386.

24. In 1918, these rates were modified to family income not exceeding $15 a week for a two-child family, $20 for three children, and $24 for four.

25. Ackerman, *George Eastman,* 391.

26. In defining and distinguishing between dental nurses, dental hygienists, and dental assistants, etc., Dr. Stanley Handleman notes these differences:

Dental assistants have the duties of chair-side assistance, instrument cleaning, and inventory.
Dental receptionists make appointments, do bookkeeping and receive patients.
Dental nurses are not employed in the U.S. In New Zealand in the 1920s they did caries removal, fillings, and simple extractions.

Dental hygienists' duties include scaling to remove calculus, cleaning, and taking radiographs.

27.   Catharine Strong Hall was given to the university by Henry Alvah Strong in memory of his mother. Henry Strong was George Eastman's business partner and the first president of the Eastman Kodak Company.

28.   Harvey J. Burkhart, *Annual Report of the Rochester Dental Dispensary,* 1920.

29.   Ibid.

30.   During World War I, Kaiser traveled to Vichy, France, and worked in a contagious disease unit. Later, during his many travels around the world, Kaiser regularly conducted free local clinics for ill children. A recipient of numerous awards, he was also the president of the Rochester Academy of Medicine and a member of the University of Rochester Board of Trustees until his death in 1955.

31.   William F. Von Dohlen to George Eastman, November 11, 1920 (INC-GEC).

32.   Roger Butterfield, "Reminiscences of George Eastman; an Introduction," *University of Rochester Library Bulletin* 26, No. 3 (Spring 1971), 53–54.

33.   Martha Gould Axelrod, "The Philanthropist: The Children Dreaded the Great George Eastman's 'Gifts,'" *Upstate Magazine,* March 9, 1986, 13.

34.   Ackerman, *George Eastman* 402.

CHAPTER 2

1.   When Miss M. Lawrence, Hangchow, China, wrote in 1919 to ask Eastman to provide financial support for a homeopathic hospital there, he responded:

> I was brought up a homoeopathist myself and have no doubt that the Hahnemann influence was a good thing in medicine. You have evidently been too long out of touch with the progress of events to realize, however, that high dilution has given way to no medicine at all and the lines between the old school and the new school have melted away by the adoption of both parties of what is best in medicine. As a separate theory of medicine, homeopathy is now dead and therefore if for no other reason I would not be interested in contributing to any institution that did not recognize this fact.

2.   In the 1850s, the Charitable Society had to sponsor concerts by Jenny Lind and lectures by P. T. Barnum to raise funds to get it started. Finally, the Common Council donated a cemetery as land, but it was 1857 before the graves were removed and 1864 before a four-story brick building opened. The first board of managers was entirely female. Tents were erected on the grounds to treat the wounded during the Civil War. Three outbuildings were added over the years—a nurses' home, a maternity building, and a children's pavilion. Eastman was approached in 1908 to help enlarge the facility. He agreed, with stipulations, to pay $500,000 of the $800,000 total. He recommended that Gordon & Madden be hired as architects and that annexes be erected to care for communicable diseases since there was at that time no place in Rochester for patients with contagious diseases other than the old pest house. The walls of the original building were allowed to stand, but they were fireproofed according to the latest Kodak techniques and incorporated into the new building. In 1910 the name of City Hospital was changed to Rochester General Hospital to reflect its private funding.

3.   Flexner's 1910 objections to the current state of medical education centered on whether faculties of medical schools should accept fees for seeing patients or should be completely salaried. This question would occupy medical reformers for a generation, roughly from 1905 to 1930, before the economics of the situation rendered it moot. In 1910, idealism was in ascendancy. "There is no inherent reason why a professor of medicine should not make something of the financial sacrifice that the professor of physics makes," Flexner declared in his Carnegie report. Even so, for salaries to be competitive, funds had to come from somewhere.

4.   Abraham Flexner, *I Remember: The Autobiography of Abraham Flexner* (New York: Simon and Schuster, 1940), 180.

5.   *Rochester Democrat and Chronicle,* June 12, 1920.

6.   George Eastman to Helen Strong Carter, June 2, 1921 (GEC-GEH).

7.   George Eastman to Rochester Dental Dispensary trustees, June 25, 1920 (GEC-GEH).

8.   Ibid.

9.   Ibid. Rhees's remark was made to Ray Ball, comptroller.

10.   George Eastman to Frank L. Babbott, August 11, 1921 (GEC-GEH).

11.   Ibid.

12.   William Gies, quoted in Marilyn J. Field, editor, *Dental Education at the Crossroads: Challenges and Change* (Committee on the Future of Dental Education, Division of Health Care Services, Institute of Medicine), 44.

13.   Ibid., 46.

14.   George Whipple, *"The First 25 Years,"* in *University of Rochester Dental Research Fellowship Program Proceedings 25th Year Celebration* (Rochester, NY: University of Rochester, June 1957), 1.

15.   Ibid., 2.

16.   Beatrice Bibby, interview with Cathy Salibian, April 14, 2004, Eastman Dental Center Interview Project (unpublished manuscript, Bibby Library).

17.   Ibid., 1.

18.   Ibid., 10.

19.   Basil Bibby, "A Note on University/Dental Center Relationships" unpublished paper apparently written in 1988, Bibby Library. The Basil Glover Bibby Library is familiarly referred to as the Bibby Library throughout. Basil Bibby is responsible for more than fifty years of often undated, sometimes untitled, and often unsigned typescripts that are held in the archives of the Bibby Library. These date from the 1940s to 1988, eighteen years after his retirement as director of the Eastman Dental Center. These typescripts are referred to as "memorandum to file" with whatever other information is known about them.

20.   Donald G. Anderson, *"The First 25 Years,"* in *University of Rochester Dental Research Fellowship Program Proceedings 25th Year Celebration* (1955) 9–11.

21.   H. C. Hodge and S. B. Finn, "Reduction in Experimental Rat Caries by Fluorine," Proceedings of the Society for Experimental Biology and Medicine 42 (1939): 318.

22.   H. C. Hodge, "Fluoride," in *Mineral Metabolism,* vol. II A, chapter 24, ed. C. L. Comar and F. Bronner (New York: Academic Press, 1964), 573–602.

23.   Gilbert B. Forbes, *Harold Hodge, Groundbreaking Pharmacologist: From a Dental Research Classic to the Manhattan Project* (Rochester, NY: The University of Rochester, 2000), 110–115.

CHAPTER 3

1.   Harvey J. Burkhart, "Centennial History of Dentistry in Rochester," vol. 4 in *The Centennial History of Rochester, New York,* vol. 13 in the Rochester Historical Society Publication Fund Series, 1934, 319.

2.   Ibid.

3.   George Eastman to Harvey Burkhart, April 4, 1927 (GEH-GEC).

4.   Ibid.

5.   George Eastman to Abraham Flexner, June 13, 1929 (GEC-GEH).

6.   George Eastman, in corresponce to Murry Guggenheim, quoted in Carl W. Ackerman, *George Eastman* (Boston: Houghton Mifflin, 1930), 385.

7.   Burkhart, "Centennial History of Dentistry in Rochester," 319.

8.   Harvey J. Burkhart, *Annual Report of the Rochester Dental Dispensary,* 1930. When the Duke of York succeeded to the throne, the Duchess of Gloucester became chairman of the board of the Royal Free Hospital and Eastman Dental Clinic in London.

9.   Harvey J. Burkhart, *Annual Report of the Rochester Dental Dispensary,* 1931.

10.   Malcolm Harris, "The Eastman Jubilee 1948–1998," lecture, December 17, 1998. Available online at http://www.eastman.ucl.ac.uk/about/inside_instit/history_edi/index.html.

11.   This section has been condensed from a transcript of the lecture noted above by Malcolm Harris, Department of Oral and Maxillofacial Surgery, Eastman Dental Institute, University College, London.

12.   Mildred L. Skinner, undated typescript of the history of the Eastman European dental clinics for the Alumnae Association, Eastman School for Dental Hygienists (Bibby Library).

13.   Harvey J. Burkhart, *Annual Report of the Rochester Dental Dispensary,* 1929.

14.   Skinner, undated typescript.

15.   George Eastman to Mary Eastman Southwick, December 8, 1927. (GEC-GEH).

16.   George Eastman to Mary Eastman Southwick, June 28, 1928 (GEC-GEH).

17.   The king was the weak Victor Emmanuel III, who in 1922 was forced to call Mussolini to form a government.

18.   Harvey J. Burkhart to George Eastman, April 16, 1930 (INC-GEC-GEH).

19.   Harvey J. Burkhart to George Eastman, April 15 and April 16, 1930 (INC-GEC-GEH).

20.   Harvey J. Burkhart to George Eastman, April 20, 1930 (INC-GEC-GEH). Eastman was on the board of directors of the Metropolitan Opera Company and often took friends and colleagues to New York City for a marathon three-day opera binge—six operas in three days.

21.   Harvey J. Burkhart to George Eastman, April and April 16, 1930 (INC-GEC-GEH).

22.   Harvey J. Burkhart to George Eastman, April 20, 1930 (INC-GEC-GEH). Burkhart is pulling Eastman's leg here in suggesting his boss might seek an audience with the Pope. By 1930, Eastman's health was deteriorating, and friends found him depressed and listless.

23.   Harvey J. Burkhart to George Eastman, May 2, 1930 (INC-GEC-GEH).

24.   Skinner, undated typescript.

25.   Ibid.

26.   Ibid.

27.   Ibid., 52.

28.   Harvey J. Burkhart, *Annual Report of the Rochester Dental Dispensary,* 1939.

29.   Skinner, undated typescript, 13–14.

30.   Harvey J. Burkhart, *Annual Report of the Rochester Dental Dispensary,* 1932.

31.   Harvey Burkhart, *Annual Report of the Rochester Dental Dispensary,* 1945.

32.   Harvey Burkhart, *Annual Report of the Rochester Dental Dispensary,* 1939.

33.   Burkhart, "Centennial History of Dentistry in Rochester," 319.

34.   The Eastman Dental Institute and Public Health Service, pamphlet, Bibby Library, 2.

35.   Ibid., 7.

36.   Ibid.

37.   Ibid., 14.

38.   Ibid., 9.

39.   Ibid., 28.

40.   Ibid., 4.

41.   Ibid.,.

42.   Harvey J. Burkhart, *Annual Report of the Rochester Dental Dispensary,* 1931.

43.   Basil Bibby, *Annual Report of the Eastman Dental Dispensary,* 1955.

44.   Malcolm Harris, "The Eastman Jubilee 1948–1998."

CHAPTER 4

1.   Milton K. Robinson, interview by Henry Nicholson, January 15, 1940, University of Rochester Library Department of Rare Books and Special Collections.

2.   Carl Ackerman, *George Eastman* (Boston: Houghton Mifflin, 1930), 389.

3.   Ibid.

4.   Harvey J. Burkhart, interview by anonymous Kodak inverviewer in preparation for an Eastman biography by Andre Marais that was never written, January 19, 1940, University of Rochester Library Department of Rare Books and Special Collections.

5.   Harvey J. Burkhart, "Centennial History of Dentistry in Rochester," vol. 4 in *The Centennial History of Rochester, New York,* vol. 13 in the Rochester Historical Society Publication Fund Series, 1934, 291.

6.   *Rochester Times Union,* June 3, 1938. From scrapbook in the Bibby Library.

7.   Typed document found in the archives of the Bibby Library and dated 1955. Unsigned but attributed to Bibby.

8.   Dr. and Mrs. Ralph Voorhis, interview by the author, ca 1980.

9.   *New York Times,* April 14, 1946. From scrapbook in the Bibby Library.

10.   *Democrat and Chronicle,* April 14, 1946. From scrapbook in the Bibby Library.

11.   *New York Herald Tribune,* April 14,1946. From scrapbook in the Bibby Library.

12.   Basil Bibby, memorandum to file, Bibby Library.

13.   Basil Bibby, memorandum to file, Bibby Library.

CHAPTER 5

1.   Beatrice Bibby, interview by Cathy Salibian, April 14, 2004, Eastman Dental Center Interview Project (unpublished manuscript, Bibby Library).

2.   Basil Bibby, memorandum to file, 1966, Basil Bibby archives, Bibby Library.

3.   Dr. Stanley Handelman contributed much written material for this research section.

4.   Martin Curzon, interview by Cathy Salibian, 2004, Eastman Dental Center Interview Project (unpublished manuscript, Bibby Library).

5.   The source of the written material on research during the Bibby years is Dr. Stanley Handelman.

6.   Basil G. Bibby, *Annual Report of the Eastman Dental Dispensary,* 1949.

7.   Ibid.

8.   Ibid.

9.   Harper Sibley to Basil G. Bibby, January 1950 (Bibby Library).

10.   According to the 1949 annual report, "Developments of the above sort are being aided by the activities of several committees of the Rochester Dental Society at the request of Dr. Kaiser and your Director."

11.   Basil Bibby, *Annual Report of the Eastman Dental Dispensary,* 1949.

12.   L. Cohen and H. Rothschild, "The Bandwagons of Medicine," *Perspectives in Biology and Medicine* 22(4) (1979): 531–38.

13.   Kaiser, A. D. "Effect of Tonsillectomy on General Health in 5,000 Children," *Journal of the Amerian Medical Association* 78 (1922):1869–73; *Children's Tonsils In or Out: A Critical Study of the End Results of Tonsillectomy* (Philadelphia: Lippincott, 1932); "Significance of Tonsils in Development of Child," *Journal of the American Medical Association* 115 (1940):1151–56.

14.   Stanley Handelman, interview by Cathy Salibian, June 16, 2004, Eastman Dental Center Interview Project (unpublished manuscript, Bibby Library).

15.   Curzon, interview by Cathy Salibian.

16.   Dental Times, "Rochester Institution Pioneered in Preventive Dentistry: Eastman Marks 50th Year as Leader in Treatment, Research, Education," *Dental Times,* November 15, 1967, 8.

17.   Ibid.

CHAPTER 6

1.   Scribbled at the top of Hein's 1953 document in Bibby's handwriting: "Presentation by Dr John Hein—circulated without BGB's approval to University Trustees. This contributed to souring Dr. Anderson on Dr Hein & perhaps BGB (who was not involved)."=

2.   John Hein, presentation to University of Rochester trustees, 1953.

3.   Dr. Donald Anderson was the person who informally started using the term University of Rochester Medical Center (URMC), perhaps to differentiate himself from his predecessor, George Whipple, who was associated with the name School of Medicine and Dentistry. From personal communication with James Stormont, MD, and others who were at the URMC in 1953 when Anderson succeeded Whipple.

4.   As with many commentators, Hein, in writing this history, confused Mr. Abraham Flexner, the author of the famous Carnegie report on the state of medical education in the United States, with his brother, Dr. Simon Flexner, the renowned bacteriologist. Hein, like many others, referred to Abraham as "Dr. Flexner."

5.   Donald Anderson, University of Rochester Dental Research Fellowship Program Proceedings 25th Year Celebration, October 8, 1955.

6.   Ibid.

7.   Basil Bibby, "Cooperation," memorandum to file, 1961, Bibby Library.

8.   Basil Bibby, memorandum to file, Basil Bibby archives, Bibby Library.

9.   Basil Bibby, memorandum to file, 1988, Bibby Library.

10.   Beatrice Bibby, interview by Cathy Salibian, April 14, 2004, Eastman Dental Center Interview Project.

CHAPTER 7

1.   "Eastman Center to Join U of R," *Democrat and Chronicle,* December 2, 1971. From scrapbook in the Bibby Library.

2.   *Campus Times,* February 1974.

3.   Eastman Dental Center Board of Trustees meeting minutes, January 12, 1993.

4.   William D. McHugh, "Where's the Dental School?" In *To Each His Farthest Star: A Book of Essays Commemorating the Fiftieth Anniversary of the University of Rochester Medical Center, 1925–1975* (Rochester, NY: University of Rochester Medical Center, 1975), 178.

5.   Erling Johansen, telephone interview by Cathy Salibian, September 2005, Eastman Dental Center Interview Project.

6.   Cyril Meyerowitz, interview by Cathy Salibian, October 11, 2004, Eastman Dental Center Interview Project.

7.   Letter to Robert L. Sproull, March 4, 1981. The letter was signed by Edward Gilda, DDS, Stanley Handelman, DDS, Helmut Zander, DDS, and Bejan Iranpour, DDS, and cosigned and sponsored by thirty-five members of the university's dental faculty.

8.   Frank E. Young to Bejan Iranpour, Ad Hoc Committee of Dental Faculty, cc. F. G. Emmings, W. McHugh, and R. L. Sproull, May 15, 1981.

9.   *Democrat and Chronicle,* June 12, 1920.

10.   William D. McHugh, "Where's the Dental School?" 178.

11.   Ibid., 176–179.

12.   City East, April 8, 1976 (newspaper clipping in scrapbook, Bibby Library).

13.   William McHugh, personal communication, ca. 2004 . . .

14.   *Campus Times,* February 1974.

15.   *Brighton Pittsford Post,* March 18, 1976.

16.   *Rochester Times Union,* February 10, 1976.

17.   *Brighton Pittsford Post.*

18.   Cyril Meyerowitz, interview by Cathy Salibian.

19.   Anonymous staff member, interview by Cathy Salibian, 2004, Eastman Dental Center Interview Project.

20.   Ibid.

21.   Ibid.

22.   Dental Products Report, July 1995.

23.   Eastman Dental Center Board of Trustees minutes, May 10, 1994.

24.   William D. McHugh "Where's the Dental School?" 164.

25.   Ronald Billings, interview by the author, May 2006.

26.   Eastman Dental Center Director's Report for 1991, 2.

27.   Ronald Billings, interview by the author.

28.   Robert Witmer, interveiw by Cathy Salibian, 2004, Eastman Dental Center Interview Project.

29.   Ibid.

30.   Ronald Billings, interview by the author.

31.   Ronald Billings, interview by the author, and Annual Reports, 1989–1998.

CHAPTER 8

1.   Basil G. Bibby, *Annual Report of the Eastman Dental Dispensary,* 1949.

2.   Cyril Meyerowitz, interview by Cathy Salibian, October 11, 2004, Eastman Dental Center Interview Project.

3.   Ibid.

4.   Ibid.

5.   Eastman Dental Center Board of Trustees meeting minutes, September 8, 1992.

6.   Ibid. University of Rochester management of endowments slipped badly for a while, perhaps due to lack of diversity in investments (for example, having too much Kodak stock), or perhaps due to simple mismanagement. The EDC endowment had no such problems, so it was natural to question turning its management over to those who were mucking up other endowments.

7.   Eastman Dental Center Board of Trustees meeting minutes, March 9, 1993.

8.   Daniel Subtelny, interview by Cathy Salibian, 2004, Eastman Dental Center Interview Project.

9.   Cyril Meyerowitz, interview by Cathy Salibian.

10.   Eastman Dental Center Board of Trustees meeting minutes, April 13, 1993.

11.   Eastman Dental Center Board of Trustees meeting minutes, May 11, 1993.

12.   Ibid.

13.   Cyril Meyerowitz, interview by Cathy Salibian.

14.   Eastman Dental Center Board of Trustees meeting minutes, November 14, 1995.

15.   Anonymous interviewee, interview by Cathy Salibian, 2004, Eastman Dental Center Interview Project.

16.   Ronald Billings, interview by the author, May 2005.

17.   The work group consisted of Ron Billings, DDS; Robert Hurlbut; Louis Langie Jr.; and Wilfred Springer, DDS, for the Eastman Dental Center and Jay Stein, MD; Richard Miller; Peter Robinson, Robert Witmer, and Betty Oppenheimer for the University of Rochester Medical Center.

18.   Cyril Meyerowitz, interview by Cathy Salibian.

19.   Ronald Billings, "Eastman Dental Center: Its History and Relation to the Medical Center," in *Teaching, Discovering, Caring: The University of Rochester Medical Center: Seventy-five Years of Achievement, 1925–2000,* ed. Jules Cohen and Robert J. Joynt (Rochester, NY: University of Rochester Press, 2000), 304.

20.   Ibid., 305.

21.   "Eastman Dental Center Becomes Part of University of Rochester Medical Center," University of Rochester press release, July 29, 1997.

22.   *Democrat and Chronicle* articles by Mark Hare, Michael Wentzel, others, and staff researchers, May 17, 18, 19, 20, and 22, 2003.

23.   Cyril Meyerowitz, interview by Cathy Salibian.

INDEX

This index refers only to the main text and consists of personal names.
Page numbers in italics refer to illustrations.